Family Practice:

Foundation of
Changing Health Care

Family Practice:

Foundation of Changing Health Care

Second Edition

John P. Geyman, M.D.
Professor and Chairman
Department of Family Medicine
School of Medicine
University of Washington
Seattle, Washington

 AC**C** APPLETON-CENTURY-CROFTS/Norwalk, Connecticut

0-8385-2538-5

Notice: The author and publisher of this volume have taken care that the information
and recommendations contained herein are accurate and compatible with the standards
generally accepted at the time of publication.

85 86 87 88 89 / 10 9 8 7 6 5 4 3 2 1

Prentice-Hall of Australia, Pty. Ltd., Sydney
Prentice-Hall Canada, Inc.
Prentice-Hall Hispanoamericana, S.A., Mexico
Prentice-Hall of India Private Limited, New Delhi
Prentice-Hall International (UK) Limited, London
Prentice-Hall of Japan, Inc., Tokyo
Prentice-Hall of Southeast Asia (Pte.) Ltd., Singapore
Whitehall Books Ltd., Wellington, New Zealand
Editora Prentice-Hall do Brasil Ltda., Rio de Janeiro

Library of Congress Cataloging-in-Publication Data

Geyman, John P., 1931–
  Family practice.

  Includes bibliographies and index.
  1. Family medicine.   2. Family medicine—United
States.   I. Title.   [DNLM: 1. Family Practice.
W 879 G397f]
R729.5.G4G46 1985   616   85-15009
ISBN 0-8385-2538-5

Design: M. Chandler Martylewski

PRINTED IN THE UNITED STATES OF AMERICA

To
the memory of my father,
a dedicated physician and contributor
to his community for 55 years

Contents

Preface

The first edition of this book appeared in 1980 shortly after the tenth anniversary of the recognition of family practice as a specialty. The goals of the book at that time were threefold: (1) to provide an overview of the specialty as it was then, including its historic context and future projections; (2) to describe progress in the field in terms of clinical, educational, research, and organizational perspectives; and (3) to show how the specialty relates to medicine as a whole and to the community. Today, just 5 years later, this second edition addresses these same goals, but because of the rapid (even revolutionary) changes now taking place in American medicine, much of the content of this edition is necessarily new.

Today the structure and process of medical practice and medical education are being stressed by rapid and unprecedented change. The expansion of various forms of prepaid medical practice is certain to realign relationships between physicians, hospitals, patients, employers, and government. Prospective payment of hospitals for the care of Medicare patients on the basis of diagnostic-related groups (DRGs) was initiated only 2 years ago and is already forcing fundamental reassessment of roles and activities of hospitals. Financing mechanisms for medical education that have been in place for 20 or more years are seriously threatened, and there is now widespread concern about a physician surplus in many specialties. The extent of these changes renders reassessment of the present role of family practice both timely and important, while making possible further future projections for the only specialty in U.S. medicine with an undivided interest and commitment to primary care.

This book is written primarily for medical students, family practice residents, family physicians, and medical educators. It will also be of value to others, both inside and outside of medicine, interested in the emerging role of family practice in modern health care and in changing trends in medical education and medical practice. An updated view of family practice should be of particular interest to the medical student considering his or her own role in medicine from 1990 into the 21st century.

Initial attention is directed to the history of general practice and the nature of family practice as a new kind of specialty. The general background of medical practice and medical education in the United States is then considered in terms of physician manpower, problems of health care delivery, the changing health care system, and changing trends in medical education. The content, objectives, and methods of education for family practice are next described for a continuum of education at predoctoral, graduate, and postgraduate levels. Subsequent chapters deal with various aspects of family practice, including clinical content, patterns of practice, research, and requisites and personal satisfactions of the family physician. Finally, an overview of progress is presented for the field since 1969, followed by a chapter focused upon future projections for primary care and family practice in a new era.

Attention is deliberately focused on changing patterns of health care delivery and the structure of medical practice, for family practice has developed in direct response to major problems within the health care system. Fundamental changes are underway in American medicine and any specific field of medicine must be examined in the context of these changes. The development of family practice and the national emphasis on expansion and improvement of primary care are important dimensions of present trends.

John P. Geyman, M.D.

Acknowledgments

This book has been made possible by the support and help of many. I am especially indebted to my family, whose continued support and encouragement have allowed me to make the time commitments needed to complete this task.

Thanks are also due to the colleagues and fellow faculty members who have reviewed manuscripts and offered helpful suggestions. The following reviewers of selected chapters contributed to their value:

Dr. Malcolm Peterson, School of Public Health and Community Medicine, University of Washington, Seattle, and American Lake Veterans' Administration Medical Center, Tacoma

Dr. Alfred Berg, Dr. Theodore Phillips, Dr. Ronald Schneeweiss, Dr. C. Kent Smith, Dr. Gabriel Smilkstein, and Dr. Roger Rosenblatt, Department of Family Medicine, University of Washington, Seattle

The generous assistance of the following individuals was helpful in updating information from their respective national organizations: Dr. Ann Crowley, Mr. Tom Gorey, and Ms. Joe Ann Jackson of the American Medical Association; Ms. Elizabeth Higgins of the Association of American Medical Colleges; Dr. Nicholas Pisacano of the American Board of Family Practice; Ms. Claudine Clinton and Mr. Gordon Schmittling of the American Academy of Family Physicians.

I would like to gratefully acknowledge the efforts of Mrs. Rowena Ramlall for her patience and care in preparing the entire manuscript.

Finally, I would particularly like to thank the staff of Appleton-Century-Crofts for their diligence and skill in publishing this book. I am especially indebted to Mr. David Stires, for his advice and continued encouragement, and for his early awareness of the importance of the specialty of family practice to the health care of the American people.

Family Practice:

Foundation of Changing Health Care

1 Family Practice as a Specialty

The adequacy of care available from the family physician, and his sense of responsibility, will in large measure determine the effectiveness with which the whole structure of medical care serves the patient.

Robert R. Huntly[1]

Since the specialty of family practice has taken root from the field of general practice, a brief review of the history of general practice provides a necessary background upon which profiles of family practice can be described and understood. There is a natural tendency today, as in previous times, to consider our problems as unique and special to our own time and place. This is usually not the case, and such a perception obscures our larger understanding of problems at hand and limits our capacity to solve these problems.

The interaction and balance between the generalist and specialist in medical practice have been the subject of continued interest and recurrent debate in many cultures for hundreds of years. The generalist/specialist interface has been a dynamic one featured by shifting trends in one or the other direction. At no time, however, has the need for the generalist disappeared from the process of medical care.

This chapter starts with a historic perspective of the generalist in medicine and then focuses on the evolution of general practice in the United States from 1900 to 1969, when family practice was recognized as the 20th specialty in American medicine. The growth of specialization will be described, including the major developments leading to the genesis of family practice as a specialty.

HISTORIC PERSPECTIVE

Herodotus, describing medical practice in the Nile valley of Egypt before 2000 BC, made the following observation: "The art of medicine is thus divided: each physician applies himself to one disease only and not more. All places abound in physicians; some are for the eyes, others for the head, others for the teeth, others for the intestines, and others for internal disorders."[2]

A similar concern was reflected in this country almost 4000 years later at the start of the 20th century. In 1900, when at least 80 percent of physicians were in general practice, the following editorial comment appeared in *The Journal of the American Medical Association*:

> In these days of specialization the field of the general practitioner is becoming greatly restricted. In fact, there is some danger that in many instances the so-called general practitioner ultimately may come to perform the functions of a mere business agent of the specialists, and to act as the local distributor for the patients in his community. At the same time, as the value and the need of genuine specialists in medicine are fully recognized and established, there cannot be too strong a warning uttered against a tendency noticeable in some quarters to carry specialization to a degree of refinement beyond all reason.[3]

At the start of this century in the United States, medical education commonly lacked both quality and content. There was a deficit of formal education, a stress on experiential training through preceptorships, and the sale of fake medical licenses and diplomas was by no means rare.[4]

The Flexner Report of 1910 was instrumental in the reform of medical education in the United States. Widespread improvements were brought about in medical schools, and many inferior schools were closed. At the same time, premedical education was introduced and postgraduate training in the form of an internship was required.[5] The Flexner Report also led to increased emphasis in the medical schools on the biomedical sciences as a foundation for medical practice. The inevitable result of these changes was the subsequent development of biomedical research, specialty boards, and formal residency training programs in the various specialties.

The first specialty to be defined and to be made official by a Board was Ophthalmology in 1917. Curiously, only 2 years later, at the 1919 meeting of the American Medical Association, a resolution was introduced recommending the encouragement of ". . . the designation of the practice of general medicine or 'family physicians' as a distinct specialty." But the proposal was defeated.[6] The reluctance of the medical profession to recognize so broad a field as a definitive specialty continued for 50 more years. It is noteworthy that in 1941, some 22 years after the initial attempt, a resolution was again introduced before the House of Delegates of the American Medical Association calling for a Board of General Practice. Once again the resolution was rejected, but in 1946, the AMA Section on General Practice was formed.

The growth of specialization has been the dominant feature of American medicine in the last 50 years, and this trend was especially accelerated after World War II. This has involved a remarkable growth of scientific, medical knowledge and the fractionation of the medical profession into many specialties and subspecialties with increasingly narrow concerns.

A look at the beginnings of the specialty boards is interesting in terms of the sequence of their appearance (Table 1–1). It can be noted that some of the specialty boards were defined by anatomy (e.g., ophthalmology and dermatology), one by sex (obstetrics–gynecology), two by age (pediatrics and internal medicine), and many by basic approach to management (e.g., most surgical specialties). It can also be seen that two of the most general of the specialties (pediatrics and internal medicine) were both established in the mid-1930s.

The university medical centers and large teaching hospitals were at the hub of increasing specialization, particularly after the 1940s. Advances in medical technology were implanted and applied in tertiary care centers, which grew more distant from the everyday practice of medicine in the community. Simultaneously, the curricula in medical schools placed major emphasis on the study of disease and technical competence, while humanistic aspects of medical care were relatively

TABLE 1-1. YEAR OF ORGANIZATION OF SPECIALTY BOARDS

Board	Year	Board	Year
Ophthalmology	1917	Surgery	1937
Otolaryngology	1924	Anesthesiology	1938
Obstetrics–gynecology	1930	Plastic surgery	1939
Dermatology	1932	Neurologic surgery	1940
Pediatrics	1933	Physical medicine and	
Orthopedic surgery	1934	rehabilitation	1947
Psychiatry–neurology	1934	Preventive medicine	1948
Radiology	1934	Thoracic surgery	1950
Colon-rectal surgery	1935	Family practice	1969
Urology	1935	Allergy and immunology	1971
Internal medicine	1936	Nuclear medicine	1971
Pathology	1936	Emergency medicine	1979

neglected.[7] The educational experiences of medical students were focused more on the clinical problems of patients referred to tertiary care centers than on the study and care of patients in primary care settings in the community.

Although specialization within the medical profession has clearly brought great benefits to the public through the possibility of increased quality of medical care, the net effects of this process are both positive and negative. In a thoughtful paper examining the division of labor within medicine. Menke summarizes the dilemma of specialization in these words:[8]

> Specialization is both a product of and a contributor to the scientific informa-
> tion explosion in medicine. It subdivides both doctor and patient, increases the
> difficulty of attaining a clear sense of medical identity for students and young
> physicians, and places additional strain on the traditional doctor–patient rela-
> tionship. Specialization emphasizes the science of medicine and its rational
> processes in the treatment of disease and contributes to depersonalization, ag-
> gravates patient anxieties, and implicitly encourages quackery. It is probably
> the major factor disturbing traditional ethical and economic patterns in medicine,
> and it dominates medical education and research and medical practice, promotes
> jurisdictional disputes within the profession, and weakens organizational strength
> and professional power.

DECLINE OF GENERAL PRACTICE

Although any discussion of general practice in recent years tends to center on its decline in numbers and influence, this discussion should not overlook the large role played by general practice in the improvement of health care in the post-Flexner era in the United States. Many well-trained physicians entered general practice and translated their knowledge and skills into nationwide quality patient care. These general practitioners brought modern surgery, obstetrics, anesthesia, medicine, and pediatrics directly to people everywhere. Most deliveries were done by general prac-titioners, and the maternal and infant mortality rates dropped sharply as modern techniques were broadly applied.

General practitioners functioned as family doctors, giving continuing care to the entire family, and establishing a public image that has been unequaled by later developments in American medicine. This type of personal care became symbolic of what people expect of the physician, and what they often fail to find in modern medicine as it grows progressively more depersonalized.

General practice probably reached its zenith in the 1930s and early 1940s. During that era, graduates of medical schools and rotating internships were able to practice a high quality of medicine. The progressive technical advances in medicine during and after World War II, however, brought with them the rise of specialist practice and the consequent decline of general practice.

In 1900, there was one general practitioner for every 600 people.[9] By the late 1960s, there was only 1 for every 3000 people. The ratio of general practitioners to specialists had been completely reversed over a period of 40 years, from about 80 percent general practitioners to 20 percent specialists in 1930 to about 20:80 percent in 1970. The shortage of generalists was even more serious since almost half of the physicians in general practice in 1969 were over 55 years old,[10] and no more than 10 percent of graduates from medical schools planned careers in general practice.

Many explanations have been advanced for the decline of general practice. The Millis Commission isolated three major reasons for the decline of general practice:[11]

1. General practice, once the mainstay of medicine, has gradually lost prestige as the specialties have risen in honor and accomplishments. In deciding upon his own career, the young physician may never see excellent examples of comprehensive, continuing care of highly qualified and prestigious primary physicians. He is certain, however, to see a variety of specialists and to observe that they usually enjoy higher prestige, greater hospital privileges, and more favorable working conditions than do general practitioners.

2. Educational opportunities that would serve to interest students in family practice and provide interns and residents with appropriate training are few in number and often poorer in quality than the programs leading to the specialties.

3. The conditions of practice for a general practitioner or a physician interested in family practice are thought to be less attractive than the conditions and privileges enjoyed by a specialist.

Although there were many reasons for the decline of general practice in past years, the four most important reasons, in my judgment, were the following:

1. Lack of definition as a specialty whereby the academic, educational, and research elements of the field could be developed for the clinical discipline.

2. De-emphasis of general practice and primary care in the medical schools, where medical students were traditionally exposed almost entirely to the model of the specialist. Most students made the decision to enter a specialty during their medical school years, although many entering freshman medical students were greatly interested at first in general practice.[12,13]

3. Value system predominating within medicine and society favoring the development and application of complex technical procedures and indepth medical knowledge in narrow areas. Students in medical schools learned

to perceive these as more interesting and of greater value than the care of common clinical problems or the uniqueness of the patient as a person.

4. Predominance of solo practice among general practitioners, who, after several years, often developed uncontrolled practices. Among those general practitioners who left general practice for a specialty residency, overwork was usually the major reason given and many were reluctant to give up the variety, interest, and personal satisfaction of general practice.

The above discussion points out the increasing separation of the medical student from the practicing family physician over a 40-year period to the end of the 1960s. At the graduate level, the record is likewise unimpressive. A small number of 2-year general practice residencies were started in community hospitals during the 1950s and 1960s. This effort, however, was a relatively minor one compared to the need, and represented a "patchwork" approach without the kinds of coordinated, fundamental changes which were required to reverse the trend away from general practice. Some exceptional programs filled their residency staffs over the years, but the average number of general practice residents was only about 400 to 500 each year, compared with totals of 20,000 specialty residents in 1960 and over 35,000 in 1968.[14,15]

IMPACT ON PRIMARY CARE

The continued decline in the numbers of general practitioners was increasingly evident to the public and to the medical profession during the 1950s and 1960s. It was becoming progressively more difficult to obtain the services provided by the family physician: first-contact care, point of entry to other health care services, and continuity of care over time with an understanding of the patient's family and social context. As a result, the public perceived health care services as increasingly fragmented, episodic, impersonal, disease-oriented, inaccessible, costly and complex.[16]

The public's demand for the services of the family physician remained strong. Medical societies throughout the country were constantly receiving calls for a physician willing to render primary care. In 1966, for example, among callers to the Chicago Medical Society's Referral Service specifically requesting a field of practice, calls for general practitioners were about four times more frequent than for internists or gynecologists, and other fields were requested to an even lesser extent.[17] The American Medical Association Placement Service's experience for 1968 showed that approximately one-third of all opportunities registered were for general practice, but only 8 percent of physician registrants were in general practice.[18]

James Bryan, a speaker at the conference of the Family Health Foundation of America in 1967, succinctly summed up the situation in these words: "What confronts us today is a societal monstrosity; a profession that is standing on its head. Its management function—its generalist coordinator—lies at the bottom of the heap—we must somehow right this pyramid and stand it on its base."[13]

By the late 1960s, only one physician in five was in general practice. Although both internal medicine and pediatrics were growing rapidly, there was a severe shortage of primary care physicians. In 1969 there was 1 internist for every 14,000 people in the United States; many of these were in subspecialty practice, while most of them practiced in the more affluent cities and over one-quarter were located in

New York or California.[19] Although the number of pediatricians rose from 1600 in 1931 to 10,500 in 1962, the child population increased at an even greater rate. In 1963, a pediatric manpower study showed a decline from 96 practitioners per 100,000 children (under 15) in 1940 to 50 per 100,000 in 1961, considering the combined effect of an increased number of pediatricians and a decreased number of general practitioners.[20]

The field of surgery was also growing rapidly during the 1960s despite the feeling by many that this was already an overcrowded field. In 1966, there were 6010 residents in surgical residencies, as compared to 494 residents in general practice residencies. At the same time, 3 percent of all opportunities reported to the American Medical Association Placement Service were for general surgeons while 38 percent of all such opportunities were for general practitioners.[21]

As of January 1, 1970, the number of residents in specialty fields showed a continuing shift away from primary care. Compared to 717 residents in general practice residencies, there were approximately 11 times as many in psychiatry, 4 times as many in obstetrics–gynecology and pediatrics, and 2 to 3 times as many in anesthesiology, ophthalmology, orthopedic surgery, pathology, and radiology.[22]

EVOLUTION OF FAMILY PRACTICE AS A SPECIALTY

In the 1950s the idea of family practice as a recognized, definable specialty was a visionary one in the minds of a few. The specialty was formally recognized by the end of the 1960s with the formation of the American Board of Family Practice in 1969.

Viewed in a larger context, the development of family practice in the late 1960s was both logical and inevitable. The growth of specialization and sub-specialization led to an increasing emphasis on the technology of medicine associated with problems of access and cost of care, fragmentation of the patient and the doctor-patient relationship, and growing confusion and even resentment by an increasing part of the population as to the role of the physician and the medical profession.

The natural climate favoring the genesis of family practice was well stated by McWhinney as follows:[23]

> It is no accident that family medicine is emerging at a time when the inter-relatedness of all things is being rediscovered, when the importance of ecology is being forced on one's awareness, when the limitations of the closed-system way of thinking are being more and more appreciated, and when scientists, especially those in the life sciences, are beginning to react to the scientific bias against integration, synthesis and teleology. Nor is it coincidence that this movement of ideas is taking place at a time when the virtues of economic growth are being questioned, when bigness for its own sake is ceasing to be considered good, when human values are being asserted over technology and when the importance of enduring and stable human relations is being discovered anew.

The shift toward family practice, with the attendant reappraisal of medical education, represents a positive step by the medical profession to respond directly to the changing needs of society. This shift can be viewed as one away from primary concern for diseases and organ systems, toward the whole patient as a person, his/her family, and the community.

Recognition of family practice as the 20th specialty in 1969 was the culmination of the work of many people, after many meetings and conferences over the years. As early as 1947, some of the leaders in the American Academy of General Practice and the AMA Section on General Practice favored board certification. One of the leading proponents in the 1950s was Dr. Ward Darley, who was especially farsighted in seeing the need for board certification and the redefinition of the modern family physician, as well as the development of more appropriate training programs.[24] It was in the 1960s, however, that support for the new specialty became widespread, and the American Academy of General Practice is to be credited with exerting strong leadership in this direction. National and regional conferences were held, and the course to certification was charted.

In a span of 100 days during 1966, four reports were released which gave the greatest thrust toward the new specialty of family practice. The most impressive thing about these reports is that they all came to very similar conclusions, yet had been prepared over a long period of time by completely independent groups. These reports called for basic changes throughout the structure of medical education.

The National Commission on Community Health Services, also known as the Folsom Commission, stressed the need for every individual to have a personal physician for easy access to health care on a coordinated, comprehensive, and continuing basis. This physician would be skilled in preventive medicine and the use of community resources.[25]

The report of the Citizens Commission on Graduate Medical Education (Millis Commission) called for a similar physician, but by the name of primary physician. This group underscored the crucial importance of comprehensive health care, and decried the lack of appreciation of this vital area in the medical schools. The following excerpts are taken from this report:[26]

> In the academic world, it is customary to put a greater premium on depth of knowledge in a specialized area than on more comprehensive wisdom covering a larger field. . . . Perhaps these attitudes are proper among scientists or in the university, where the men most honored are the ones who are extending the frontiers of knowledge. But medicine, although intimately based upon science, is not science. It is an application of science.

Specific recommendations made by the Millis Commission include the following:[26]

1. Simple rotation among several services, in the manner of the classic rotating internship, though extending over a longer period of time, will not be sufficient. Knowledge and skill in several areas are essential, but the teaching should stress continuing and comprehensive patient responsibility rather than the episodic handling of acute conditions in the several areas.
2. Experience in the management of emergency cases and knowledge of specialized care required before and following surgery should be included.
3. A new body of knowledge should be taught in addition to the medical specialties that constitute the bulk of the program.
4. There should be ample opportunities for individual variation in the graduate program.
5. The level of training should be on a par with that of other specialties. A 2-year graduate program is not sufficient.

6. Each teaching hospital should organize its staff, through an educational council, a committee on graduate education, or some similar means, so as to make its programs of graduate medical education a corporate responsibility rather than the individual responsibilities of particular medical or surgical services or heads of services.

7. The internship, as a separate and distinct portion of medical education, should be abandoned, and the internship and residency years should be combined into a single period of graduate medical education called a residency and planned as a unified whole.

8. State licensure acts and statements of certification requirements should be amended to eliminate the requirement of a separate internship and an appropriately described period of graduate medical education should be substituted therefore.

9. Graduation from medical school should be recognized as the end of general medical education, and specialized training should begin with the start of graduate medical education.

The Millis Commission viewed national health priorities in this way:[28]

What is wanted is comprehensive and continuing health care, including not only the diagnosis and treatment of illness, but also its prevention and the supportive and rehabilitative care that helps a person to maintain, or return to, as high a level of physical and mental health and well being as he can attain.

The report of the Ad Hoc Committee on Education for Family Practice of the Council on Medical Education (Willard Report) labeled the new specialist in comprehensive health care the family physician. The committee recognized the need for " . . . significant reorientation of medical education and change in the attitudes of the medical profession." Seeing the preparation of a large number of family physicians as the first order of business for American medicine at this time, the committee felt that " . . . a major national need exists, that such an approach is justified, and that it should be initiated promptly."[27]

The Ad Hoc Committee felt that family practice is truly a specialty because both the composite body of knowledge used by the family practitioner and his function are significantly different from other specialists. The Willard Report made the following further recommendations:[27]

1. Keynotes in family practice programs should be excellence comparable to programs in other specialties and flexibility to permit the design of training programs which will meet the needs and interests of individual physicians.

2. Medical schools and teaching hospitals should explore the possibility of developing models of family practice in cooperation with the practicing profession.

3. Recognition and status equivalent to other specialties should be accorded to family practice.

4. Study should be made of the effect of premedical programs and the admission procedures, curricula, and student evaluation policies of medical schools upon the production of family physicians.

5. An adequate graduate training program in family practice can be provided in 3 years if it is properly designed and incorporates experience in a suitable model of practice, under the supervision of family practice physicians.

The report of the Committee on Requirements for Certification of the American Academy of General Practice was the fourth major report of 1966 which was of special importance to the new specialty of family practice.[28] This Committee formulated the core content of family medicine, which served as the take-off point for emerging residency programs in family practice.

As a logical subsequent step in the evolution of family practice, the American Academy of General Practice became the American Academy of Family Physicians in 1971. The Academy has continued to play a vital role in the development of the new specialty, particularly in the facilitation of education programs at all levels and through liaison with other specialties and various levels of government.

THE AMERICAN BOARD OF FAMILY PRACTICE

The American Board of Family Practice since 1969 has been responsible for development and implementation of certification and recertification procedures. The Board thereby has an important responsibility for setting and maintaining high standards of performance in the field.

The American Board of Family Practice is noteworthy from several standpoints. Most important, perhaps, is that it has provided recognition for the specialized knowledge and skills of the generalist as a family physician. Secondly, this was the first board to require recertification by examination, which was established at 6-year intervals. Thirdly, this Board was the first to include specialists from other clinical fields in its membership.* Finally, no grandfather clause was permitted. Initially, to be eligible for examination, a candidate must have completed an approved family practice residency program or have been in active family practice for a minimum of 6 years and completed at least 300 hours of continuing study acceptable to the Board. This kind of practice eligibility was permitted only until 1978. Since then all candidates have been required to satisfactorily complete a 3-year family practice residency program.

Examinations have been given annually since 1970, and there are now over 32,000 diplomates of the American Board of Family Practice.

The certification examination is a 1-day examination which covers the breadth of family practice and tests both clinical knowledge and problem-solving skills. Two basic kinds of questions are included: multiple choice (including pictorial material), and clinical set problems, which focus on diagnosis, treatment, and/or management. The recertification examination involves a 1-day cognitive examination one-half of which includes three modular examinations selected by the candidate from the following eight modules: internal medicine, surgery, obstetrics, community medicine, pediatrics, psychiatry, gerontology, and gynecology. The recertification process also involves Office Record Review of 20 of the physician's actual patients. This audit is subject to review by the Board, and involves the indepth self-audit of patients' records selected from the following categories:

---

*The membership of the American Board of Family Practice is constituted as follows: five members representing the American Academy of Family Physicians; five members representing the AMA Section on General/Family Practice; five members representing other specialty boards (one representative each from Internal Medicine, Pediatrics, Psychiatry and Neurology, Obstetrics-Gynecology, and Surgery).

1. Abnormal vaginal bleeding
2. Acute appendicitis
3. Alcoholism and alcohol abuse
4. Allergy
5. Arthritis
6. Carcinoma of the breast
7. Chronic heart failure
8. Chronic obstructive pulmonary disease
9. Coronary artery disease
10. Depression
11. Diabetes mellitus
12. Duodenal ulcer
13. Geriatric patient
14. Hypertension
15. Irritable bowel syndrome
16. Low back pain
17. Normal pregnancy
18. Urethral discharge
19. Urinary tract infection
20. Well-child care

In addition to the cognitive examination and Office Record Review requirements, recertification candidates must hold a valid and unrestricted license to practice medicine and surgery in the United States and Canada, and have completed 300 hours of documented approvable continuing medical education during the preceding 6 years (this requirement is similar to that of the AAFP, so that continuous active membership in the AAFP satisfies this requirement).

SOME BASIC DEFINITIONS

Family Physician
The American Academy of Family Physicians (AAFP) and the American Board of Family Practice (ABFP) defined the family physician as one who:

> . . . provides health care in the discipline of family practice. His training and experience qualify him to practice in the several fields of medicine and surgery.
> The family physician is educated and trained to develop and bring to bear in practice unique attitudes and skills which qualify him or her to provide continuing, comprehensive health maintenance and medical care to the entire family regardless of sex, age, or type of problems, be it biologic, behavioral, or social. This physician serves as the patient's or family's advocate in all health-related matters, including the appropriate use of consultants and community resources.

A closely related definition has been developed by the American Medical Association, which views the family physician as one who:

> . . . serves the public as a physician of first contact and means of entry into the health care system; evaluates his patients' total health care needs; assumes responsibility for his patients' comprehensive and continuing health care and acts as coordinator of his patients' health services; and accepts responsibility for his pa-

tients' total health care, including the use of consultants, within the context of their environment, including the community and the family or comparable social unit.

Family Practice
The definition by the ABFP for family practice is as follows:

> Family practice is comprehensive medical care with particular emphasis on the family unit, in which the physician's continuing responsibility for health care is not limited by the patient's age or sex nor by a particular organ system or disease entity.
>   Family practice is the specialty in breadth which builds upon a core of knowledge from other disciplines—drawing most heavily on internal medicine, pediatrics, obstetrics and gynecology, surgery and psychiatry—and which establishes a cohesive unit, combining the behavioral sciences with the traditional biological and clinical sciences. The core of knowledge encompassed by the discipline of family practice prepares the family physician for a unique role in patient management, problem solving, counseling and as a personal physician who coordinates total health care delivery.

Family Medicine
There was early agreement that family medicine constitutes the academic discipline which is applied in family practice. In the first several years of family practice development, however, there was considerable controversy on the more specific definition of the academic discipline. Some felt that family medicine should be defined only in terms of its unique content, as different from all other clinical disciplines. For some this approach tended to focus principally on the behavioral and ecologic interactions of the family as a unit. Recent years, however, have seen a consensus that a functional definition of family medicine is required. In functional terms, family medicine can be satisfactorily defined as that body of knowledge and skills applied by the family physician as he/she provides primary, continuing and comprehensive health care to patients and their families regardless of their age, sex, or presenting complaint. It is a horizontal discipline, sharing portions of all other clinical and related disciplines from which it is derived but applying these derivative portions in a unique way to families. In addition, family medicine includes new, incompletely developed elements stemming from its own areas of developing research.

FUNCTIONAL ELEMENTS OF FAMILY PRACTICE

Family practice is thus the broadest of clinical specialties in medicine by inclusion of portions of the other clinical disciplines and other areas related to the ongoing care of the whole patient and his/her family. All other specialties have defined their areas by exclusion, on the basis of anatomy, organ system, age, sex, or basic kind of management (i.e., most surgical fields). Family practice cuts across the territorial boundaries of all of the traditional specialties, and varies somewhat in its application by each family physician based upon his/her own training, interests and skills, as well as the community of practice and the proximity to other medical resources.

Millis had called this a horizontal kind of specialization, and has seen the need for all physicians not only to specialize but also to remain open to future changes in their specialized areas. In his words: "It is inevitable that as time runs, we must deal with greater amounts of knowledge and that choices will have to be made as to that portion of knowledge that we will make our own."[29]

Family practice can be further described as: (1) including an area of clinical competency to deal definitively with those common clinical problems which constitute approximately 95 percent of all patient visits to primary care physicians;[30–32] (2) including responsibility for continuity of patient care both in and out of the hospital, with the emphasis on more effective ambulatory care; (3) involving the responsibility to arrange and coordinate consultation or referral to other specialists and community resources as indicated; and (4) requiring teamwork with other members of the health care team. Although there may be some differences between the actual practices of individual family physicians in different parts of the country and different community settings, the sine qua non of family practice, as Stephens suggests, is "the knowledge and skills which allow the family physician to confront relatively large numbers of unselected patients with unselected conditions and to carry on therapeutic relationships with patients over time."[33]

As is true of other primary care physicians (i.e., general pediatrics and general internal medicine), the family physician's practice is featured by five key elements: (1) accessibility; (2) continuity of care; (3) comprehensiveness of services; (4) coordination of total health care; and (5) accountability, or ongoing responsibility for the patient's welfare. One of these elements, comprehensive health care, has been the subject of some attention as to the appropriate range of the physician's concerns. Dr. George James, as Commissioner of Health in New York City, in 1963 suggested the following four basic categories of health care which held to clarify this issue.[34]

- Stage I: The Foundations of Disease. This stage includes many factors which individually or in combination may later be responsible for disease, and which are subject to preventive care of the individual or his family. Examples of such factors include: genetic heritage of the individual, dietary patterns, activity habits, smoking, housing conditions.
- Stage II: Preclinical Disease. Defined as "the stage when a health problem is developing but is not yet far enough advanced to make the victim aware."[34] In this stage detection is possible but often neglected. Examples include prediabetes, premalignant lesions, asymptomatic glaucoma.
- Stage III: Treatment of Symptomatic Disease. Third stage medicine constitutes the bulk of traditional clinical medicine, and forms the basis for existing patterns of medical practice.
- Stage IV: Rehabilitation and Management of Medical Conditions for Which Biologic Cure Is Not Possible. James calls this stage the "control of disability,"[34] and stresses rehabilitation during this stage. Examples are individuals with chronic disease, stable posttraumatic sequelae, and other handicapping problems.

On the basis of such a framework as the James stages, comprehensive health care can then be viewed as including:

- Health education
- Assessment of foundations of disease and the degree of risk for individual patients and their families, with planning of appropriate follow-up care
- Periodic physical examinations and laboratory screening, multiphasic screening as indicated
- Emergency care

- Care of acute symptomatic disease
- Care of chronic conditions, including rehabilitation
- Counseling, on an individual or family basis, for such conditions as marital or family problems, individual emotional problems, genetic problems, and nutritional problems

It is obvious that there are environmental factors important in Stage I which need attention by society in general and by the community in particular (e.g., air pollution, housing, poverty), but which are usually beyond the capability of the physician himself. It is also clear that the individual family physician's practice will vary in the mix of emphasis by James stage and by clinical content based upon many variables, such as the demography of the practice and community, the health beliefs and behavior of the community, third-party reimbursement policies, and many other related factors.

The foregoing discussion of the functional elements of family practice is not complete without reemphasis of the centrality of the individual patient as person and the family itself as patient. As McWhinney points out, the personal commitment of the family physician to his/her patient "involves 'staying with' the patient whatever his problem may be." To the family physician, "problems become interesting and important not only for their own sake but because they are Mr. Smith's or Mrs. Jones' problem. Very often in such relations there is not even a very clear distinction between a medical problem and a nonmedical one. The patient defines the problem.[23]

The family as the unit of care is important for many reasons. Perhaps the major reason is that the physician needs to apply health care to the smallest unit which at the same time allows optimal results of health care. Many individual illnesses are illnesses of the family as well, ranging from communicable disease to behavioral problems. The management of the individual patient with a disease must involve the understanding and assistance of other members of the family. Though the family as a unit has undergone evolutionary changes in recent decades, it remains the primary social group out of which all other social groupings are formed. Dennis has brought this perspective to the subject:[35]

> It is within the family milieu, and very early in life, that we find the genesis of social or antisocial human behavior, mental health or illness, many communicable diseases, and the nutritional and other factors that ultimately lead to many of the chronic degenerative and disabling disorders of later life. It is not possible to separate poor mental and physical health, ignorance, and poverty from the pathology of the family.

COMMENT

Having traced the progressive decline of general practice over the last 40 years, it is logical to ask why we can expect family practice to grow and develop as a foundation of future primary health care in the United States. Some of the reasons which allow us to project a bright future for family practice are:

1. Increased realization that the quality and quantity of health care actually delivered in this country fall far short of the public's needs and medicine's potential
2. Disenchantment with increasing specialism among many medical students

3. Commitment of today's medical student to improved delivery of health care
4. Development of Departments of Family Practice in a majority of the nation's medical schools
5. Development of residencies in family practice
6. Progress toward development of an active research base in the field
7. Board certification in family practice
8. Growing emphasis on group practice, which can afford family physicians an opportunity for a full family and personal life outside of medicine

As new graduates from the expanding number of family practice residencies have joined the ranks of board-certified family physicians drawn from general practice, the pendulum is starting to swing back toward a more desirable balance with the other specialties.

We are surrounded daily with ample evidence that modern health care in this country is excessively fragmented, uncoordinated, wasteful, impersonal, and confusing to the public. There is an urgent need for synthesis amidst this disarray. As Magraw has said in his pleas for synthesis in medicine:[36] "Integration and synthesis does not occur in an institution—it only occurs within a man and not between men." And to James, the family physician is "the man responsible for the navigation of human beings through the problems and difficulties involved in the maintenance of their health through each of the four stages of the natural history of disease. He is the key generalist of the future of medicine, and is the most indispensable of all."[34]

REFERENCES

1. Huntly RR: Epidemiology of family practice. JAMA 185:175, 1963
2. Margotta R: The Story of Medicine. New York, Golden Press, 1968, p 25
3. Editorial, JAMA 232:1420, 1900
4. Canfield PR: Family medicine: An historical perspective. J Med Educ 51:904, 1976
5. Shaw WJ: Evolution of a specialty. JAMA 186:575, 1963
6. Greenwood G, Frederickson RF: Specialization in the Medical and Legal Professions. Chicago, Callaghan & Company, 1964, p 45
7. Engel G: Care and feeding of the medical student. JAMA 215:1135, 1971
8. Menke WG: Divided labor: The doctor as specialist. Ann Int Med 72:943, 1970
9. Silver GA: Family practice: Resuscitation or reform? JAMA 185:188, 1963
10. What's ahead? Med Economics, Sept. 2, 1969, p 16
11. The Graduate Education of Physicians: The Report of the Citizens Commission on Graduate Medical Education (Millis Commission). Chicago, American Medical Association, 1966, p 179
12. Haggerty RJ: Etiology of decline of general practice. JAMA 185:180, 1963, p 179
13. Bryan JE: A summary report on the regional conferences on comprehensive medical care for the American family. GP (suppl) 1967, p 17
14. Angrist A: Plea for two-year mixed internship for family physician and specialist. JAMA 173:1642, 1960
15. Editorial: Annual report on graduate medical education in the United States. JAMA 210:1498, 1969
16. Lewis CE: Family practice: The primary care specialty. In Lewis CE, Fein R, Mechanic D (ed): A Right to Health: The Problem of Access to Primary Medical Care. New York, John Wiley & Sons, 1976, p 77

17. Marchmont-Robinson H: Today's challenge. JAMA 204:247, 1968
18. Annual Report on Graduate Medical Education in the United States. JAMA 210: 1508, 1969
19. Rutstein DD: The Coming Revolution in Medicine. Cambridge, Mass., The M.I.T. Press, 1967, p 66
20. Knowles JH: The quantity and quality of medical manpower: A review of medicine's current efforts. J Med Educ 44:102, 1969
21. Editorial: More and better GP's, fewer and better surgeons. Calif GP 18:15, 1967
22. AMA Mailing Service; personal communication, Dec., 1969
23. McWhinney IR: Family medicine in perspective. N Engl J Med 293(4): 180, 1975
24. Darley W: An educator's approach to training for comprehensive medical care. GP (suppl) Aug. 1967, p 22
25. Health Is a Community Affair. The Report of the National Commission on Community Health Services. Cambridge, Mass., Harvard University Press, 1966
26. The Graduate Education of Physicians: The Report of the Citizens Commission of Graduate Medical Education. Chicago, American Medical Association, 1966, p 40
27. Meeting the Challenge of Family Practice. The Report of the Ad Hoc Committee on Education for Family Practice of the Council on Medical Education. Chicago, American Medical Association, 1966, p 1
28. Editorial: The core content of family medicine, report of the committee on requirements for certification. GP 34:225, 1966
29. Millis JS: A re-examination of assumptions in medical education. GP (suppl), Aug. 1967, p 46
30. Schmidt DD: Referral patterns in an individual family practice. J Fam Pract 5:401, 1977
31. Geyman JP, Brown TC, Rivers K: Referrals in family practice: A comparative study by geographic region and practice setting. J Fam Pract 3:163, 1976
32. Metcalfe DH, Sishy D: Patterns of referral from family practice. J Fam Pract 1:34, 1974
33. Stephens GG: The intellectual basis of family practice. J Fam Pract 2:423, 1975
34. James G: The general practitioner of the future. N Engl J Med 27:1287, 1963
35. Dennis JL: Medical education, physician manpower, the state and community. J Med Educ 44:21, 1969
36. Magraw RM: The increasing ferment in medicine in comprehensive medical care. GP (suppl), 1967, p 33

2 | Supply and Distribution of Physicians

The intersection in the 1980's and 1990's of a plentiful supply of physicians, the introduction of underwriting systems based on prepayment and shared risk, and the development of large corporations for health care is bringing about a fundamental restructuring of the health services system and a transformation of the practice of medicine. Actions of this order that restructure a system, taken for the greater good, always have some unintended, unanticipated, and undesirable effects. But the actions are forceful and rarely reversed, at least in the near term. We should understand the roots of these changes, be outwardly directed, and assist society in achieving its goals within the context of the social purposes for which the health care system exists.

Alvin R. Tarlov[1]

Since the development of family practice represents a direct response to systemic problems in the health care system in the United States, it is useful to examine the general context of these problems to better understand the future role of family practice in this country. This is the first of four chapters which will deal with general background issues. We will focus first on trends and problems related to the supply and distribution of physicians.

The supply of physicians has been important and controversial subject especially during the last 30 years in the United States. Although there was general agreement throughout the 1950s and 1960s that a physician shortage existed as a serious problem, there was considerable debate as to how to relieve this shortage and the number of physicians needed. The 1970s saw increasing pessimism among health planners and policy makers that simply increasing the total number of physicians would effectively address the problems of delivery of health care, and there was some evidence that these problems were even aggravated by the growing supply of physicians. The end of the 1970s saw a growing consensus that the physician shortage of earlier years would become a physician surplus in the 1980s, and that the real problems of physician supply involved geographic and specialty maldistribution.

The purpose of this chapter is fourfold: (1) to discuss briefly the various factors affecting the adequacy of physician supply, (2) to summarize the basic features of various approaches to measure and make projections of the physician supply, (3) to outline the trends in total numbers of physicians, together with their geographic and specialty distribution, and (4) to review past and current approaches to the problems of physician supply and distribution.

VARIABLES AFFECTING PHYSICIAN SUPPLY

It is now apparent that the total number of physicians available to provide health care is only one of many factors important in any analysis of the relation between supply and demand of health care services.

In a comprehensive review of medicine's efforts concerning the quantity and quality of medical manpower in this country, Knowles in 1969 listed the following variables in connection with any appraisal of the physician supply:[2]

1. Specification of the type of physician involved (by field), the actual use of his time (practice, research, administration), and in what location (rural–urban, hospital, medical school)
2. Effectiveness of recruitment of workers into the field
3. The training capacity of hospitals and medical schools
4. The restraining or facilitating functions of state and specialty board licensure
5. Analysis of training expense
6. Degree of retention of physicians once in school, hospital, or practice
7. The productivity of the physician
8. The accessibility and availability of physicians
9. The ability to substitute other health workers in roles previously assumed by the physician

In 1975, Howard Stambler, as Chief of the Manpower Analysis Branch of the Bureau of Health Manpower, suggested four additional important variables influencing the adequacy of physician supply:[3]

1. Changes in the organization and delivery of health care (e.g., introduction and expansion of prepaid group practice plans)
2. Changes in the financial structure of the health care delivery system (e.g., Medicare, Medicaid, a possible future National Health Insurance)
3. Effects of technologic breakthroughs of virtually unknown dimensions
4. Major legislation or policy changes, such as those related to licensing and credentialing of health manpower, changes affecting immigration of foreign medical graduates, or unforeseen state and federal laws

Certainly many other factors can have important effects on the adequacy (or lack thereof) of the physician supply, but the range of the factors listed above points to the complexity of any analysis of physician manpower needs and projections.

The demand for health care services is likewise subject to many variables, such as:[2]

1. Age, sex, race, geographic location, education, cultural and attitudinal perspectives, and income of the population being considered
2. The extent of health information
3. Availability of physician and other health workers, equipment, and facilities
4. Social legislation and financing mechanisms

Knowles has pointed out the important observation that "demand" is by no means synonymous with "need" for health care services.[2] It is clear that many needs for health care are not being demanded by certain segments of our population. On the other side of the coin, it can likewise be argued that the "demand," as represented by health services delivered, may also exceed genuine needs. Mechanic has observed that: "Medical care is a highly discretionary activity; and physicians can generate considerable work that they would not be inclined to do if there were more demand for their services."[4] McNerney has documented that the more hospital beds or surgeons in a community, the higher the rates of hospital admissions and of surgical procedures.[5]

Pursuing the definition of "medical needs" further, Mechanic suggests that they include the following three components:[4]

1. Those needs recognized by medical personnel and also by the recipients as requiring care
2. Those needs recognized by medical personnel as needing care but not so recognized by the recipients (e.g., outreach work and health education)
3. Those needs defined by the consumer but not evident in medical screening or community assessments

MEASUREMENT OF PHYSICIAN SUPPLY

Measurement and forecasting of the physician supply unavoidably involve myriad complexities which to date have frustrated all attempts to develop consensus around any given method. The simplest measurement is to project the total number of physicians as a ratio to poulation, and indeed the physician–population ratio has been analyzed and discussed on many occasions over the years. Today most observers place little stock in this figure except as a crude descriptor of the overall physician supply. One needs to clarify many other factors before any sense can be made of the extent to which the physician supply meets the population's needs for health care. These factors range from the distribution of physicians by specialty and geographic location to biomedical, psychosocial, and socioeconomic influences on the need for health care services. In addition, it has been conclusively demonstrated that the physician–population ratio per se bears no direct relation to indices of health status.[6]

Although there are variations with either approach, there are two basic approaches for forecasting the supply of any health provider group—the demand-utilization model and the needs model.

The demand-based approach is illustrated by the study of U.S. physician manpower reported in 1959 by the Bane Committee. Assuming that the demand for health services by the population at that time was satisfactory, this study projected the number of physicians that would be needed in future years in order to keep the nation's supply of physicians constant at the level of 141 physicians per 100,000 people. The inherent problem with this model, of course, is that demand may be quite different from need for health services and even if they were equivalent, interactions between patients, physicians, and third-party payers are unlikely to remain unchanged in a changing health care system, especially as new knowledge and technology develops. The demand-based model can be modified by adjustments for various determinants of utilization of health care services, such as predicted demographic changes of the population or expected changes in the reimbursement system, but there is still ample room for forecasting error with this approach.

The needs-based approach assumes that the incidence and prevalence of disease and illness can be calculated for the population and extrapolated to the volume and types of health care services needed in the future. These services are then translated into units of service based on accepted norms of care for specific clinical problems. Finally, the number of physicians needed at some future time can be estimated by dividing the volume of required health care services by predicted average productivity of physicians providing care for patients with these problems. Here again, there are inherent problems with the needs-based approach, as illustrated by the following comment by Reinhardt:[7]

> The needs-based approach makes sense when it is realistic to assume that panels of experts now can develop plausible normative standards for health care utilization 10 to 20 years hence and when there is a reasonable hope that the future financing and delivery of health care will be so rearranged as to lead to a faithful translation of the normative "needs" standards into effective demand. Whether these assumptions are plausible depends, in the first instance, on whether individual consumers 10 to 20 years hence will share the experts' current perceptions of a need for medical intervention. It also depends on the political and economic climate of the future period. That climate will dictate whether the individual's perception of a need for medical intervention will actually translate itself into effective demand. If these two sets of conditions are not met, then the authors of needs-based forecasts run the risk of having egg on their face, for it is always effective demand, and not perceived need, that interacts with the effective supply to determine the actual utilization of health services and of health manpower. For that reason, economists generally prefer to develop their forecasts on the basis of effective demand and not need, even at the risk of being accused of insensitivity to human needs. It is simply a question of realism.

The most recent major study of physician manpower in this country is the *Report of the Graduate Medical Education National Advisory Committee* (GMENAC).[8] Since this report has been widely discussed and debated within medicine and health policy circles and is likely to have considerable influence on future health policy, its methods will be briefly summarized here. Because of the difficulty of projecting future physician manpower needs based upon present rates of utilization of physicians' services, which would perpetuate current inadequacies of health care for many, GMENAC selected the needs-based approach for its studies. Figure 2–1 displays the process of this study in arriving at future physician manpower requirements by specialty on an adjusted needs-based model. Expert panels for each specialty were charged with four tasks:[9]

1. Review data from various data bases relevant to each specialty and accept, increase, or decrease the Survey's findings to estimate future needs for health services.
2. Estimate the share of that group likely to visit a given specialty physician.
3. Estimate volume of services from norms of care (i.e., number of visits per year or per illness).
4. Estimate the proportion of visits to be delegated to nonphysician providers.

The panels included practitioners and academicians; they were specialty-specific, but included some representatives from other specialties and, in some cases, consumer representatives. A modified Delphi technique was used by each of 32 expert panels, and the recommendations of the panels were then reviewed and modified as needed by the Committee in order to compensate for differences or incongruities across specialties. In addition, GMENAC made extrapolations from the experience over the last 20 years concerning inter- and intraspecialty shifts of physicians during graduate medical education. GMENAC's final recommendations included con-

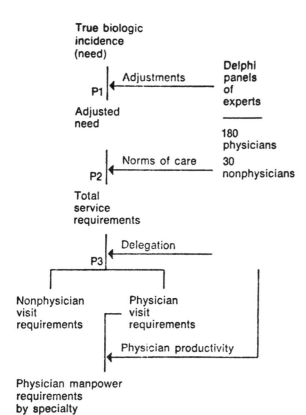

Figure 2-1. Physician requirements model. *(From Jacoby I: Physician manpower: GMENAC and afterwards. Public Health Rep 96(4):295, 1981, with permission.)*

sideration of socioeconomic and political factors related to future physician requirements.

It can readily be seen that there are substantial problems with either demand-based or needs-based projections of the future need for physicians, with or without adjustments. As Peterson points out:[10]

> The needs-based model relies on the opinions of panels of physician experts. Their viewpoints may not be tempered by the realities of patients' behaviors and expectations, interprofessional differences about who should give care, economic and social influences on the availability of resources for health care, etc. Gastroenterologists and general surgeons might apply quite different norms of care for detection and treatment of polyps of the colon. . . . In contrast, the demand-based model has the inherent risk of incorporating current inequities, inefficiencies, and ineffectiveness of the health care system. . . . Unmet needs are not reflected in the projections because they are either unrecognized or the strategies for meeting them have not been developed.

AGGREGATE NUMBER OF PHYSICIANS

At this writing, there are about 212 physicians per 100,000 people in the United States, compared to 140 per 100,000 in 1950. The United States now has more physicians per capita than almost all other nations (exceptions include the Soviet Union,

Israel, Belgium, and West Germany). This increase in the aggregate number of physicians is the inevitable result of the concerted efforts of government, medical schools, and other groups which focused primarily on the number of physicians as the principal factor to consider.

Much of the increase in numbers of physicians is due to rapid expansion of enrollments in United States allopathic and osteopathic schools; current first-year enrollments are more than double 1966 levels. A second major part of the growth in the aggregate number of physicians is the influx of foreign medical graduates. By 1973, active foreign medical graduates numbered 68,000, or one-fifth of all practicing physicians.[3] Between 1965 and 1982, foreign medical graduates filled about 25 to 30 percent of first-year residency positions in the United States.[1] Most of these have been non-U.S. citizens, and most have remained in this country after completing their training.

By 1990 the projected number of physicians in the United States will almost double.[1] GMENAC estimates a surplus of 62,750 and 137,200 physicians in 1990 and 2000 (Table 2–1), at which time the physician-to-population ratios are projected to be 215 and 240 per 100,000 population, respectively.[11]

GEOGRAPHIC DISTRIBUTION

It has been generally recognized that geographic maldistribution among physicians has existed for years both in total numbers of physicians and in specialty distribution by region, state, or size of community. The data show extreme variations by geographic area. In 1976, for example, it was estimated by the Macy Commission that over 45 million Americans lived in areas where the delivery of health services was inadequate or nonexistent.[12] The federal government presently designates more

TABLE 2-1. AGGREGATE PHYSICIAN SUPPLY AND REQUIREMENTS 1978, AND ESTIMATES FOR 1990 AND 2000[a]

	1978	1990	2000
Physician supply[b]	374,800	535,750	642,950
Physician requirements[c]	424,850	437,000	505,750
Surplus (shortage)	(50,050)	62,750	137,200

[a]This table has been revised from Table 1 of original Graduate Medical Education National Advisory Committee Summary Final Report (1980) to incorporate results of revised requirements for six specialties. Estimates have been rounded to the nearest 50.

[b]Includes all professionally active physicians (M.D.s and D.O.s) together with 0.35 of all residents in training in year indicated. 1990 and 2000 figures assume that US allopathic medical school first-year enrollment will increase 2.5 percent per year until 1982–1983 for a total increase of 10 percent over 1978–1979 enrollment of 16,501, and then will remain level at 18,151, that US osteopathic medical school enrollment will increase 4.6 percent per year until 1987–1988 for total increase of 41 percent over 1978–1979 number of 1322, and then will remain level at 1868, and that foreign medical graduates will be added to residency pool at the rate of 3100 per year in 1979–1980, increase to 4100 per year by 1983, and then remain level. All supply data in following tables have been calculated using these assumptions.

[c]1978 and 2000 figures on requirements extrapolated from 1990 calculated requirements simply on basis of population differences in 3 years.

(From Bowman MA, Katzoff JM, Garrison LP, et al.: Estimates of physician requirements for 1990 for the specialties of neurology, anesthesiology, nuclear medicine, pathology, physical medicine and rehabilitation, and radiology: A further application of the GMENAC methodology. JAMA 250:2623, 1983, with permission. Copyright 1983, American Medical Association.)

than 1200 counties, portions of counties, and inner-city neighborhoods as critical health manpower shortage areas. The major criterion for these designations is a physician–population ratio greater than 1:3500 (compared to current national average of 1:600). Modifiers of this definition include high mortality rates (more than 1 in 25), impacted poverty areas (more than 30 percent of the population with incomes below the poverty level), high annual visits (more than 8000 per physician per year), high waiting times, and high rates of physician refusal to see patients.[13] Five states and the District of Columbia have more than 180 patient care physicians per 100,000 people (New York, Massachusetts, Connecticut, Maryland, and California), whereas five states have less than 100 patient care physicians per 100,000 people (South Dakota, Mississippi, Wyoming, Idaho, and Arkansas).[14] In New York City, there is now one physician for every 315 people, although many residents of that city have major barriers to health care.

Two recent studies of the distribution trends of physicians in the United States during the 1970s have suggested that the increasing supply of physicians is beginning to improve the problem of their geographic maldistribution. Schwartz and his colleagues studied the changing geographic distribution of board-certified specialists in 8 specialties in 23 states between 1960 and 1977. The 23 states comprised almost one-half of the country's nonmetropolitan population in 1976. "Nonmetropolitan" was defined as areas outside Standard Metropolitan Statistical Areas (SMSAs), which are counties containing cities of more than 50,000 people. They found an outward movement of all specialties studied to smaller communities. Surgeons and radiologists were most likely of the consultant specialties to disperse to smaller communities. Table 2–2 shows an increasing proportion of smaller communities by 1977 with the five largest consulting specialties (i.e., internal medicine, surgery, pediatrics, obstetrics–gynecology, and radiology). As expected, family physicians were found in communities of all sizes, including 37 percent of towns with populations of 2500 to 5000 people.

In a similar study, Newhouse and his colleagues extended the above study to include noncertified physicians, together with previously omitted specialties, again in 23 states from 1970 to 1979. They utilized physicians' self-reported specialty designations, using aggregated AMA specialty codes (e.g., medical and pediatric subspecialists categorized as internists and pediatricians, respectively). They also documented an increasing percentage of self-reported specialists in smaller communities. By 1979, only 57 towns out of a total 1426 towns of more than 2500 peo-

TABLE 2-2. PERCENTAGE OF COMMUNITIES IN WHICH THE FIVE LARGEST SPECIALTIES ARE ALL REPRESENTED.[a]

Year	Population in Thousands						
	2.5–5	5–10	10–20	20–30	30–50	50–200	>200
1960	0	1	3	30	58	85	100
1970	0	1	11	44	80	92	100
1977	0	4	18	71	95	95	100

[a]Internal medicine, surgery, pediatrics, obstetrics/gynecology, and radiology. Data are drawn from the 23 states listed in the text.

(From Schwartz WB, Newhouse JP, Bennett BW, et al.: The changing geographic distribution of board-certified physicians. N. Engl J Med 303:1032, 1980, with permission.)

ple were without a nonfederal physician, and 16 of these had ready access to medical care in adjacent urban areas.[16]

Despite the findings of these two studies, however, there is evidence that considerable geographic maldistribution of physicians persists as a chronic problem. A recent study by the National Center for Health Services Research involving all states over the period 1950 to 1978 showed continued disparity in population–physician ratios. During that period the population–physician ratios dropped from 721 people per physician in 1970 to 498 in 1978 for all SMSAs and from 1443 people per physician in 1960 to 1165 in 1978 in non-SMSAs. They noted that the growth in nonfederal physician supply remains slowest in counties with less than 25,000 people, and concluded that little actual spillover has yet occurred from physician-saturated SMSAs into rural areas.[17] In addition, a recent statewide study in Kentucky found that the more urban counties are increasing their physician supply at a rate ten times greater than the more rural counties.[18]

GMENAC has recognized the difficulties in using geopolitical units, such as states, counties, cities, or towns, for analysis of health care services. The Committee recommends the development of functional medical service areas for analysis and planning on a service-by-service basis. It proposes two criteria for the designation of an area as medically underserved: (1) physician–population ratio less than one-half that recommended for the country as a whole, or (2) maximum travel time required to gain access to medical care is not feasible for 95 percent of the population. In addition, GMENAC proposed the following specific minimum standards of adequacy for each type of service:[19]

- Child medical: 24.6 physicians for 100,000 children under 17 years of age and a maximum of 30 minutes travel time
- Adult medical: 15.2 physicians per 100,000 total population and 30 minutes travel time
- General surgical: 4.8 physicians per 100,000 total population and 90 minutes travel time
- Obstetrical: 9.6 physicians per 100,000 women of all ages and 45 minutes travel time
- Emergency medical: 2.8 physicians per 100,000 total population and 30 minutes travel time

The above proposal presumes that specific standards could be established for each type of service in terms of the minimal number of physicians involved in that type of service (e.g., pediatricians and general/family physicians in the area of child health care).

SPECIALTY DISTRIBUTION

There is ample evidence that maldistribution of physicians by specialty has been an increasing problem during the last several decades which has now reached serious proportions. Examples of the magnitude of this problem are plentiful. Most of the imbalance by specialty has resulted from the rapid growth in the surgical specialties and the medical subspecialties. For example, whereas there was an 8.4 percent reduction in the total number of physicians in general/family practice, internal medicine, and pediatrics between 1965 and 1972, there was an increase of 19.6 percent in the number of surgical specialists and an increase of 33.6 percent in the number of other specialists during the same period.[20] Between 1971 and 1975, the growth rate of active, Board-certified surgeons was about seven times as fast as the population growth rate.[21] Between 1976 and 1983, there was a 23 percent increase in the number of residents training in internal medicine, but a very large proportion of these are subspecializing, as demonstrated in Table 2–3.[22] The impact of specialty maldistribution has been colorfully stated by Petersdorf as follows:[23]

> In the communities with which I am familiar, there are few echocardiograms in search of cardiologists to read them, there is only a rare belch wanting a gastroenterologist, and there is not a single, even slightly plugged coronary that does not have three surgeons waiting in the wings. Moreover, the specialists are young, since specialty training programs are, for the most part, a creation of the 1960's and 1970's, and most of them will be in practice a long time.

The rapid growth in subspecialization has had a severe impact on the number of practitioners in the primary care specialties. Although family practice grew rapidly in the early 1970s, its growth stabilized between 1976 and 1980, as did primary care internal medicine and pediatrics. Thus, as shown in Table 2–4, the total proportion of U.S. medical school graduates projected to be in the primary care specialties remained stable at appoximately 30 percent for graduates in 1974, 1976, and 1980.[24]

GMENAC's final projections for physician supply by specialty for 1990 are shown in Table 2–5. The Committee viewed any supply between 80 and 120 percent as being near balance. It further recommended that any change in a particular specialty not exceed a 20 percent increase or decrease in that specialty, even though it realized that balance by specialty is in no way achievable by 1990.[9]

As is the case for geographic maldistribution of physicians, graduate medical education so far has contributed to the increasing specialty maldistribution of physi-

TABLE 2-3. SUBSPECIALIZATION RATES: 1977-1978 THROUGH 1982-1983[a]

Year	Total (%)	USMGs[b] (%)	USFMGs (%)	FMGs (%)	Women (%)	Men (%)	Blacks (%)
1977–1978	75	69	55				
1978–1979	69	65	50	93			
1979–1980	63	59	45	96			
1980–1981	58	54	41	86			
1981–1982	56	54	35	79	44	59	
1982–1983	58	57	31	79	47	61	34

[a]Percentage of internal medicine residents who enter subspecialty fellowship training after completing residency—(fellowship entrants of the given year) / (residency completers of the previous year) × 100. The residency completers are the sum of the third-, fourth- and fifth-year residents of the previous year minus the fourth- and fifth-year residents of the given year. Only the 11 traditional subspecialty fields were used for the calculations in this table. Clinical pharmacology, critical care medicine, geriatric medicine, nutrition, and general internal medicine fellowship positions were not included. The 1982–1983 total subspecialization rate calculated with the new subspecialty fields included (but general internal medicine excluded) was 62 percent.
[b]USMG = graduates of U.S., Canadian, or Puerto Rican medical schools; USFMG = U.S. or Canadian citizens who graduated from medical schools outside the United States, Canada, or Puerto Rico; FMG = graduates of foreign medical schools who are not U.S. citizens.
(From Schleiter MK, Tarlov AR: National study of internal medicine manpower. VII. Internal medicine residency and fellowship training: 1983 update. Ann Intern Med 99:380, 1983, with permission.)

TABLE 2-4. PROJECTED SPECIALTY OF U.S. MEDICAL SCHOOL GRADUATES, ACCORD-ING TO YEAR OF STARTING GRADUATE MEDICAL EDUCATION[a]

Category	1970		1974		1976		1980	
	%	No.	%	No.	%	No.	%	No.
Total	100.0	8070	100.0	10,933	100.0	12,904	100.0	14,930
Internship or flex year only	6.8	551	3.3	360	2.0	253	1.6	243
Primary care	21.3	1721	29.5	3229	32.2	4156	31.8	4747
Internal medicine	11.2	904	13.4	1465	14.0	1801	13.2	1975
Pediatrics	7.0	568	7.1	779	6.6	855	6.3	948
Family practice	3.1	249	9.0	985	11.6	1501	12.2	1824
Medical specialties	14.3	1156	17.0	1861	17.6	2277	16.7	2489
Pediatric specialties	2.0	163	2.3	251	2.2	289	2.2	321
Surgical specialties	29.3	2361	27.0	2952	25.1	3233	27.0	4041
General surgery	5.9	480	5.4	592	4.2	541	4.4	664
Obstetrics/gynecology	5.4	436	6.5	716	6.5	838	7.2	1073
Other specialties	17.9	1445	15.0	1644	14.4	1854	15.4	2304
Hospital-based specialties	13.3	1072	10.4	1136	10.8	1392	11.4	1700
Anesthesiology	3.2	255	2.2	243	2.8	367	3.4	514
Pathology	2.9	236	3.2	349	2.9	380	2.7	402
Radiology	7.2	582	5.0	544	5.0	645	5.3	784
Other specialties	13.0	1046	10.5	1143	10.1	1303	9.3	1389
Psychiatry	7.6	610	6.8	740	5.9	761	5.1	758
Neurology	2.0	165	1.5	169	1.6	206	1.4	214
Other	3.4	271	2.1	234	2.6	388	2.8	418

[a]Percentages and numbers do not total exactly because of rounding off.

(From Steinwachs DM, Levine DM, Elymga DT, et al.: Changing patterns of graduate medical education: Analyzing recent trends and projecting their impact. N Engl J Med 306:10, 1982, with permission.)

cians, rather than helping to alleviate the problem. To date, the number and type of residency positions in the various specialties has been determined solely by the respective specialties without a coordinated effort to "rationalize the mix" at any level. The "territorial imperative" often operates at the level of the individual residency program, whereby programs are unnecessarily expanded or continued at the same level past a time when a clear need exists for more graduates in the field. Many hospitals have relied on residents for their service function, which may be considered cheaper than hiring staff physicians. Residents have also been depended upon for teaching by clinical departments in medical schools and the larger teaching hospitals.

The influx of foreign medical graduates is again part of the specialty maldistribution problem. The number of foreign medical graduates in this country increased from 36,569 in 1963 to 77,660 in 1973, an increase of 112.3 percent, compared with a growth rate of 21 percent for U.S. medical graduates over the same period.[25] As a result, the annual growth of licensed foreign medical graduates became almost as large as the increase U.S.-trained licensed physicians and by 1973 represented one-fifth of all practicing physicians.[3] In the mid-1970s it was observed

TABLE 2-5. RATIO PERCENTAGE OF PROJECTED SUPPLY TO ESTIMATED REQUIREMENTS, 1990[a]

	Ratio (%)	Requirements	Surplus (Shortage)
Shortages			
Child psychiatry	45	9,000	(4,900)
Physical medicine and rehabilitation	60	4,050	(1,650)
Emergency medicine	70	13,600	(4,250)
Preventive medicine	75	7,300	(1,750)
General psychiatry	80	38,500	(8,000)
Near balance			
Therapeutic radiology	85	2,560	(400)
Anesthesiology	90	22,150	(2,000)
Hematology/oncology-internal medicine	90	9,000	(700)
Dermatology	105	8,950	400
Gastroenterology-internal medicine	105	8,500	400
Osteopathic general practice	105	22,750	1,150
Family practice	105	81,300	3,100
General internal medicine	105	70,250	3,550
Otolaryngology	105	8,000	500
Pathology	105	15,900	950
Neurology	105	8,350	300
General pediatrics and subspecialties	115	38,400	4,950
Surpluses			
Urology	120	7,700	1,650
Diagnostic radiology	135	19,200	6,450
Orthopedic surgery	135	15,100	5,000
Ophthalmology	140	11,600	4,700
Thoracic surgery	140	2,050	880
Infectious disease-internal medicine	145	2,250	1,000
Obstetrics-gynecology	145	24,000	10,450
Plastic surgery	145	2,700	1,200
Allergy/immunology-internal medicine	150	2,050	1,000
General surgery	150	23,500	11,800
Nephrology-internal medicine	175	2,750	2,100
Rheumatology-internal medicine	175	1,700	1,300
Cardiology-internal medicine	190	7,750	7,150
Endocrinology-internal medicine	190	2,050	1,800
Neurosurgery	190	2,650	2,450
Pulmonary-internal medicine	195	3,800	3,350
Nuclear medicine	Not available	4,300	Not available

[a]*This table has been revised from Figure 1 of the original Graduate Medical Education National Advisory Committee Summary Final Report (1980) to incorporate results of revised requirements for six specialties. Estimates have been rounded to the nearest 50.*
(From Bowman MA, Katzoff JM, Garrison LP, et al.: Estimates of physician requirements for 1990 for the specialties of neurology, anesthesiology, nuclear medicine, pathology, physical medicine and rehabilitation, and radiology: A further application of the GMENAC methodology. JAMA 250:2623, 1983, with permission. Copyright 1983, American Medical Association.)

that of the approximately 2000 foreign medical graduates entering the United States each year for surgical training, 1500 were remaining as surgeons and only about 400 becoming board certified.[26] There were more than 13,000 foreign medical graduates in U.S. residency programs in 1983 (18.4 percent of all residents in training), with considerable variation by specialty (e.g., physical medicine and rehabilitation—40.4 percent; psychiatry—28.6 percent; pediatrics—27 percent; internal medicine—21.3 percent; surgery—15.1 percent; obstetrics-gynecology—14.7 percent; and family practice—12.9 percent).[27] Table 2–3 shows extremely high rates of subspecialization among foreign medical graduates trained in internal medicine, and only a very small number enter the primary care specialties. In addition, the quality of care provided by many foreign medical graduates has been seriously questioned by a number of observers. Weiss and colleagues, for example, observed that "a large number of FMG's are functioning in a medical underground delivering patient care in an unsupervised and unregulated fashion."[28] Some estimates have been made that the number of unlicensed FMGs may exceed 10,000.[29]

Dr. Robert Knouss, while serving as Director of the Division of Medicine of the Bureau of Health Manpower, in 1976 summarized the end result of these trends in these words:[30]

> Specialization, which has been stimulated by shifts toward hospital care and uncontrolled because of a lack of adequate planning, has also been accompanied by an increased fragmentation of medical care. Furthermore, specialization as a general phenomenon appears to have been associated with observable inefficiencies in the delivery of services. Underutilization, overtraining, duplication, and varying levels of compensation for the performance of similar tasks have all been cited as factors in rising health care costs, the forces of inflation aside. . . . this should not be interpreted as an argument for despecialization, it is, instead, a plea for achieving a balance between generalism and specialism, for improved efficiency in the delivery of services, and for a move away from fragmentation.

APPROACHES TO PHYSICIAN MANPOWER PROBLEMS

The foregoing makes it clear that the main theme in most thinking and responses to address physician manpower problems during recent years in this country focused primarily on efforts to increase the total number of physicians. By the mid-1970s, however, there was general consensus that these efforts had failed and that other kinds of intervention to address geographic and specialty maldistribution were needed. Some new initiatives have been taken at several levels since the mid-1970s which have especially involved organized medicine, academic medicine, and government in an increasingly collaborative manner. An overall perspective of these new initiatives can be developed by brief review of some of the policy statements of several of the major organizations.

The Association of American Medical Colleges (AAMC) Task Force on Foreign Medical Graduates in 1974 proposed a series of actions that would reduce the influx of foreign medical graduates without adopting discriminatory policies. The following steps were recommended:[31]

1. Limit the number of first-year positions in approved residency programs of graduate medical education "so as to exceed only slightly the expected

number of graduates from domestic medical schools and to provide sufficient opportunities to highly qualified FMGs."

2. Apply the same standards of admission to residency programs to FMGs and U.S. graduates.
3. Close the loopholes in licensure of FMGs by state medical boards.

The mid-1970s saw the formation of two new bodies with broad responsibilities for improving the coordination of medical education—the Coordinating Council on Medical Education (CCME), now renamed the Accrediting Council on Medical Education, and the Liaison Committee on Graduate Medical Education (LCGME), renamed the Accrediting Committee for Graduate Medical Education.* These groups included wide representation within medicine in the hope that the overall needs of medical education could be better served, particularly through accreditation decisions. In 1975, the CCME recommended:[32]

> As a national goal, schools of medicine should be encouraged to accept voluntarily the responsibility for providing an appropriate environment that will motivate students to select careers related to the teaching and practice of primary care. An initial national target of having 50% of graduating medical students choose careers as primary care specialists appears reasonable.

This goal had the support of the House of Delegates of the American Medical Association, many professional organizations, and the federal government.

At the federal level, the Health Professions Educational Assistance Act of 1976 (Public Law 94-484) also established new directions from previous legislation. This act extended federal support for the training of physicians, dentists, and other health personnel with new provisions to more directly affect the kinds of health professionals being trained and where they will practice. Among the various provisions of the law were the following:[33]

1. Capitation grants to medical schools provided that percentages of filled first-year residency positions in direct or affiliated residency programs in primary care (family medicine, general internal medicine, and general pediatrics) exceeded 35 percent in 1978, 40 percent in 1979, and 50 percent in 1980.
2. Project grants provided to help establish academic administrative units in family medicine in medical and osteopathic schools.
3. Matching construction grants for ambulatory primary care teaching facilities.
4. Revision of the Immigration and Naturalization Act to restrict the entry of foreign medical graduates.
5. New student assistance programs of insured loans and scholarships for needy health professions students.
6. Increased authorizations for National Health Service Corps (NHSC) scholarships with obligated service conditions broadened to include private practice.

---

*The Liaison Committee for Graduate Medical Education includes representatives from the AMA, AAMC, the American Hospital Association (AHA), the Council of Medical Specialty Societies (CMSS), and the American Board of Medical Specialties (ABMS).

7. Categorical support for teaching programs in general dentistry, since a problem of excess specialization has taken place in dentistry as in medicine.

After intensive study, the Institute of Medicine of the National Academy of Sciences in 1978 released a comprehensive report, *An Integrated Manpower Policy for Primary Care.* Among its specific recommendations were the following:[34]

1. For the present, the number of entrants to medical school should remain at the current annual level.
2. For the present, the number of nurse practitioners and physician assistants trained should remain at the current annual level.
3. A substantial increase should be made in the national goal for percentage distribution of first-year residents in primary care fields (although a definite level was not recommended, there was a general feeling that 60 to 70 percent of first-year residency positions in primary care specialties may be indicated instead of the 50 percent figure called for in Public Law 94-484).
4. Third-party reimbursement by federal and state programs and private insurers to all physicians should be at the same level of payment for the same primary care service, and consideration should be given to narrowing the differentials in payment levels between primary care and nonprimary care procedures.
5. Medical schools should provide all students with some clinical experience in a primary care setting.
6. The curriculum of undergraduate medical education should include epidemiology and the behavioral and social sciences.
7. In selecting among applicants for admission, medical schools should give weight to likely indicators of primary care selections.

Another important contribution to physician manpower planning during the late 1970s was the excellent report of the Macy Commission, *Physicians for the Future.* This group made the following observations:[12]

> [The] responsibility for the nation's health programs is so fragmented that the programs are not being carried out with maximal effectiveness. It also became clear, after careful review of existing professional organizations; that no one agency is at this time "putting it all together"—coordinating and giving unified direction to the numerous current efforts aimed at the improvement of health.

The Commission noted further that "Differences of opinion among the parent organizations and the lack of independent status and staff have thus far limited the CCME's effectiveness in dealing with current problems."

The Macy Commission therefore called for the formation of an independent, broadly representative National Commission of Medical Education, Manpower, and Services, which would concern itself with:[12]

1. The nation's need for physicians
2. The expansion of existing medical schools and the number and location of new schools
3. The apportionment of graduates among the various specialties and their geographic distribution
4. The flow of foreign medical graduates and United States foreign medical graduates

5. The financing of medical education, so that federal support will meet reasonable needs
6. The nation's need for nurse practitioners and physicians' assistants

COMMENT

Although it is clear that redistribution of residency positions in graduate medical education (GME) cannot as an isolated measure solve complex physician manpower problems, it is generally agreed that this is a vital and indispensable part of any effective response to these problems. Yet, after more than a decade of concerted efforts by government and concerned professional organizations, little headway has been made in reversing medicine's headlong rush to subspecialization and fragmentation of health care. Only 32 percent of all U.S. residency positions are in bona fide primary care. Family practice has plateaued at about 13 percent of these positions, and the other 19 percent represent physicians trained in internal medicine and pediatrics who do not subspecialize. Tracking studies of residents in training have demonstrated a high frequency of changes in career choice with many residents abandoning primary care in favor of nonprimary care specialties. Jacoby applied a GME flow model and found that only 47 and 65 percent of first-year residents in general internal medicine and general pediatrics, respectively, ended up practicing in those specialties.[35]

In order to effectively address the imbalance between primary care and the consulting specialties, reform in graduate medical education is required, together with other changes in the health care system. A variety of important issues must be addressed simultaneously, such as financing mechanisms for medical education, reimbursement policies, and remodeling of the existing health care delivery system around a stronger primary care base. As Petersdorf observes:[26]

> We should aim to make the practice of primary care medicine—whether it be by family practitioners, general internists, or pediatricians—as attractive, prestigious and rewarding as subspecialty practice. This should be the major goal of medical schools, professional organizations, accrediting bodies, and government. If it can be reached, many of our health manpower problems will be relieved.

Although some will say that we do not yet have the information or capability to "fine-tune" the mix of physicians by specialty, this is not the issue at this point. The pendulum has swung so far in this country toward subspecialization that the problems are major and call for "rough-tuning" or equally major actions to rebalance the health care delivery system. Stevens has observed that two revolutionary periods have already occurred in American medicine during the 20th century—the revolution in undergraduate medical education between 1905 and 1910, and that involving the development of specialist education and certification in the 1930s. In 1971 she saw the inevitable need for a "third period of radical education and manpower reform in the 1970's and 1980's in response to organizational and economic pressures, whether through national health insurance or government financing of medical education."[36]

Only time will tell whether the currently accepted target of 50 percent for the three primary care specialties will meet the needs of the public. In my view, this is well short of the mark, and a target at or above 60 or 70 percent will probably be required. The critical question concerning the effectiveness of any such target, however, is the extent to which the long-standing trend toward subspecialization in internal medicine and pediatrics can be altered toward primary care roles. Academic departments and faculty in internal medicine and pediatrics are predominantly oriented to the subspecialties, and there is considerable evidence that the trends toward subspecialization remain strong. As Somers observes:[37]

> The primary care issue is not just a matter of numbers or how the doctor is listed in the medical directories. It involves the physician's basic value system, his philosophy of patient care, and his personal professional priorities. The effective primary care physician must be prepared—not only technically, but philosophically and temperamentally—to assume continuing responsibility for the patient's overall health needs, including health maintenance. Medical school and residency training, and attitudes inculcated in those settings, must be reasonably consistent with the end-product that Congress and the public are demanding, or avoidable conflict and frustrations will continue to plague the profession and its educational institutions.

While recent recommendations for total numbers of primary care physicians have become quite specific, there has been less specificity with respect to the balance among the primary care disciplines themselves. In 1973, the American Academy of Family Physicians adopted a goal that sufficient family practice residency positions be developed to accommodate at least 25 percent of medical school graduates each year. At a recent reunion meeting of the Willard Committee, which in 1966 drafted the landmark Willard Report on Education for Family Practice, the group recommended that a goal be established for 25 percent of American medical school graduates to enter residency training in family practice by 1985.[38] Other health manpower experts have likewise recommended this level for family practice.[39] This goal appears logical and even minimal, particularly since family practice is the only specialty in American medicine with an exclusive mission in primary care, whereas the other primary care disciplines have divided goals and practice styles involving both primary care and subspecialty care. In order to reach a 25 percent goal, however, family practice will have to double its present proportion of U.S. residents in training, which should probably be achieved by concurrent reduction in surplus fields and expansion of graduate training in family practice. In any event, GMENAC's recommended limit of 20 percent change in the numbers of any specialty appear to be inappropriate in this instance if a strong primary care base is to be established for the future health care system. Indeed, the work by Jacoby on graduate medical education and ultimate specialty distribution provides solid support for the nation's investment in family practice as the most effective way to strengthen the primary care base.[35]

It is clear from the foregoing that physician manpower problems are complex, and their resolution inextricable from broader issues in medical education and clinical practice. There is an urgent need to formulate a cohesive and effective national policy for physician manpower issues. Ginzberg challenges medicine as follows:[40]

> There are many important questions about the future supply of physicians that warrant attention by members of the profession and its leaders. These include the determination of whether an oversupply threatens or is already here; the criteria for reaching a judgment about the adequacy of the supply; the extent

to which factors on the demand side, e.g., pressures to reduce reimbursement or the growing number of the elderly, will affect physicians' work loads; conflicts with nurse practitioners and nonmedical providers over "turf"; the rate at which the corporate practice of medicine is likely to expand as a result of the availability of young physicians looking for employment opportunities; the long-term effects on the profession of the growing proportion of women graduates of medical schools; and still other questions involving recruitment, education, residency training, and practice modes.

In this connection, the recent observation by Bloom and Peterson is on target:[41]

> There may be some reluctance to reverse policies for physician manpower that are based on opinion and poor information, but inaction because appropriate data are lacking is no longer justified.

REFERENCES

1. Tarlov AR: Shattuck lecture—The increasing supply of physicians, the changing structure of the health-services system, and the future practice of medicine. N Engl J Med 308:(20):1235, 1983
2. Knowles JH: The quantity and quality of medical manpower: A review of medicine's current efforts. J Med Educ 44:84, 1969
3. Stambler HV: Health manpower—the right number. In: Health Manpower Issues. DHEW Publication No. (HRA) 76–40, Government Printing Office, 1976, pp 12–13
4. Mechanic D: Relationships between medical need and responsiveness of care: A framework for developing policy options. In Lewis CE, Fein R, Mechanic D (ed): A Right to Health: The Problem of Access to Primary Medical Care. New York, John Wiley & Sons, 1976, p 21
5. McNerney W: Why does medical care cost so much? N Engl J Med 282:1458, 1970
6. Peterson ML: Planning for the appropriate number of physicians. University of Washington Medicine 8(1):3, 1981
7. Reinhardt UE: The GMENAC forecast: An alternative view. Am J Public Health 71(10):1149, 1981
8. U.S. Department of Health and Human Services: Report of the Graduate Medical Education National Advisory Committee to the Secretary, Vol. 1, Sept. 1980. Hyattsville, Md., DHHS Pub. No. 81–651, 1981
9. Jacoby I: Physician manpower: GMENAC and afterwards. Public Health Rep 96(4):295, 1981
10. Peterson ML: Planning for the appropriate number of physicians. University of Washington Medicine 8(1):3, 1981
11. Bowman MA, Katzoff JM, Garrison LP, et al.: Estimates of physician requirements for 1990 for the specialties of neurology, anesthesiology, nuclear medicine, pathology, physical medicine and rehabilitation, and radiology: A further application of the GMENAC methodology. JAMA 250:2623, 1983
12. Physicians for the Future. Report of the Macy Commission. New York, Josiah Macy, Jr. Foundation, 1976, p 80
13. Wise DA, Zook CJ: Physician shortage areas and policies to influence practice location. Health Serv Res 18(2):251, 1983
14. Profile of Medical Practice, 1980. Chicago, American Medical Association, 1980, p 166
15. Schwartz WB, Newhouse JP, Bennett BW, et al.: The changing geographic distribution of board-certified physicians. N Engl J Med 303:1032, 1980

16. Newhouse JP, Williams AP, Bennett BW, et al.: Where have all the doctors gone? JAMA 247:2392, 1982

17. Fruen MA, Cantwell JR: Geographic distribution of physicians: Past trends and future influences. Inquiry 19:44, 1982

18. Cooper JK, Johnson TP: Physician distribution—Will it get worse instead of better? AM J Med 75:4, 1983

19. Tarlov AR: The increasing dispersion of specialists. N Engl J Med 303:1058, 1980

20. Holden WD: Attitudes of the Coordinating Council on Medical Education toward physician manpower. Bull NY Acad Med 52:1078, Nov. 1976

21. Moore FD, Zuidema GD, Ballinger WF: Surgical manpower and public policy. Surgery 83:116, 1978

22. Schleiter MK, Tarlov AR: National study of internal medicine manpower. VII. Internal medicine residency and fellowship training: 1983 update. Ann Intern Med 99:380, 1983

23. Petersdorf RG: Is the establishment defensible? N Engl J Med 309:1053, 1983

24. Steinwachs DM, Levine DM, Elymga DT, et al.: Changing patterns of graduate medical education: Analyzing recent trends and projecting their impact. N Engl J Med 306:10, 1982

25. Distribution of Physicians in the United States, 1973. Chicago, American Medical Association, Center for Health Services Research and Development, 1974, p 42

26. Petersdorf RG: Health manpower: Numbers, distribution, quality. Ann Intern Med 82:696, 1975

27. Summary statistics on graduate medical education in the United States. JAMA 252:1550, 1984

28. Weiss RJ, et al.: Foreign medical graduates and the medical underground. N Engl J Med 290:1408, 1974

29. Holden WD: Developments in graduate medical education. In Purcell EF (ed): Recent Trends in Medical Education. New York, Josiah Macy, Jr. Foundation, 1976, p 257

30. Knouss RF: Health manpower—the right kind. In: Health Manpower Issues. DHEW Publication No. (HRA) 76-40, Government Printing Office, 1976, pp 17–18

31. Graduates of foreign medical schools in the United States: A challenge to medical education. J Med Educ 49:809, 1974

32. Coordinating Council on Medical Education: Physician Manpower and Distribution: The Primary Care Physician. Chicago, Coordinating Council on Medical Education, 1975, p 6

33. Whiteside DF: Training the nation's health manpower—the next 4 years. Public Health Rep 92(2):99, 1977

34. Institute of Medicine of the National Academy of Sciences: An Integrated Manpower Policy for Primary Care. Washington, D.C., 1978

35. Jacoby I: Graduate medical education: Its impact on specialty distribution. JAMA 245:1046, 1981

36. Stevens R: Trends in medical specialization in the United States. Inquiry 8(1):18, 1971

37. Somers AR, Somers HM: Health and Health Care: Policies in Perspective. Germantown, Md., Aspen Systems Corporation, 1977, p 441

38. Willard WA, Ruhe CHW: The challenge of family practice reconsidered. JAMA 240:454, 1978

39. Morrow JH, Edwards AB: U.S. health manpower policy: Will the benefits justify the costs? J Med Educ 51:792, 1976

40. Ginzberg E. A new physician supply policy is needed. JAMA 250:2621, 1983

41. Bloom BS, Peterson OL: Changing the number of surgeons. N Engl J Med 303:1227, 1980

3 The Changing Health Care System

Equal access to high-quality health services in all geographic areas at an affordable cost is the nation's primary health-policy objective. Attainment requires an adequate supply of physicians in each specialty, an equitable geographic distribution of physicians related to population density, and mechanisms for financial payment that do not deny needed services for any reason.

Alvin R. Tarlov[1]

A majority of the people in the United States believe that there is a "crisis" in health care in this country. About three-fourths of the population feel that basic changes are needed in the delivery of medical services. According to a Harris poll taken in the fall of 1983, for example, two-thirds of physicians felt that the present health care system "works pretty well and needs only minor changes," but only a small minority of other respondent groups agreed with that view (i.e., 21 percent of the public, 19 percent of union leaders, and 16 percent of insurance executives). The predominant public view is that health care is too costly and for many inaccessible, that "policies that benefit physicians are a source of health care inflation, and that a broad range of cost containment policies are needed."[2]

The overriding health care priority 10 and 15 years ago involved the need to improve the population's access to health care. Today, cost containment has become far and away the highest priority in U.S. health care. This is by no means unexpected, since national health expenditures have increased almost tenfold in the past 20 years to $310 billion in 1982, mostly as a result of skyrocketing hospital outlays (up 700 percent since 1965.)[3] Moreover, it has become widely recognized that past cost containment strategies have not been effective, and that the projected increase in the physician supply described in the last chapter will further aggravate the cost problem.

Accompanying the widespread public concern over the escalating cost of health care has been an increasingly vocal expression questioning the benefits of health care and the extent to which the nation's investment in health care is justified. Criticism of medical care has ranged from rates of hospitalization and surgery, to the effectiveness of psychotherapy. The 1970s spawned such books as Illich's *Medical Nemesis*[4] and Maxmen's *The Post Physician Era.*[5] The well-known health economist, Victor Fuchs concluded that the addition of more medical care to the system would reduce neither mortality nor disease.[6] The mood of the mid-1970s is well characterized by the following observations of Holman:[7]

For years, as medical care expenditures have risen beyond the rate of inflation, there has been no direct relationship between expense and outcome. Longevity has changed little, and the major illnesses such as malignancy and cardiovascular disease remain unimpeded. Heralded preventive measures, such as multiphasic screening and modification of risk factors for cardiovascular disease yield limited benefit. Illnesses disproportionately affect the poor, major environmental and occupational causes of illness receive little attention and less action, and malpractice charges intensify. Clearly, there is a crisis in health care, both in its effect upon health and in its cost.

In response to these perceptions, major changes are now in process and the health care system is being reshaped into quite a different system at a faster rate that has yet been seen. This chapter will take a macroview of the changing health care system, with three objectives: (1) to describe briefly the magnitude of the expanding health care industry; (2) to outline four major problems of today's health care system; and (3) to present an overview of recent trends and approaches to these problems.

THE HEALTH CARE INDUSTRY: A GROWING MONOLITH

The health care industry is one of the largest, most diverse, and fastest growing industries in the country. Over 5 million people were employed by the industry by 1978 in more than 100 discrete occupations representing over 600 different titles. This number included well over 410,000 (today 520,000) active physicians and more than 1.5 million registered nurses and practical nurses.[8]

National health expenditures have more than doubled during the last 20 years, and now total almost 11 percent of the Gross National Product (GNP).[8] This accelerating rate of growth reflects inflation in medical care costs, technologic and other quality changes, population growth, and increased utilization. This represents a higher expenditure for health care than almost any other country in the world. For comparison, Britain devoted 6.3 percent of its GNP to health care in 1982.[9] At the beginning of the 1970s, Canada and the United States were each spending about the same proportion of their GNPs on health care (7.3 percent). By 1980, after Canada had established a negotiated rate plan with providers while the United States continued with a cost-based reimbursement system, Canada and the United States were expending 7.5 and 9.4 percent of their GNPs on health care.

Health care expenditures in the United States reached an estimated $313 billion in 1983, compared with $12 billion in 1950 and $74 billion in 1970.[8] Recent increases in total annual national health expenditures (15.3 percent in 1980, 15.1 percent in 1981, and 12.5 percent in 1982) are the highest annual increases since 1929, when this kind of information monitoring was started.[11] By 1982 per capita health expenditures in the United States were $1265, compared with $863 just 4 years earlier and $386 in Britain in 1982.[9] While the proportion spent for physicians' services has remained relatively stable at about one-fifth of total expenditures, expenditures for hospital care have shown a marked increase. In the 10-year period from 1968 to 1978, expenditures for hospital care increased from $103 per capita to $341 per capita, about 36 and 40 percent, respectively, of total annual health expenditures.[8] These accelerating per capita health care costs are well beyond inflationary increases.[8]

Expenditures for personal health care, including hospitalization, physicians' and dentists' services, drugs, and other services and supplies provided to individuals, more than tripled between 1970 and 1980, increasing at an average annual rate of 13 percent. Third-party payers, including government and private health insurance, paid for two-thirds of these expenditures. The steadily increasing role played by third-party payers since 1950 is reflected by the fact that out-of-pocket personal health care expenditures decreased from two-thirds to one-third of personal health care payments between 1950 and 1980.[12] Hospital care represents the largest single part of national health expenditures (today about 42 percent of the health care dollar). Although the average length of stay has been reduced in recent years, the numbers of hospital admissions and hospital days per 1000 people per year have increased.

The number of people covered by private health insurance has grown rapidly since 1940 to its present level of about 80 percent of the population. In 1977 mean health insurance premiums were about $600 per eligible employee, with employers paying for about 80 percent of these premiums. Public programs, however, paid for about 40 percent of the country's personal health care bill in 1980, compared with 27 percent for private health insurance.[12]

In addition to the increasing role of government in paying for health care services over the last 20 years, other major trends have been especially important in recent years—the consolidation of the hospital system and the emergence of a growing for-profit sector, termed the medical-industrial complex by Relman.[13] Over the 19-year period from 1961 to 1980, the number of hospital consolidations in the United States increased from 5 to 245. In 1980 almost three-fifths of the beds in multihospital systems were in the nonprofit sector, but for-profit companies have shown the more rapid growth since then. In 1980, there were more than 1000 proprietary hospitals[10] in the country, comprising more than 15 percent of nongovernmental acute general care hospitals and more than one-half of the nongovernmental psychiatric hospitals in the country.[13]

The impressive growth of the health care industry in recent years is not a sign of health, and in fact masks fundamental and severe problems reflecting the paradox of modern medicine in this country. This has been summed up by Somers and Somers in their recent book, *Health and Health Care: Policies in Perspective* in the following way:

> As America entered the last quarter of the twentieth century, following three decades of unprecedented expansion in medical services—in volume and technical quality of care—many of the premises underlying national health policies were falling under increasing challenge. The major ongoing controversies of past and present—regarding methods of financing, strengthening delivery systems, quality protection, the appropriate role of government, etc.—were rooted in a context of commonly accepted assumptions as to the overriding importance of maximum acces to ever-rising levels of scientific medicine and the central place of medical care in individual and national health.
>
> By 1975 the consensus was breaking up. Views were segmented in various graduations of rejection and defense of traditional assumptions. The conviction was growing that the Western societies' reliance on medical care had become excessive; that it was not, in fact, a primary determinant of health status, and that diversion of resources to more exotic high-technology procedures was socially wasteful.

Starr describes the paradox of today's medicine in these terms:[15]

> American medicine today contains a paradox. Outwardly, its institutions, prosperous and authoritative, show imposing strength, yet their social and economic structure is fundamentally unstable, and long-standing assumptions that have governed their operation are in danger of breaking down. A fundamental intellectual reassessment of medicine is taking place; a sense of impending change fills the air . . . . Controlling costs will mean redrawing the "contract," if you will, between the medical profession and the society . . . .

MAJOR PROBLEMS OF THE HEALTH CARE SYSTEM

Although it is somewhat arbitrary and risky to identify any small number of problems as the major problems of an organism as complex as the expanding health care system, this is useful in developing an overall perspective within which specific developments, such as changing approaches to primary care, can be better understood. Four major problems will be presented in brief, with full recognition that their interrelatedness prevents sharp dissection from each other, and surely there are other significant problems which will escape mention by this approach.

Barriers to Health Care
Examination of various barriers between the patient and the health provider is useful to a clearer understanding of present deficiencies of medical practice. Obviously, many often exist concurrently and consideration of each alone is somewhat artificial.

Consumer Related

Socioeconomic Barrier. This barrier can be looked on as a twofold problem involving (1) the large part of the population which is poor, or has difficulty in paying the costs of medical care, and (2) the spiraling costs of health care services.

Although well over 80 percent of Americans have some kind of health insurance for general hospital care, many do not have coverage for drugs, diagnostic studies, nursing home, and dental expenses. Moreover, for the family just above poverty levels by existing formulas, health care is difficult to purchase. Often such families have no insurance coverage, and can afford only the rudiments of acute care.

A recent study by the National Center for Health Services Research estimates that one of four Americans under age 65 is without health insurance coverage at least part of the year or has inadequate coverage (e.g., as defined by uncovered health care outlays exceeding 10 percent of income or lack of protection for catastrophic illness).[16] Most likely to be uninsured are the poor, minorities, young adults, and residents of rural areas.[17]

Major improvements have been made over the last 20 years in improving access to health care by disadvantaged people in the United States. Largely as a result of federal programs in the 1960s and the 1970s, utilization of services increased markedly among the poor, minorities, and rural residents. By the 1970s the poor even visited physicians more often than the nonpoor.[18]

Elimination of the financial barrier to services, however, has been shown not to be effective in itself for improving the health of the concerned group. Thus, in Buffalo, New York, among children 5 to 9 years old, 73 percent of children in the upper class had obtained measles immunization as compared to only 19 percent in the lower economic stratum, despite the free availability of the vaccine through Health Department clinics.[19] Similar observations were made after 15 years of experience in England with the National Health Service, where the high income groups have made better use of available health services both in and out of the hospital, including psychiatric care.[20,21]

The poor have been observed to behave differently from people in higher socioeconomic strata. They often define illness in different terms, and tend to seek health care on an episodic basis and relatively late after the onset of illness. They are more likely to seek care from subprofessionals or marginal practitioners often available in their neighborhoods.[19]

Income and educational level have shown to correlate adversely with such outcomes of care as infant mortality rate. Likewise, the number of some types of visits to physicians are negatively related to income levels, particularly with respect to visits for preventive care.[22]

Educational Barrier. Increasing levels of education are correlated with utilization of a wider breadth of health services. People with more education use more preventive services, and show a higher average use of medical facilities than people with less education.[23] For example, a nationwide study of patterns of prenatal care has shown that the amount of prenatal care was even more closely related to educational level than income. College graduates recorded almost twice as many prenatal visits, on the average, than mothers with an elementary education or less, and sought care at an earlier time.[24] The value of prenatal care has been amply demonstrated in many studies, and a higher infant mortality rate has been shown to correlate with lower levels of the mother's education.[25]

Informational Barrier. This is, of course, often related to the educational barrier, but may be influential in limiting utilization of available services even in well-educated groups. In a time of proliferating agencies, medical, and community resources, an individual family often does not know where to seek appropriate help for a particular health problem. Language differences often constitute additional problems. Serious illnesses with innocuous-appearing initial symptoms may frequently be ignored. We are seeing increasing emphasis today on patient education in response to these problems.

Psychological Barrier. All practicing physicians can recount many examples of patients who either delayed or failed entirely to seek medical care for a multitude of psychological reasons. We all have seen patients who have avoided seeing a physician because of fear of a disease such as cancer, anxiety about particular diagnostic or therapeutic procedures, apprehension of seeing the physician, and a variety of other reasons. McWhinney has suggested that many patients do not seek medical attention until their limits to tolerate anxiety are reached.[26]

Cultural Barrier. It is incumbent on health professionals to understand the cultural and religious beliefs of the people in their communities. Beyond the frequently coexistent language barrier, there are often widely disparate interpretations of disease or method of treatment on a cultural basis. In order to extend adequate care to such groups, physicians should be able to make their services acceptable to the people involved, and understandable in terms of their own culture. In some ethnic groups, for instance, it may be considered "weak" for a man and head of a household to seek psychiatric counseling, or even any preventive medical care. Sickness may be interpreted as a threat to his male self-image.

Racial Barrier. Certain racial groups regularly have lower income and educational levels than whites, and have not always been accorded ready access to first-class medical care even if these barriers were not present. Unemployment tends to be higher and salaries lower in minority groups.

Although substantial improvement has been made in access to health care for minority groups in recent years, life expectancy at birth is still significantly longer for whites than nonwhites. Age adjusted mortality rates were 48 percent higher for blacks than whites in 1978, and the mortality rate for black infants is still almost twice as high as for white infants.[12]

Geographic Barrier. Most studies show that the utilization of health services (especially preventive services) decreases with increasing distance from medical resources.[27] This is easy to comprehend in view of the sometimes great distances and poor roads which must be negotiated to get to a medical facility in many rural areas. But the geographic alienation from medical care can be just as great in the urban ghetto where transportation is often not available though distances are short.

Provider Related

Lack of Facilities and Manpower. The lack of uniform distribution of physician manpower has been seen in the last chapter. A similar situation exists for other health personnel and facilities.

Operational Features of Services. The physical and operational features of medical facilities, especially for the poor, often discourage their use. Such aspects as inconvenient clinic hours, disrespectful eligibility procedure, long waits, frequent changes of physicians and nurses, and impersonal care tend to work against comprehensive family health care and to meet only basic needs for the more acute illnesses.

Fragmented Care. Fragmentation of health care services, a severe problem for the poverty group, also permeates much of the population. Patients without a family physician often see multiple physicians for a given illness and never receive comprehensive evaluation or care.

Over the years, county Public Health Departments have developed many programs to meet specific needs within their locales, but few such services are comprehensive. Thus we have the Well-Baby Clinic, where immunizations are also provided, but no sick care; or the Family Planning Clinic where the postpartum mother is seen, but not her baby.

Dollar Shortage. A report by the Committee on the Role of Medicine in Society of the California Medical Association in 1970 made the following observations which summarize this barrier well, and are equally true today:

> It is unreasonable to expect that all the dollars needed can ever be assigned to health care and their comparative lack will therefore always be a barrier to the quality as well as the quantity and availability of services.[28]

Special Problems of the Poor, Elderly, and Rural Inhabitants

The Poor. Many, if not all, of the barriers to health care which have been described often are operating at the interface between the poor patient and the health provider. Extension of health care to this large part of the population represents a most difficult challenge to our health care system. Whatever progress is made in this direction should be helpful in reducing barriers to care for other neglected segments of the population.

The higher prevalence of serious chronic health problems in the poor compared with the nonpoor has been documented by many studies. Figure 3–1 shows striking examples of these differences for various disease categories.[29]

Although the Medicaid program has improved the access to medical care for many poor people in recent years, many of the poor do not qualify for Medicaid or live in states where the benefits are minimal. Two-parent families are usually ineligible for Medicaid and single adults are covered only if they are disabled or elderly.[17] In addition, many states have set income eligibility cutoffs well below the poverty level. In 1979, for example, the income eligibility level was set as low as $2000 per year for a family of four in Texas, Alabama, and Tennessee. Because of these restrictions, only about 40 percent of the poor are covered by Medicaid.[30]

English has graphically described the health problems of the poor in these terms:[31]

Being poor means more than simply being without money—or without enough money. It means living, as most low income families do, under conditions that undermine both physical and mental health. Residents of poverty areas struggle with malnutrition, with inadequate housing, heating, and sanitary facilities, with substandard working conditions—sometimes, with rats. These unsatisfactory liv-

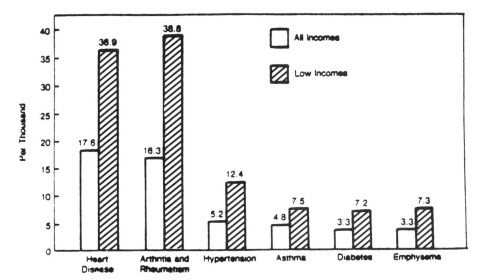

Figure 3-1. Prevalence of serious chronic health conditions by income. *(From Newacheck PW, Butter LH, Harper AK, et al.: Income and Illness. Med Care 18:1165, 1980, with permission.)*

ing conditions breed illness or make it worse. And the vicious cycle continues, since the poor who are also sick are handicapped in their efforts to take advantage of the educational and employment opportunities that might lift them above the poverty threshold.

The Elderly. People over 65 years of age represent a steadily increasing proportion of the population. Since 1900 this age group has increased from 3 million people to about 30 million people today. The age group over 65 years of age currently represents about 11 percent of the population, and this proportion is projected to increase to between 18 and 23 percent by the year 2035.[32] The fastest growth is in the group over 75 years of age, which is expected to reach 5 percent of the population by 1990.[33] In 1940, only 13 percent of people over 65 years of age were 80 years of age and over; by 1979, this figure was 21 percent.[12]

The elderly have special problems with respect to health care. In 1978, people over 65 years of age comprised 11 percent of the total population in the United States, but accounted for 29 percent of the total expenditures for health care.[12] This age group requires a broad range of services including acute care, long-term care of chronic and mental illness, rehabilitation and support services, and care of terminal illness. The per capita hospital expenditures for people over 65 years of age is 3-1/2 times that of people under the age of 65.[34] Five percent of today's elderly live in nursing homes (22 percent of those over 85 years of age), and this number is expected to double by the year 2000.[12]

The economic barrier to health care is a major one for many older people. Their postretirement incomes are sharply reduced at a time when their needs for health care tend to increase considerably. Medicare is of some help, but by no means covers the costs. In 1969, for example, Medicare paid for 50 percent of the total national bill for senior citizens, but this figure fell to 38 percent by 1980.[35] Medicare imposes higher cost sharing and other limitations on ambulatory care than on hospital care, and covers only 2 percent of nursing home expenditures.[36]

Rural Inhabitants. In 1980, about one-quarter of the U.S. population lived outside towns or in towns with populations of 25,000 or less that are not in metropolitan areas.[36] This number is projected to increase in future years as the population continues to disperse to rural areas.[31]

Inhabitants of rural areas encounter special problems with respect to health care. The following observations suggest the complexity of those interrelated problems and the extent to which they act as barriers to health care:[37]

- Twenty-one percent of rural inhabitants have incomes below federally defined poverty levels (double the urban figure).
- There are nine dependents for every ten working age adults in rural areas compared to seven dependents in urban settings.
- Rural areas experience special environmental, occupational, and social health hazards (e.g., 60 percent of all substandard housing in the United States is in rural areas).
- Rural areas have fewer health care resources despite their critical needs.
- Regulatory and reimbursement policies tend to disregard the special problems of rural hospitals.
- Rates of reimbursement for rural Medicare and Medicaid patients are substantially below those for urban providers.

- Transportation costs are often barriers to health care in rural areas due to poor roads and inadequate public and private transportation.
- The number of physician visits per person-year for rural farm inhabitants is lower than that of central city dwellers.

Increasing Cost of Health Care

The causes that fuel the spiraling costs of health care as already described are varied and complex. New technology is partly accountable for increased costs through the widespread application of new techniques often requiring hospitalization and complicated, expensive equipment. Examples include computerized tomography (CT) scanning, renal dialysis, coronary bypass surgery, organ transplants, and advances in various kinds of intensive care. Although estimates vary considerably of the effect of technology on increased per diem hospital costs, 50 percent is an average ball-park figure.[38] The prevailing attitude that these services are "covered" by third-party payers has merely delayed full recognition of the cost problem. Indeed, the costs of coronary bypass procedures and hemodialysis of end-stage renal disease have been doubling every few years.[39]

As Larson points out, the cost of "big ticket" technologies can be cost effective or inflationary depending on whether they are substitutive or additive to other interventions.[38] Thus, CT scanning has been found to decrease the cost of diagnostic evaluation of patients with suspected brain tumor (by eliminating the need for some hospital admissions) whereas the use of CT scanning increased the costs of care for patients with suspected cerebrovascular accident (i.e., no other studies or interventions were replaced).[40,41]

Initial interest in the cost problem focused particularly on the newer, more complex technologies as the main culprit. More recently, however, the importance of "little ticket" items (especially laboratory tests and x-rays) has been recognized for their cumulative effect on costs. One national study, for example, showed that the total cost of clinical laboratory tests alone far exceeded the costs of capital equipment purchased by hospitals.[42] Indeed, clinical laboratory testing accounts for about one-quarter of hospital charges, and their utilization steadily increases. The average number of laboratory tests for a patient with perforated appendicitis rose from 5.3 per case in 1951 to 31 in 1971.[43] Moreover, in just 3 years between 1975 and 1978, the use of clinical laboratory services increased by 27 percent.[44]

Many factors aside from advancing technology contribute to escalating costs of health care, including inflation, population growth, patient and physician preferences, the potential threat of malpractice claims, and related factors. Among these, however, it is likely that physicians, in one way or another influence, or directly control, at least 70 percent of health care expenditures.[45] Many studies have been carried out, especially during the last few years in an attempt to better understand the extent to which cost savings might be possible without compromising the quality of care. The following examples highlight some of the complexities and dimensions of the cost-containment problem:

1. In a careful analysis of data drawn from the recent National Medical Care Expenditures Study (NMCES), Wilensky and Rossiter report these findings:[46]
   a. In 1977, about 39 percent of all ambulatory physician visits were physician-initiated, were more expensive than patient-initiated visits, and represented about 45 percent of the costs of ambulatory physician care.

    b. In areas of increased physician density, there was an increase in physician-initiated ambulatory care (i.e., in both the number and costs of visits), but did not effect the likelihood of surgery or total physician-initiated expenditures when insurance coverage and other factors were taken into account.

    c. Older physicians initiated visits less often than younger physicians, but generated higher expenditures.

    d. The more complete the patient's insurance coverage, the higher the number of physician-initiated visits and related expenditures.

2. Wertman and colleagues studied the reasons of physicians in ordering the 11 most frequently requested laboratory tests in a large teaching hospital. Their findings include:[47]

    a. The four most common reasons for requesting these tests were for diagnosis (37 percent), screening (32 percent), monitoring (33 percent), and to follow-up on a previously abnormal result (12 percent).

    b. Two-thirds of responses indicated that test results were useful in diagnosis, therapy, prognosis, or understanding of the disease.

    c. Less than 7 percent of physicians would not have ordered particular tests if the patient had to pay for them directly.

3. Other studies have shown that many laboratory tests are ordered which are not clinically useful; for example, one such study found that only 5 percent of laboratory data were actually used in diagnosis and treatment of patients on a general medical service in one teaching hospital.[48]

4. In one group of 33 faculty internists providing care for a relatively homogeneous population of patients, Schroeder and colleagues noted a 17-fold variation in the use of laboratory tests.[49]

5. Many studies show that physicians are not well informed about the costs of the services which they generate, and there is even one study showing that cost awareness does not improve after periodic education and feedback.[50]

6. In one study of the extent of defensive medicine reflected in physicians use of diagnostic tests, Garg and colleagues found that:[51]

    a. X-rays were more often ordered for defensive reasons than laboratory tests (14 percent versus 9 percent).

    b. High-risk patients (i.e., apparent psychoneurotic tendencies, low socioeconomic group, belligerent attitude) accounted for 41 percent of x-rays and 29 percent of laboratory tests ordered for defensive reasons.

With respect to the potential impact of physician-induced demand, it has been solidly demonstrated that the higher the level of professional uncertainty or disagreement about a particular diagnostic or therapeutic intervention, the higher the rate of variation from physician to physician. For example, Wennberg and Gittelsoln studied statewide patterns of surgical care in Vermont, and found wide variations from one hospital area to another in the rate of common surgical procedures not related to the health needs of the population. They also found higher total surgery rates in areas with more surgeons. Figure 3–2 illustrates the extent of differences observed for hysterectomy.[52] Based upon their findings, they offer the following comment:

> We suggest that the failure of planning and regulatory programs to contain health costs is in part because they have assumed that the regulatory problem is deviant physician behavior rather than the more central problem of difference

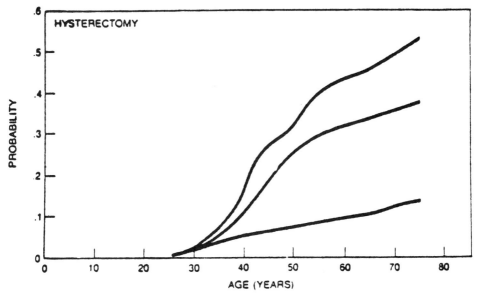

Figure 3-2. Variations in medical care among small areas. *(From Wennberg JE, Gittelsohn A: Variations in medical care among small areas. Scientific American 246(4):120, 1982, with permission.)*

among physicians concerning their beliefs about disease and the outcomes of alternative therapies—(We therefore) stress the importance of a policy that promotes improved information on health care outcomes and more uniform professional decision making in the future.[53]

Marginal Outcomes of Health Care

When one looks at the outcomes of health care, one sees a mixed picture. On the one hand, the United States has clearly seen remarkable improvements in mortality and morbidity in recent years. Between 1968 and 1980, for example, overall adjusted death rates for Americans declined by 20 percent, there were reductions in deaths from 10 of the 15 leading causes of death, and the infant mortality rate for black newborns decreased by 45 percent.[12,54] On the other hand, it is not clear to what extent these gains result from improved medical care, and a growing body of evidence supports the notion that more medical care per se may not only fail to be cost effective in a new era of limits but may also be hazardous.

Fuchs sums up the problem in this way:[55]

. . . health status (as measured by mortality, morbidity, or other indices), depends on many things besides medical care. . . . Current variations in health among individuals and groups are determined largely by genetic factors, environment, and lifestyle (including diet, smoking, stability of family life, and similar variables). To be sure, changes in the health of the population over time are influenced by medical care—but mainly through scientific advances, not through changes in the quantity of care. The most rapid of these gains occurred between 1930 and 1955, largely due to the development of relatively inexpensive, highly effective drugs for the prevention or treatment of influenza and pneumonia, tuber-culosis, and other infectious disease. The current major health problems—heart disease, cancer, accidents, emotional illness, and viral infections—are more diffi-cult to solve with the available medical technology.

The law of diminishing returns with more health care services is illustrated by Figure 3–3; for example, a chest x-ray early in a patient's hospitalization is highly useful and even essential to diagnosis and management, whereas it is of little or no benefit later in the hospitalization.[56] Enthoven terms the marginal or negative part of the curve (points 3 and 4) as "flat of the curve medicine."[57]

Beyond the problems of cost and waste of unnecessary health care services, there is abundant evidence that they may contribute to iatrogenic morbidity and mortality. Several examples attest to the importance of the problem. Wennberg and colleagues have documented a fivefold difference in the mortality of seven com-mon surgical procedures as observed in northern New England and the United Kingdom.[53] It is estimated that 2 million nosocomial infections (7 percent of hospital admissions) occur in U.S. hospitals each year; resulting in 150,000 deaths.[58] Three percent of hospital admissions to general medical services are due to adverse drug reactions, and almost one-third of hospitalized patients have at least one adverse drug reaction during their hospitalization.[59] One study of iatrogenic illness on a general medical service of a university hospital revealed that 36 percent of patients had such an illness, which contributed to mortality in 2 percent of pa-tients.[60]

Kane notes that every decision in medicine (including that to avoid an interven-tion) involves some risk. He observes that iatrogenic illness may occur on the basis of four basic mechanisms: conscious risk, unexpected complications, inept care, and overzealous care.[61] In any event, continuous education is required based on monitoring of patient care outcomes and evaluation of the efficacy and safety of medical interventions. In this connection more refined measures of patient care out-come are needed than mortality or morbidity. Still needed are more effective measures of health status. As Mechanic points out:[62]

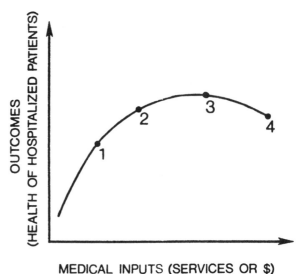

Figure 3-3. Marginal benefit curve showing relation between medical services or expenditures (inputs) and patient health (outcomes). At point 1, provision of a specific ser-vice will produce a certain and dramatic improvement in health. At point 2, additional services do not add greatly to the patient's health. At point 3, no gain in health results from additional services. Finally, at point 4, additional care does more harm than good. *(From Myers LP, Schroeder SA: Physician use of ser-vices for the hospitalized patient: A review with implications for cost containment. Milbank Mem Fund Quarterly/Health and Society 59(4):481, 1981, with permission.)*

OUTCOMES (HEALTH OF HOSPITALIZED PATIENTS)

MEDICAL INPUTS (SERVICES OR $)

None of the indicators used to measure health status, for example, take into account the essential contribution medical care makes toward relieving worry and uncertainty, alleviating pain and discomfort, providing support and reassurance, and facilitating the ability of individuals to make a better adjustment to their environment. Although attention to the impact of medical care on illness and death is crucial to an overall evaluation of how best to allocate resources, this perspective should not detract from the caring function of medical service. We must begin to focus more accurately on the extent to which medicine aids a person in using his capacities and fulfilling his aspirations within the limits of physical and psychological handicaps. We must try to ascertain how varying modes of delivering medical services differentially affect the patient who is worried and distressed and to learn the extent to which different models provide support and hope. In short, if medicine exists to enhance the quality of life and to lengthen it, we must examine how successfully its technology and mode of organization fulfill these purposes.

CURRENT APPROACHES AND TRENDS

It is beyond the scope of this chapter to deal with the myriad of approaches being taken to address today's problems in the health care system. Four selected approaches will be touched on, however, as examples of several important directions toward remodeling the system.

Cost Containment

Medicare and Medicaid Cutbacks. Two decades after its adoption in 1965, the Medicare program is in serious financial straits. Its trust fund for hospital insurance, financed from payroll taxes, has been projected to be bankrupt in 1988. The fund's deficit is expected to reach $300 billion by 1995 as a result of estimated annual increases in hospital costs of 13 percent.[63]

Medicare was never designed as a program of comprehensive care. Its principal purpose was to provide payments for acute, short-term illnesses. In its first 10 years of operation, the costs of health services for the elderly increased threefold. The result has been that Medicare has covered a decreasing portion of the total costs of care for the elderly, dropping from 50 percent of the total national bill for this care in 1969 to only 38 percent in 1980.[64]

Faced with declining assistance with their health care bills, 70 percent of Medicare recipients have purchased some form of supplemental insurance. A wide variety of policies are marketed as Medigap policies and abuses are common in terms of misrepresentation, false claims, and exclusions. Elderly patients have been confronted with escalating cost-sharing requirements under Medicare. Moreover, they have found that many physicians do not accept assignment as full payment of their professional fees, and that Medicare fails to provide coverage for many of their needs (e.g., drugs prescribed as outpatients, eye examinations and eye glasses, preventive services, and long-term institutional services).[64]

In order to deal with the impending financial crisis of the Medicare program, the federal government has made periodic cuts in this appropriation and has recently inaugurated a major reimbursement change based on diagnostic-related groups (DRGs) Possible future changes are reflected in the following recommendations made by the Social Security Advisory Panel in late 1983:[65]

1. Establish fee schedules for reimbursing physician services that would be adjusted for the cost of living and costs of maintaining a practice.
2. Require that physicians either accept all claims on assignment or no claims on assignment, and provide incentives for the acceptance of assignment.
3. Enact a voluntary Medicare voucher option.
4. Raise the age of Medicare disability from 65 to 67 over a 6-year period starting in 1985.

Medicaid, which finances health care for more than 21 million Americans, has been faced with similar cost problems. As observed earlier, this program has been plagued with many inequities varying from one state to another. In an effort to contain costs, Medicaid is increasingly shifting from fee-for-fee service reimbursement to prepayment mechanisms.[66] Based upon their recent analysis of current Medicaid coverage and exclusions, Davis and Rowland have proposed the following corrective approaches:[30]

1. Medicaid coverage should be expanded to provide basic insurance coverage for all low-income individuals as defined by a reasonable minimum income standard.
2. Medicaid coverage should be broadened to include children and adults in two-parent families, as well as catastrophic coverage.

Diagnostic-Related Groups (DRGs). The DRG system of prospective payment of hospital costs incurred by Medicare recipients is being widely hailed as the most important and fundamental change in U.S. health care since the adoption of Medicare and Medicaid in 1965. It seems certain to have a profound impact on reshaping the health care system. Medicare outlays have been increasing at an average annual rate of 17.7 percent since 1970.[67] The DRG system signals an end to uncontrolled, retrospective cost-based reimbursement of hospitals, and shifts the risk of cost overruns to hospitals.

DRGs are a patient classification system developed in the late 1960s at the Yale University School of Organization and Management by Thompson and Fetter for the purpose of utilization review and quality assessment.[68] Hospital administrators later began using this system for case mix adjustments in cross-institutional comparisons, and now DRGs are linked to cost and payment in the new system of Medicare reimbursement. There are 467 DRGs, representing subdivisions of the 23 major diagnostic categories of ICD-9-CM on the basis of principal and secondary diagnoses, surgical procedure, complications and comorbidities, age, and discharge status. The DRG system is therefore patient based rather than dependent on characteristics of providers. Hospitals are reimbursed at fixed rates, set in advance, for discharges classified into 467 diagnosis-related groups to cover all hospital services for Medicare recipients. This program took effect on October 1, 1983, on a 3-year phase-in basis; regional cost variations will be accounted for during this transition, but a single national rate per DRG will be set in place by October 1986. Reimbursement rates will be adjusted for wage differences in metropolitan and nonmetropolitan areas. In addition, between 5 and 6 percent of Medicare payments will be allocated on a marginal cost basis for "outliers," patients exceeding length of stay or costs for their DRG; the intent of this provision is to assist some institutions in meeting the cost burden of treating particularly complicated patients, especially in teaching hospitals.[69]

All nonfederal hospitals participating in the Medicare program are affected by prospective DRG reimbursement except psychiatric hospitals, long-term care and rehabilitation hospitals, and childrens' hospitals. Payment for each case is based on the product of four factors: (1) the relative costliness weight for the patient's DRG (set by the Health Care Financing Administration); (2) the average price per case price; (3) a wage index comparing labor and supply costs in different urban and rural areas; and (4) the hospital's indirect medical education adjustment.[68] The DRG system has been in effect in New Jersey since 1980. Analysis of the experience with this system for 1981 has shown that 28 DRGs comprised one-half of all cases, with the 10 DRGs listed in Table 3–1 accounting for 28.6 percent of almost 2 million sample cases.[70]

The DRG system abruptly changes the incentives to hospitals and providers in a fundamental way.[71] Under cost-based reimbursement policies, hospitals were paid on the basis of services provided. Under the DRG system hospitals will be penalized by exceeding a set rate in terms of length of stay or services. The incentives now are toward shorter length of stay and use of minimal diagnostic and therapeutic services consistent with quality of care for the patient's needs.

TABLE 3–1. TOP 10 HOSPITAL DRGs IN 1981[a]

DRG	Title	Relative Weights	Mean Length of Stay in Days	Becomes Outlier at Day	% of 1981 Sample Cases in the DRG
127	Heart failure plus shock	1.0408	7.8	28	3.92
182	Esophagitis, gastroenteritis, plus miscellaneous digestive disease, patient older than 69; and/or complicating condition	0.6185	5.4	22	3.79
132	Atherosclerosis, older than age 69, and/or complicating condition	0.9182	6.7	27	3.61
39	Lens procedure	0.5010	2.8	6	3.40
88	Chronic obstructive pulmonary disease	1.0412	7.5	28	2.69
14	Specific cerebrovascular disorders, except transient ischemic attacks	1.3527	9.9	30	2.66
89	Simple pneumonia plus pleurisy, age older than 69, and/or complicating condition	1.1029	8.5	29	2.37
46	Other disorders of the eye, age older than 17, with complicating condition	0.5964	4.1	23	2.22
122	Circulatory disorders with acute myocardial infarction without cardiovascular complications, dishcarged alive	1.3651	9.8	30	2.05
294	diabetes, aged 36 or older	0.8087	7.7	28	2.04

[a]In 1981, these 10 DRGs accounted for 28.6 percent of the 1.95 million sample cases on which the new Medicare payment system is based. They are listed in order of the frequency of occurrence. Twenty–eight DRGs comprised 50.14 percent of all cases in the sample. Payment is determined by multiplying the base payment rate by the relative weight assigned to the DRG.

(From Are DRGs for physicians advisable? Am Med News, Oct. 7, 1983, p 2, with permission. Copyright 1983, American Medical News.)

It can readily be seen that hospitals can "win or lose" on particular DRGs. Figures 3–4 and 3–5 illustrate these points in terms of analysis in one institution by hospital and by physician.[69]

DRGs are likely to encourage ambulatory and home care and could lead to increasing specialization among hospitals for certain kinds of care. A Prospective Payment Assessment Commission has recently been established to advise the Department of Health and Human Services (HHS) on needed modifications or additions to the DRG system and to recommend an appropriate annual increase in DRG reimbursement. The Congressional Office of Technology Assessment (OTA) has proposed the following guidelines for monitoring this program:[72]

1. The quality and appropriate use of technologies should be monitored to assure that hospitals do not underprovide services or inappropriately admit and discharge patients.
2. DRG rates will need to be reevaluated regularly, perhaps annually.
3. Further research is needed on the effectiveness, risks, and costs of new techniques as they relate to utilization and reimbursement patterns

Critics of the DRG system are already pointing out several potential problems with this method of reimbursement. Concern is raised that DRGs are not sufficiently sensitive to distinguish between differing severity of illness within the same DRG. This system may also encourage an increased rate of surgical procedures since these surgical DRGs receive higher reimbursement levels than medical DRGs. In addition, there may be some possibility for hospitals to manipulate the sequence

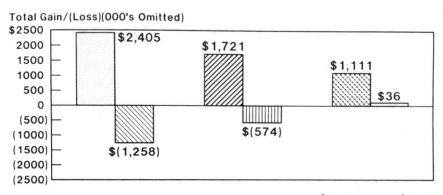

	Number of Cases	Average DRG Payment	Average DRG Cost
Surgical DRG's	802	$15,649	$12,651
Medical DRG's	932	4,789	6,139
High Priced DRG's	1137	12,686	11,173
Low Priced DRG's	597	4,339	5,300
High Volume DRG's	1645	9,827	9,152
Low Volume DRG's	89	9,532	9,136

Figure 3-4. Medicare prospective payment—analysis of major diagnostic category 5—diseases and disorders of the circulatory system. *(From Medicare Prospective Payment System: Implications for the Medical Schools and Faculties. Washington, D.C., Association of American Medical Colleges, 1983, with permission.)*

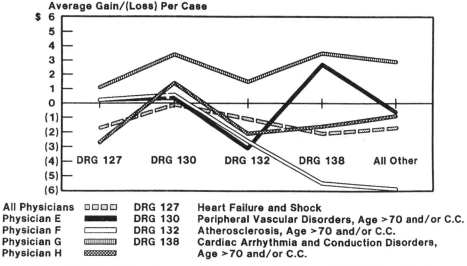

Figure 3–5. Circulatory system performance by physician and DRG (000s omitted). *(From Medicare Prospective Payment System: Implications for the Medical Schools and Faculties. Washington, D.C., Association of American Medical Colleges, 1983, with permission.)*

of diagnoses in order to maximize reimbursement based on the most favorable DRG.[73]

The Veterans Administration will start using DRGs as an internal management tool in 1985.[74] Medicaid, Blue Cross, and other third-party payers are considering DRG-based prospective reimbursement, and Congress has directed HHS to advise Congress by 1985 concerning the advisability and feasibility of extending DRGs to physicians' services to hospitalized patients. Although it is premature to assess the ultimate impact of DRG reimbursement, it seems certain that this system will have a profound and enduring influence on the health care system. After just 1 year under DRG-based prospective reimbursement, behavior changes were clearly demonstrated in U.S. hospitals, including reductions in hospital staffs, capital expansion, and laboratory testing, as well as new initiatives to contract with less costly providers of health care and to "specialize" in selected hospital services.[75]

Other Cost Containment Efforts. Brief mention of other cost containment measures is useful as an illustration of their varied types and their effectiveness.

Hospital Rate Regulation. About one-half of the states initiated one form or another of statewide rate setting for hospital charges during the 1970s. The American Hospital Association categorizes these programs under four distinct types: mandatory–regulatory, mandatory–advisory, voluntary–regulatory, and voluntary–advisory. Regulatory programs may invoke penalties for noncompliance, while advisory programs serve only in an educational or informational feedback capacity.[76] Table 3–2 lists 27 participating states by type of program. States with mandatory-regulatory rate-setting programs have been effective in decreasing expenditures per patient day and per admission, whereas the other three types have been largely ineffective in reducing costs.[77]

TABLE 3-2 RATE REGULATION PROGRAMS BY STATE, 1980

Mandatory–Regulatory	Mandatory–Advisory	Voluntary–Regulatory	Voluntary–Advisory
Connecticut	Arizona	Arkansas	Pennsylvania[a]
Illinois	Minnesota	Delaware	Wyoming
Maryland	Oregon	Florida	
Massachusetts	Virginia	Indiana	
New Jersey		Kansas	
New York		Kentucky	
Washington		Michigan	
Wisconsin		Missouri[a]	
		Montana	
		New Hampshire	
		Ohio[a]	
		Rhode Island	
		Vermont	

[a]Only part of state covered by rate regulation: Missouri—Blue Cross of Kansas City Plan Area; Ohio—Blue Cross of Southwest Ohio Plain Area; Pennsylvania—Blue Cross of Western Pennsylvania Plan Area.
(From Sloan FA: Rate regulation as a strategy for hospital cost control: Evidence from the last decade. Milbank Mem Fund Quarterly/Health and Society 61(2):195, 1983, with permission.)

Certificate-of-need. Certificate-of-need regulation has been implemented in all but one state since its beginning in the early 1970s in an effort to prevent duplication of facilities. Review and approval is required for a capital expenditure exceeding $100,000 or $150,000 per year. Studies have shown that this program has retarded the expansion of hospital beds, but has been ineffective in reducing total dollar investments by hospitals—capital funds have been shifted into new services and equipment.[78,79]

Professional Standards Review Organizations (PSROs). The PSRO program was established in 1972 for the purpose of containing costs and assuring quality of care for beneficiaries of the Medicare, Medicaid, and Maternal and Child Health programs. The program has focused primarily on cost containment by controlling hospital expenditures by monitoring the length of stay in short-term hospitals.[71] Based largely on studies of the experience of the PSRO program with Medicare, the program appears to have minimal impact on cost containment. In 1977 and 1978, the PSRO program accounted for only a 1.5 to 2 percent decrease in days of hospitalization for the entire country. Since hospitals often merely shift costs to other patients when Medicare payments are reduced, however, the PSRO program may well have had a net loss.[80] Little is yet known about PSRO's effect on costs of nursing home care, ancillary services, and ambulatory care, or on quality of care.

Second-Opinion Program. Mandatory second-opinion programs have been found to be cost effective in reducing rates of surgical procedures, but little is known about the consequences of these programs on the health status of the populations where they have been applied. It appears that second-opinion programs deter both needed and unneeded surgery.[81] In one recent study in Massachusetts, for example, a non-confirmation rate of 14.5 percent was found; 85 percent of the confirmed patients had their operation, while only 31 percent of the nonconfirmed patients underwent the proposed operation. Almost one-half of nonconfirmed patients sought a third opinion, and two-thirds of these patients went ahead with their surgery. The largest percentage declines by procedure were for hysterectomy, meniscectomy, hemorrhoidectomy, and tonsillectomy/adenoidectomy.[82] There is a considerable body of evidence suggesting that much surgery is discretionary and unnecessary. In a recent national study, for example, total surgery rates were found to vary between 11 and 153 surgical procedures per 1000 people; only 9 percent of variation could be explained for all procedures, and only 5 percent for elective surgery.[83]

Foundations for Medical Care. Foundations for medical care began to appear in the late 1950s as an alternative to health maintenance organizations in an effort to contain costs and preserve the patients' free choice of physician. By 1982 there were more than 100 such foundations in the United States representing about 27,000 physicians and 1.5 million patients. These organizations are operated by physicians through oversight and administration of private health care insurance plans and peer review regulating physicians' fees. The largest of these foundations, the United Foundation for Medical Care in California, has demonstrated an 8 to 12 percent savings from peer review activities alone, and a reduction in physicians' billings in 1 year of one third.[84]

Alternative Delivery Systems

The last decade has seen the proliferation of various alternatives to the traditional fee-for-service and cost-based reimbursement system in the United States. Lest one think that this is a new idea (especially prepayment), the following recommendations of the Committee on the Costs of Medical Care (CCMC), made more than 50 years ago in 1932, are of interest:[85]

1. Medical service should be furnished largely by organized groups.
2. Basic public health services should be extended so that they will be available to the entire population according to its needs.
3. The costs of medical care should be placed on a group payment basis through the use of insurance or taxation or both.[85]

Three major types of alternative delivery systems have evolved—the health maintenance organization (HMO), independent practitioner association (IPA), and the preferred provider organization (PPO). Table 3–3 summarizes the basic features of each type.

Health Maintenance Organizations. Proponents of HMOs believe that such organized systems of care which emphasize the delivery of a broad range of ambulatory care services can decrease hospital utilization and costs of health care. In actual fact, the nation's largest HMO, Kaiser Health Plan (2.2 million members, 21 hospitals, and over 2000 physicians),[14] has demonstrated that adequate health care can be provided to its membership with 1.8 hospital beds per 1000 people,[86] compared to the availability of 4.5 beds in the nation's community hospitals per 1000 population in 1975.[87]

TABLE 3-3. ALTERNATIVE DELIVERY SYSTEMS

	Health Maintenance Organization	Independant Practitioner Association	Preferred Provider Organization
Purchaser payment	Capitation	Capitation	Fee-for-service
Relation to purchaser	Health plan	Health plan	Vendor
State regulation	Insurance plan	Insurance plan	Provider licensure
Consumer incentives	Broader scope of services and minimal copay/deductibles	Broader choice of providers	Reduction or waiver of copay and deductibles
Scope of services	Comprehensive only	Physicians and hospitals	Physicians and hospitals
Consumer choice	HMO providers only	Provider panel	PPO or non-PB providers
Provider reimbursement	Capitation	Fee-for-service	Fee-for-service
Provider risk sharing	Yes	Yes/no	No
Marketing and claims management	Internal	Internal or 3rd party	3rd parties
Organization costs	Moderate/high	Low/moderate	Low
Startup time	Medium/long	Short/medium	Short
Service location	Centralized few outlets	Decentralized many outlets	Decentralized many outlets

(From M. Stensager, Health Care Purchasers Association, Suite 741, 1111 Third Avenue, Seattle, Washington 98101, with permission.)

The 1973 HMO Bill (P.L. 93–222), as amended in 1976, established the basic requirements for HMOs, which are expected to provide a comprehensive range of health services with high levels of availability, accessibility, and continuity. HMOs must assume full financial risk on a prospective basis for provision of basic health services to the enrollee population, must have a quality assurance mechanism, and must enroll broadly representative population groups. Many feel that an enrollment of 30,000 people is needed for a sound and viable plan.[14]

The following range of services are provided by HMOs:[88]

Basic Range of Necessary Services

- Physician services, including consultation and referral
- Inpatient and outpatient hospital services
- Medically necessary emergency services, both inside and outside of the service area

- Short-term outpatient mental-health services (20-visit maximum)
- Drug and alcohol abuse treatment and referral services
- Diagnostic laboratory, and diagnostic and therapeutic radiology services
- Home health services
- Preventive health services, including voluntary family planning, infertility studies, preventive dental care for children, and corrective eye examinations for children

Supplemental Health Services (Optional Inclusion in Enrollee Contract)

- Intermediate and long-term facilities services
- Vision, dental, and mental-health services not included in the basic range of services
- Provision of prescription drugs required in conjunction with services provided under contract

By 1984 there were 323 HMOs operating in the United States serving about 13.6 million members,[89] compared with 30 HMOs serving 3.5 million people 10 years earlier.[90] Although federal funding has facilitated the development of many HMOs, a majority of their support has come from the private sector.[90] The HMO concept is growing rapidly (18 percent growth in 1983),[91] has now become well accepted, and larger organizations are beginning to dominate the field. In fact, HMOs have become the major growth area for Blue Cross and Blue Shield, which now account for about 10 percent of all HMO enrollees in the country.[92] Blue Cross and Blue Shield HMOs experienced a membership increase of 26 percent in 1983.[93]

Independent Practitioner Associations. IPAs were initiated by organized medicine in response to competition from "closed panel" HMOs with the intent to help preserve the traditional physician–patient relationship. They are organized networks of physicians based on an established physician–patient relationship with a primary care physician. The IPA may be considered "open panel" compared to the HMO, but each IPA has specific criteria by which physicians are accepted or excluded from participation in the plan.

IPAs are usually tied to HMOs on a contractual basis, but as separate legal entities may provide health services on their own. IPA physicians practice in their usual locations, and are usually reimbursed on a discounted fee-for-service basis. Incentives for cost-effective practice involve various forms of risk sharing with participating physicians. Some large corporations have started IPAs as a way of providing their employees with prepaid health care through community based physicians. In general, IPAs still do not yet have a major share of the market, and have been shown to be more expensive than HMOs.[94]

Preferred Provider Organizations. The PPO is the newest type of alternative delivery system to appear on the scene. It differs from the HMO and IPA in not being prepaid on a capitation basis and not being a legal entity of its own. Instead the PPO is a negotiated arrangement between providers and purchasers of health care services. Purchasers may include employers, insurance carriers, or third-party administrators. In a recent study by the American Medical Association, the typical operational PPO involves about 380 physicians and 8 hospitals. Most PPOs share the following characteristics:[95]

- A designated panel of health care professionals and/or institutions which are the preferred providers.
- An established fee schedule (usually discounted about 15 to 20 percent from usual and customary fees).
- Fee-for-service reimbursement for medical services.
- Strong emphasis on utilization review and control.
- No "lock-in" of the patient to specific providers, although incentives (e.g., reduced copayments or deductibles) are often used to encourage use of preferred providers.
- No financial risk sharing by physicians.

Pro-Competition and Emerging Corporate Practice

The two major options to control health care expenditures which have been debated at length in recent years fall roughly into regulatory or competitive approaches. The present administration and political climate favors a pro-competition approach. Ginzberg identifies the following building blocks in the pro-competition strategy:[96]

- Increased choice of consumers at the point where they purchase health insurance or select a prepaid plan
- Ceiling on the maximum amount of tax-free health benefits that the employer can cover
- Higher deductibles and copayments for consumers, with back-up catastrophic coverage for large expenses (e.g., over $2500 to $35,000 per year)
- A Medicare voucher, initially voluntary, set at 95 percent of average adjusted per capita cost and indexed for inflation
- Reduction and elimination of many regulatory approaches to cost containment
- New forms of prepaid health care

The advent of the competitive strategy has been associated with a rapid movement toward various forms of corporate health care. As Starr observes:[10]

> Corporations have begun to integrate a hitherto decentralized hospital system, enter a variety of other health care businesses, and consolidate ownership and control in what may eventually become an industry dominated by huge health care conglomerates.

The trend toward the new medical–industrial complex in the for-profit sector has already been pointed out.[13] The potential extent of this trend is well illustrated by the fact that one-third of all long-term renal dialysis services in the United States are now provided by one corporation.[97] Starr describes five dimensions currently at work in the shift toward corporate practice:[10]

1. Change in type of ownership and control: the shift from nonprofit and governmental organizations to for-profit companies in health care
2. Horizontal integration: the decline of freestanding institutions and rise of multi-institutional systems (consortium of acute care hospitals), and the consequent shift in the locus of control from the community boards to regional and national health care corporations
3. Diversification and corporate restructuring: the shift from single-unit organizations operating in one market to "poly corporate" and con-

glomerate enterprises, often organized under holding companies, sometimes with both nonprofit and for-profit subsidiaries involved in a variety of different health care markets

4. Vertical integration: the shift from single-level-of-care organizations, such as acute care hospitals, to organizations that embrace the various phases and levels of care (e.g., consortium of acute care hospitals, rehabilitation facilities, nursing homes, etc.)

5. Industry concentration: the increasing concentration of ownership and control of health services in regional markets and the nation as a whole.

Perhaps the greatest diversity and intensity of the pro-competition approach is best illustrated by events in California. Plagued by recurrent cost overruns in the Medicaid programs and an 18 percent increase in hospital costs in 1981, the legislature passed legislation authorizing both the government and private insurance companies to negotiate prepaid contracts with hospitals and providers in an effort to contain costs. In a recent analysis of what some have called California's "health care revolution," Melia and colleagues include the following as unresolved issues and questions concerning access, equity, and quality of care:[98]

- What influence will Medicaid negotiations have on the programs of private insurance carriers?
- What roles will organized medicine and medical staffs of hospitals play in negotiations involving hospitals and providers?
- Will HMOs, IPAs, and PPOs become the predominant forms of medical practice?
- Will prepayment replace fee-for-service as the main type of reimbursement?
- What will be the impact on hospitals and their medical staffs of current pressures to reduce hospital services in favor of increased ambulatory services?
- How will physician–patient and physician–hospital relationships be changed?
- What behaviors will follow among business–labor coalitions and the public?

Equity, Rationing, and Quality of Care

The diverse spectrum of health care plans with various kinds of cost sharing now available to the public are certain to influence access and quality of care. A certain amount of "rationing" of services will no doubt take place either directly or indirectly. Table 3–4 displays the likely impacts of differences in price, accessibility, and practice styles on utilization of services in different settings as projected by Luft.[99]

It is clear that the demand for and costs of health care services in the United States are pushing the economic limits of the society more than ever before, and that structured changes are needed in the system in order to control costs. Other nations have already been forced to deal with these constraints in more systematic ways than have yet taken place in this country. The goals of equity and access of health care for the population at once raises questions which are medical, ethical, economic, moral, legal, social, and political in nature.[100]

Mechanic identifies three general approaches to rationing of medical care:[101]

1. Market approach: Through manipulation of coinsurance and deductibles, forcing patients to share in the costs of health services and to consider the marginal value of purchasing more medical care

TABLE 3-4. PROBABLE EFFECTS ON UTILIZATION OF SERVICES OF VARIOUS FACTORS IN DIFFERENT PRACTICE SETTINGS

Type of Medical Care/ Rationing Factors	Conventional Fee-for-Service and Insurance	IPA–HMOs: Fee-for-Service Practitioners at Risk		PGP–HMOs	
Patient-initiated visits					
Price to consumer	Initial and preventive visits often not covered	−	Comprehensive coverage of all visits	+	Comprehensive coverage of all visits
Knowledge of provider	Often a local physician with a longstanding relationship	+	Often a local physician with a longstanding relationship	−	Often a local physician with no prior contact with patient
Appointment lag	Typically short, urgent visits "squeezed in"	+	Typically short, urgent visits "squeezed in"	−	Typically long, urgent visits routed to separate clinic
Accessibility to provider	Decentralized, likely one close to patient	+	Decentralized, likely one close to patient	−	Centralized, generally further from patient
Waiting time in office	Variable, often long because patients "squeezed in"	−	Variable, often long because patients "squeezed in"	+	Typically short if appointment made in advance
Physician initiated visits					
Physician incentives	Follow-up increases revenue	+	Follow-up increases revenue more than risk sharing	+/−	Follow-up reduces net income; substitute call-backs
Other factors similar to above				−	

Physician-initiated referral					
Physician incentives	Reciprocal referrals among different specialists encouraged by professional network, discouraged by prohibitions on fee splitting	+	Referrals encouraged by professional network but discouraged by risk sharing	+/−	Referral attractive to "dump" a problem patient, but collegial and financial costs if frequent	−
Price to consumer	More likely covered than initial visit, still not complete	+/−	Comprehensive coverage of all visits	+	Comprehensive coverage of all visits	+
Accessibility of provider	Typically at a different location	−	Typically at a different location	−	Centralized—"one stop care"	+
Incentives to "return patient to primary care physician"	Depends on nature of referral network	+	Depends on referral network, sometimes encouraged by HMO	+/−	Typically encouraged by the system	−
Hospitalization					
Price to patient	Often fairly comprehensive coverage but some copayments	−	Comprehensive coverage pays in full	+	Comprehensive coverage pays in full	+
Incentives for physician	Hourly income higher in hospital	+	Hourly income higher, but risk sharing tends to counter	+/−	No additional income, costs are borne by plan	+/−

+ = Tends to increase utilization; − = tends to decrease utilization; +/− = mixed effects.

(From Luft HS: Health maintenance organizations and the rationing of medical care. Milbank Mem Fund Quarterly 60(2):268, 1982, with permission.)

2. Explicit rationing: Through imposition of administrative constraints (e.g., exclusion of certain services from payment, predetermined interrelated between services in order to be covered)
3. Implicit rationing: Through use of fixed budgets, capitation arrangements, and limitations on providers (e.g., prepaid group practice); this alternative allows more latitude for professional autonomy and clinical decision making than the explicit approach

The word rationing has become a value-laden word, prompting Evans to propose the term allocation as a more appropriate word for describing the distribution of unequal resources which is unavoidably required.[102]

As the demand for health services and the advances of biomedical technology collide head on with fixed economic limits, a dilemma immediately arises involving the interest of the individual patient versus the interest of the system as a whole. Dorsey frames this issue well from the physician's perspective:[103]

> More and more, physicians are being asked to define quality care in measurable terms. Physicians are, frankly, ill equipped to deal with much of the challenge society is presenting them. In their training, the value system they learn emphasizes their responsibility to the individual patient in their care. Balancing of likely costs and benefits is mainly an exercise relative to the individual patient. The costs they consider are the morbidity associated with diagnostic procedures, the side effects of therapies, loss of time from work, and out-of-pocket payments for services not covered by third-party insurance coverage. Benefits include relief of symptoms, prolongation of life, and enhancement of functional capacity. . . . What physicians will find themselves pressed to do in the future will be population-based analyses. How much will a particular approach (e.g., wider use of thallium scintigraphy, coronary arteriography, and bypass surgery) cost for a defined population, i.e., not only what is the unit cost for one patient but the multiplier effect of the utilization rate prescribing practices generate.

Quality of care has proven to be an elusive and complex subject resisting easy definition. Donabedian points out that quality of care relates to both technical and interpersonal components of patient care. He observes that the quality of technical care depends on the balance of expected benefits and risks, whereas the quality of the interpersonal component involves conformity to legitimate patient expectations and to social and professional norms. In connection with a social definition of quality of care (i.e., related to a population, not to an individual patient), he recognizes that the physician trying to do the most for each patient may be in conflict with the best social outcome.[104] Reinhardt divides quality of care into two dimensions:[105]

1. Macro quality of care: Impact of the entire health care system on the population it serves
2. Micro quality of care: Efficacy and effectiveness of the management of particular health problems or of particular clinical procedures

For the purpose of considering the cost–benefit of any particular element of health care, Hemenway observes that the optimal benefit from an economic standpoint occurs at the point where the difference between total costs and total benefits are the greatest (e.g., point C in Figure 3–6, not point A where benefits are maximized at great costs or point B where benefits and costs are equal).[106]

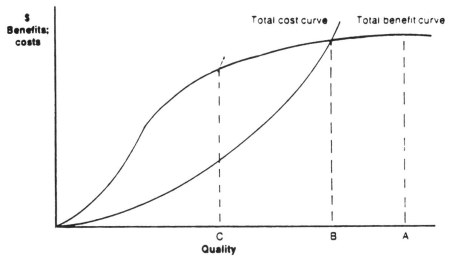

Figure 3-6. Total benefits and total costs of higher quality. *(From Hemenway D: Thinking about quality: An economic perspective. QRB 9(11):321, November 1983, with permission.)*

COMMENT

The health care system in the United States is undergoing rapid and virtually revolutionary changes. The cost crisis is not at some future time—it is now, and fundamental changes are taking place which are certain to reshape the traditional system. The pro-competition approach is being taken in a time of limited resources, which Starr has labeled a "zero-sum game."[10] A predominant theme of the 1970s, health care planning has for many become health care marketing. There is now a legitimate concern that the for-profit sector of health care could further disenfranchise certain groups of the population whose access to the system is already suboptimal. Cunningham's comments on the potential harmful effects of competition are squarely on target:[107]

> Care of the disadvantaged is a central problem in the health care system, and it is getting worse. It may not be upper most among current concerns of the health professions, government, or industry, but it should be, because it could be the critical weakness in the whole structure. For all that may be developed in the competitive environment, all the marketing, reorganizing, diversifying, and maneuvering of hospitals, unless some combination of the resources of hospitals, doctors, industry, and government can be used to accommodate the needs of the unserved and underserved, our health-care system will be overturned—no matter how efficiently it may serve those who can afford it.

The medical profession shares some responsibility for today's problems in health care and likewise must accept responsibility for sharing in their resolution. In order to contribute to future improvements in health care in this country, physicians will have to take off the "blinders" which may limit their interest to their own specialty, and focus their efforts on relating their respective specialties and roles to the real needs of the public.

The observations of two experienced health policy analysts speak directly to the challenges facing American medicine at this juncture. As Hiatt notes:[108]

> The critical question confronting the medical professions is not whether society will find ways to govern access to and control the use of the medical commons. The question, rather, is how physicians will participate in the creation of control mechanisms in a manner that reflects both enlightened self-interest and the public interest.

Finally, in Iglehart's words:[92]

> The message to organized medicine, it seems to me, is not that the government's efforts will obliterate the fee-for-service mode, but that they will test it in many different ways. The challenge for American medicine is to face up to these tests rather than steadfastly cling to the status quo, and to develop new variations on the traditional theme that more efficiently reconcile the intensifying conflict between infinite demand and limited resources.

REFERENCES

1.   Tarlov AR: The increasing dispersion of specialists. N Engl J Med 303:1058, 1980
2.   Public favors major restructuring of health care systems: Harris poll. Am Med News, Oct. 21, 1983, pp 1,8
3.   Rosenberg H: Investing in specialized health care. Financial World, Oct. 15, 1983, p 16
4.   Illich I: Medical Nemesis: The Expropriation of Health. New York, Pantheon, 1976
5.   Maxmen JS: The Post-Physician Era. New York, John Wiley & Sons, 1976
6.   Fuchs VR: Who Shall Live? Health, Economics and Social Choice. New York, Basic Books, 1974
7.   Holman HR: The "excellence" deception in medicine. Hosp Pract 11, April 1976
8.   Hough DE, Misek GI (eds): Socioeconomic Issues of Health 1980. Chicago, American Medical Association, 1980, p 148
9.   Iglehart JK: The British National Health Service under the Conservatives. N Engl J Med 309:1264, 1983
10.   Starr P: The Social Transformation of American Medicine. New York, Basic Books, 1982, p 412
11.   Falk IS: Some lessons from the fifty years since the CCMC Final Report, 1932. J Publ Health Policy 4(2):156, 1983
12.   Health—United States 1981. Hyattsville, Md., U.S. Department of Health and Human Services, DHHS Publication No. (PHS) 82-1232, Government Printing Office, 1981, p 2
13.   Relman AS: The new medical–industrial complex. N Engl J Med 303:963, 1980
14.   Somers AR, Somers HM: Health and Health Care: Policies in Perspective. Germantown, Md, Aspen Systems Corporation, 1977, p 1
15.   Starr P: Medicine and the waning of professional sovereignty. Daedalus 107(1):176, 1978
16.   Farley PJ: Study by National Center for Health Services Research. Washington Post, Nov. 12, 1984
17.   Wilensky GR, Walden DC: Minorities, poverty, and the uninsured. Paper presented

at the 109th meeting of the American Public Health Association, Los Angeles, National Center for Health Service Research, November. Hyattsville, Md., 1981

18. Davis K, Schoen C: Health and the War on Poverty: A Ten Year Appraisal. Washington, D.C., Brookings Institution, 1978

19. Bergner L. Yerby AS: Low income and barriers to use of health services. N Engl J Med 278:541, 1968

20. Morris JN: Uses of Epidemiology. Edinburgh, E. & S. Livingstone, 1957

21. Titmuss RM: Role of redistribution in social policy. Soc Sec Bull 28:14 (No. 6), June, 1965

22. U.S. National Center for Health Statistics. Physician Visits—Volume and Interval Since Last Visit: U.S.—1971. Public Health Service, Series 10, No. 97, Rockville, Md., 1975

23. Mechanic D: Relationships between medical need and responsiveness of care. In Lewis CE, Fein R, Mechanic D (eds): A Right to Health: The Problem of Access to Primary Medical Care. New York, John Wiley & Sons, 1976, p 17

24. Socio-Economic Report: San Francisco, Bureau of Research and Planning, Calif Med Assoc, 8(12), Nov. 1968

25. U.S. National Center for Health Statistics. Infant Mortality Rates: Socioeconomic Factors, United States. Washington, D.C., Series 22, No. 14, DHEW Publication No. (HSM) 72-1045, Government Printing Office, 1972

26. McWhinney IR: Beyond diagnosis—An approach to the integration of behavioral science and clinical medicine. N Engl J Med 287:384, 1972

27. Weiss JE, Greenlick MR, Jones JF: Determinants of medical care utilization: The impact of spatial factors. Inquiry 8:50, 1971

28. Fifth progress report of Committee on The Role of Medicine in Society, Part I. Calif Med 112:68, 1970

29. Newacheck PW, Butter LH, Harper AK, et al.: Income and illness. Med Care 18:1165, 1980

30. Davis K, Rowland D: Uninsured and underserved: Inequities in health care in the United States. Milbank Mem Fund Quarterly 61(2):149, 1983

31. English JT: The dimensions of poverty. Amer J Nurs 69:2426, 1969

32. Ostow M, Millman ML: The demographic dimensions of health policy. Publ Health Rpts 96:304, 1981

33. McNerney WJ: Control of health care costs in the 1980s. N Engl J Med 303:1088, 1980

34. Environmental analysis of the hospital industry (appendix). Chicago, American Hospital Association, 1979

35. Van Ellet T: Medigap: State responses to problems with health insurance for the elderly. The Intergovernmental Health Policy Project, 1979, p 3

36. Feder J, Scanlon W: The underused benefit: Medicare's coverage of nursing home care. Milbank Mem Fund Quarterly 60(4):604, 1982

37. Williams AP, Schwartz W, Newhouse JP, et al.: How many miles to the doctor? N Engl J Med 309:958, 1983

38. Larson EB: Consequences of medical technology: Controversies and dilemmas. Univ of Washington Medicine 8(4):2, 1981

39. Relman AS: Technology costs and evaluation. N Engl J Med 301:1444, 1979

40. Larson EB, Omenn GS: The impact of computed tomography on the care of patients with suspected brain tumor. Med Care 15:543, 1977

41. Larson EB, Omenn GS, Loop JW: Computed tomography in patients with cerebrovascular disease: Impact of a new technology on patient care. Am J Roentgenol 131:35, 1978

42.   Fineberg HV: Clinical chemistries: The high cost of low-cost diagnostic tests. In Altman SH, Blendon R (eds): Medical Technology: The Culprit Behind Health Care Costs? (DHEW Publication No. [PHS] 79-3216). Washington, D.C., Government Printing Office, 1979, p 144

43.   Scitovsky AA, McCall N: Changes in the costs of treatment of selected illnesses. 1951–1964–1971. San Francisco: Health Policy Program. University of California, School of Medicine, Sept. 1975

44.   National survey of hospital and nonhospital clinical laboratories. Laboratory Management 17:33, 1979

45.   Relman AS: The allocation of medical resources by physicians. J Med Educ 55:99, 1980

46.   Wilensky GR, Rossiter LF: The relative importance of physician-induced demand in the demand for medical care. Milbank Mem Fund Quarterly/Health and Society 61(2):252, 1983

47.   Wertman BG, Sostrim SV, Pavlova Z, et al.: Why do physicians order laboratory tests? A study of laboratory test request and use patterns. JAMA 243:2080, 1980

48.   Dixon RH, Laszlo J: Utilization of clinical chemistry services by medical house staff. Arch Intern Med 134:1064, 1974

49.   Schroeder SA, Kenders K, Cooper J, et al.: Use of laboratory tests and pharmaceuticals—Variation among physicians and the effect of a cost audit on subsequent use. JAMA 225:969, 1973

50.   Robertson WO: Costs of diagnostic tests: Estimates by health professionals. Med Care 18:556, 1980

51.   Garg ML, Gliebe WA, Elkhatib MB: The extent of defensive medicine: Some imperial evidence. Legal Aspects of Medical Practice. Feb. 1978, p 25

52.   Wennberg JE, Gittelsohn A: Variations in medical care among small areas. Scientific American 246(4):120, 1982

53.   Wennberg JE, Barnes BA, Zubkoff M: Professional uncertainty and the problem of supplier-induced demand. Soc Sci & Med 16:811, 1982

54.   Rogers DE, Blendon RJ, Moloney TW: Who needs Medicaid? N Engl J Med 307:13, 1982

55.   Fuchs VR: Who Shall Live? Health Economics and Social Choice. New York, Basic Books, 1974, p 144

56.   Myers LP, Schroeder SA: Physician use of services for the hospitalized patient: A review with implications for cost containment. Milbank Mem Fund Quarterly/Health and Society 59(4):481, 1981

57.   Enthoven AC: Cutting cost without cutting the quality of care. N Engl J Med 298:1229, 1978

58.   Bennett JV: Human infections: Economic implications and prevention. Ann Int Med 89 (part 2):761, 1978

59.   Jack H: The discovery of drug-induced illness. N Engl J Med 296:481, 1977

60.   Steel K, Gertman PM, Orescengi C, et al.: Iatrogenic illness on a general medical service at a university hospital. N Engl J Med 304:638, 1981

61.   Kane R: Iatrogenesis: Just what the doctor ordered. J Comm Health 5(3):149, 1980

62.   Mechanic D: The problem of access to medical care. In Lewis CE, Fein R, Mechanic D (eds): A Right to Health: The Problem of Access to Primary Care. New York, John Wiley & Sons, 1976, p 9

63.   Winsten IA: Bailing out Medicare. New York Times, May 5, 1983

64.   Stettner M: Medigap: Are we cheating the nation's elderly? West J Med 139:742, 1983

65.   Legislative Roundup. Chicago, Council on Legislation, American Medical Association, Nov. 11, 1983, p 3

66. Iglehart JK: Medicaid in transition. N Engl J Med 309:868, 1983
67. Iglehart JK: Medicare begins prospective payment of hospitals. N Engl J Med 308:1428, 1983
68. Thompson JD, Fetter RB, Moss CD: Case mix and resource use. Inquiry 12:300, 1975
69. Medicare Prospective Payment System: Implications for the Medical Schools and Faculties. Washington, D.C., Association of American Medical Colleges, 1983
70. Are DRGs for physicians advisable? Am Med News, Oct. 7, 1983, p 2
71. Rosenthal M: DRGs: Why should corporations care? Health Cost Containment 1:5, 1983
72. OTA Press Release, July 29, 1983
73. Schwartz WB: The regulation strategy for controlling hospital costs. N Engl J Med 305:1249, 1981
74. VA to use DRGs in '85. Am Med News, May 4, 1984, p 18
75. Medical groups foresee a powerful role in future. Am Med News, Nov. 23/30, 1984, p 9
76. Rate review: A look at state programs. Hospitals 54:99, 1980
77. Sloan FA: Rate regulation as a strategy for hospital cost control: Evidence from the last decade. Milbank Mem Fund Quarterly/Health and Society 61(2):195, 1983
78. Salkever DS, Bice TW: The impact of certificate-of-need controls on hospital investment. Milbank Mem Fund Quarterly 54:185, 1976
79. Hellinger FJ: The effect of certificate-of-need legislation on hospital investment. Inquiry 13:187, 1976
80. Congress of the United States, Congressional Budget Office. The impact of PSROs on health-care costs: Update of CBO's 1979 evaluation. Washington, D.C., Government Printing Office, 1981
81. Brook RH, Lohr KN: Second-opinion programs: Beyond cost-benefit analysis. Med Care 20(1):1, 1982
82. Martin SG, Schwartz M, Whalen BJ, et al.: Impact of a mandatory second-opinion program in Medicaid surgery rates. Med Care 20(1):21, 1982
83. Mitchell JB, Cromwell J: Variations in surgery rates and the supply surgeons. Health Care Financing Administration Grant No. 95-P-97245/2-01, 1980
84. Sandrick KM: United Foundation for Medical Care: Reducing physicians fees. QRB 9(10):304, 1983
85. Falk IS: Some lessons from the fifty years since the CCMC Final Report, 1932. J Publ Health Policy 4(2):139, 1983
86. Boardman JJ: Utilization data and the planning process. In Somers AR (ed): The Kaiser-Permanente Medical Care Program: A Symposium. New York, The Commonwealth Fund, 1971, p 65
87. American Hospital Association, Hospital Statistics, 1976 ed, Table 1, p 4, 1976
88. Appendix B, Summary of Main Features of 1973 HMO Bill (P.L. 93-222). In Lewis CE, Fein R, Mechanic D (eds): A Right to Health: The Problem of Access to Primary Medical Care. New York, John Wiley & Sons, 1976, p 325
89. Iglehart JK: HMOs (For-profit and not-for-profit) on the move. N Engl J Med 310:1203, 1984
90. December 1981 HMO enrollment in the United States: A mid-year census. Excelsior, Minnesota, Inter Study, 1982
91. Half of metropolitan areas offer HMOs. Am Med News, Sept. 28, 1984, p 17
92. Igelhart JK: The future of HMOs. N Engl J Med 307:451, 1982
93. HMOs proliferating rapidly:265 plans. Fam Pract News, May, 1983, p 1
94. Legislative Roundup. Chicago, Council on Legislation, American Medical Association, Sept. 28, 1984, p 2

95. A Physician's Guide to Preferred Provider Organizations. Chicago, American Medical Association, 1983

96. Ginzberg E: Procompetition in health care: Policy or fantasy? Milbank Mem Fund Quarterly/Health and Society 60(3):386, 1982

97. Seward EW, Gallagher EK: Reflections on change in medical practice: The current trend to large-scale medical organizations. JAMA 250:2820, 1983

98. Melia EP, Aucoin LM, Duhl LJ, et al.: Competition in the health care marketplace: A beginning in California. N Engl J Med 308:788, 1983

99. Luft HS: Health maintenance organizations and the rationing of medical care. Milbank Mem Fund Quarterly 60(2):268, 1982

100. Lundberg GD: Rationing human life. JAMA 249:2223, 1983

101. Mechanic D: Rationing of medical care and the preservation of clinical judgment. J Fam Pract 11:431, 1980

102. Evans RW: Health care technology and the inevitability of resource allocation and rationing decisions. JAMA 249:2208, 1983

103. Dorsey JL: Use of diagnostic resources in health maintenance organizations and fee-for-service practice settings. Arch Int Med 143:1863, 1983

104. Donabedian A: The quality of medical care: A concept in search of a definition. J Fam Pract 9(2):277, 1979

105. Reinhardt UE: Quality assessment of medical care: An economist's perspective. QRB 9(9):252, 1983

106. Hemenway D: Thinking about quality: An economic perspective. QRB 9(11):321, November 1983

107. Cunningham RM Jr.: Entrepreneurialism in medicine. N Engl J Med 309:1313, 1983

108. Hiatt HH: Protecting the medical commons: Who is responsible? N Engl J Med 293:235, 1975

4 Issues and Perspectives in Primary Care

Primary care cannot be grafted onto the health-care system without affecting the structure and the power relationships of that system. More effective delivery of primary care cannot be attained while leaving all other parts of medicine as they are today . . . . Effective primary care is more than just another specialty, more than just a group of dedicated physicians and other health professionals, more than just another body of knowledge. An effective primary care sector, linked into the rest of medicine, cannot coexist with the rest of medicine without having its important impact on all that is linked to and that is linked to it.

Rashi Fein[1]

The last two chapters have traced the major trends of the last 20 years which have led to an exponential increase in expectations and demand for health services, together with a concurrent recognition of the need for a more coherent health care policy emphasizing a strong primary care base.

As the interest in primary care has grown at various levels both within and outside of medicine, so has confusion been generated on a number of basic issues related to its definition, content, and process. The purpose of this chapter is threefold: (1) to outline various definitions of primary care, (2) to describe briefly the basic elements of primary care, and (3) to discuss seven current issues with respect to primary care in this country.

DEFINITIONS OF PRIMARY CARE

One of the most debated of terms in recent years is that of "primary care" itself. There has been a tendency by many disciplines and groups to claim major investments in primary care from their various perspectives, and the issues become cloudy in short order unless some basic definitions are established. We have seen a number of definitions proposed, and it is now possible to clarify the fundamental issues.

The following definition suggested by Alpert draws from the contributions of many[2-6] and represents a general consensus within medicine.[7]

> Primary care can be defined as being within the personal rather than the public health system, and is therefore focused on the health needs of individuals and families—it is family-oriented. Primary care is "first-contact" care, and thus should be separated from secondary care and tertiary care, which are based on referral rather than initial contact.

Primary care assumes longitudinal responsibility for the patient regardless of the presence or absence of disease. The primary care physician holds the contract for providing personal health services over a period of time. Specifically, primary care is neither limited to the course of a single episode of illness nor confined to the ambulatory setting. It serves as the "integrationist" for the patient. When other health resources are involved, the primary care physician retains the coordinating role. He or she cares for as many of the patient's problems as possible, and, where referral is indicated, fulfills his longitudinal responsibility as the integrationist.

Although much of primary care takes place in ambulatory settings, primary care is not synonymous with ambulatory care. For example, many hospitalized patients will remain under the continuing primary care of the primary care physician, while many ambulatory patients may be receiving secondary care services (e.g., radiation therapy).

Primary care is defined by the American Academy of Family Physicians (AAFP) and the American Board of Family Practice (ABFP) as:

. . . a form of medical care delivery which emphasizes first contact care and assumes ongoing responsibility for the patient in both health maintenance and therapy of illness. It is personal care involving a unique interaction and communication between the patient and the physician. It is comprehensive in scope, and includes the overall coordination of the care of the patient's health problems, be they biological, behavioral or social. The appropriate use of consultants and community resources is an important part of effective primary care.

A further description of the functions of primary care is added by the ABFP.

1. It is "first-contact" care serving as point-of-entry for the patient into the health-care system;
2. It includes continuity by virtue of caring for patients over a period of time in both sickness and in health;
3. It is comprehensive care, drawing from all the traditional major disciplines for its functional content;
4. It serves a coordinative function for all the health-care needs of the patient;
5. It assumes continuing responsibility for individual patient follow-up and community health problems; and
6. It is a highly personalized type of care.

ELEMENTS OF PRIMARY CARE

These definitions are broad and leave room for various interpretations of the precise nature of primary care. In an attempt to introduce greater specificity to the definition of primary care, the Institute of Medicine has developed a checklist for primary care (Table 4–1) which categorizes desirable indicators of good primary care under its five major elements: (1) accessibility, (2) comprehensiveness, (3) coordination, (4) continuity, and (5) accountability.[8]

Accessibility
Ready access to primary care is obviously essential to the first contact and continuity dimensions of primary care. As noted in the preceding chapter, adequate ac-

TABLE 4-1. A CHECKLIST FOR PRIMARY CARE

A. Are services accessible?
   1. Are services available to patients?
      a. Is access to primary care services provided 24 hours a day, 7 days a week?[a]
      b. Is there an opportunity for a patient to schedule an appointment?[a]
      c. Are scheduled office hours compatible with the work and way of life of most of the patients?
      d. Can most (90 percent) medically urgent cases be seen within 1 hour?
      e. Can most patients (90 percent) with acute but not urgent problems be seen within 1 day?
      f. Can most (90 percent) appropriate requests for routine appointments, such as preventive exams, be met within 1 week?
   2. Are services convenient to patients?
      a. Is the practice unit conveniently located, so that most patients can reach it by public or private transportation?
      b. Is the practice unit so designed that handicapped or elderly patients are not inconvenienced?
      c. Does the practice unit accept patients who have a means of payment, regardless of source (Medicare, Medicaid)?
   3. Are services acceptable to patients?
      a. Is the waiting time for most (90 percent) of the scheduled appointments less than one-half hour?[a]
      b. If a substantial minority (25 percent) of patients have a special language or other communication barrier, does the office staff include people who can deal with this problem?[a]
      c. Are waiting accommodations comfortable and uncrowded?
      d. Does the practice staff consistently demonstrate an interest in and appreciation of the culture, background, socioeconomic status, work environment, and living circumstances of patients?
      e. Is simple, understandable information provided to patients about fees, billing procedures, scheduling of appointments, contacting the unit after hours, and grievance procedures?
      f. Are patients encouraged to ask questions about their illness and their care, to discuss their health problems freely, and to review their records, if desired?
      g. Does the practice unit accept patients without regard to race, religion, or ethnic origin?
B. Are services comprehensive?
   1. Within the patient population served, and realizing that this might be restricted to a certain age (pediatrics) or sex (obstetrics/gynecology), is the practice unit willing to handle, without referral, the great majority (over 90 percent) of the problems arising in this population (for example, general complaints such as fever or fatigue, minor trauma, sore throat, cough, and chest pain)?[a]
   2. Are appropriate primary and secondary preventive measures used for those people at risk (for example, immunizations for tetanus, polio; early detection of hypertension; control of risk factors for coronary disease)?[a]
   3. Are the practitioners in the unit willing, if appropriate, to admit and care for patients in hospitals?[a]

(continued)

TABLE 4-1. *(cont.)*

4. Are the practitioners in the unit willing to admit and care for patients in nursing homes or convalescent homes?[a]

5. Are the practitioners in the unit willing, if appropriate, to visit the patient at home?[a]

6. Are patients encouraged and assisted in providing for their own care and participating as allies in their own health care plan (for example, through instruction in nutrition, diet, exercise, accident prevention, family planning, and adolescent problems)?[a]

7. Do the practitioners in the unit provide support to those agencies and organizations promoting community health (for example, health education programs for the public; disease detection programs; school health and sports medicine programs; emergency care training)?

C. Are services coordinated?
   1. Do the practitioners in the unit furnish pertinent information to other providers serving the patient, actively seek relevant feedback from consultants and other providers, and serve as the patient's ombudsmen in contacts with other providers?[a]

   2. Is a summary or abstract of the patient's record provided to other physicians when needed?[a]

   3. Do the practitioners in the unit develop a treatment plan with the patient that reflects consideration of the patient's understanding? Do the practitioners use a variety of tactics to ensure that the patient will cooperate in the treatment? Does the plan of treatment reflect the patient's physical, emotional, and financial ability to carry it out?[a]

   4. Is another source of care recommended when a patient moves to another geographic area?

D. Are services continuous?
   1. Can a patient who desires to do so make subsequent appointments with the same provider?[a]

   2. Are complete records maintained in a form that is easily retrievable and accessible?[a]

   3. Are relevant items or problems in the patient's record highlighted, regularly reviewed, and used in planning care?[a]

   4. Is each patient reminded of his or her next appointment?

E. Is the unit accountable?
   1. Do the practitioners in the unit assume responsibility for alerting proper authorities if a patient problem reveals a health hazard that may affect others in the community (for example, discovery of exposure to toxic chemicals in an industrial plant; discovery of a communicable disease)?[a]

   2. Is there a patient–disease and age–sex registry maintained that can provide the basis of a practice audit?

   3. Is there a system for regular review of the quality of the process of medical care (for example, reviews for completeness of therapeutic programs and follow-up of acute illnesses)?

   4. Is there a system for regular assessment of the outcomes of the care offered (for example, review of outcome of treatment of specific illnesses; review of level of satisfaction of patients with the services provided; review of compliance with recommendations)?

TABLE 4-1. *(cont.)*

5. Is there evidence that the unit regularly assesses the capability of the staff and provides opportunity for continuing education?

6. Are patients appropriately informed about the nature of their condition, the benefits and risks of available treatments, and the expected outcomes? Are they provided the opportunity to ask questions and discuss their medical record?

7. If unexpected or undesired outcomes occur, are they made known and adequately explained to patients, and is a method established for responding to any expressed dissatisfaction (such as conferences, counseling, arbitration, adjustment of billing, or referral)?

8. Does the provider maintain financial accountability by keeping accurate records and by having adequate professional liability coverage?

[a]Essential to provision of primary care.
(From Institute of Medicine. Primary Care in Medicine: A Definition. Washington, D.C., National Academy of Sciences, 1977, pp 8–14.)

cessibility includes geographic and around-the-clock availability as well as reduction of the various barriers to primary care. Concern for the patient and sensitivity to the sociocultural dimensions of illness comprise necessary attributes of availability.

Comprehensiveness

Comprehensiveness relates to the ability, interest, and willingness of the primary care provider to definitively manage the large majority of health problems occurring in the population served. This is the feature of primary care which most effectively helps to classify health care services as primary care or nonprimary care. For example, a subspecialist may provide readily available first contact and continuity care for some patients with selected problems, but does not provide a sufficient range of services to be considered a primary care physician.

Coordination

The primary care provider coordinates the patient's total care, including that provided by other specialists. The patient's plan of care is individualized to the patient's family and occupational environment, preferences, way of life, and financial circumstances.[8] The primary care provider serves as the patient's advocate for care by other specialists or community resources, and helps to interpret the patient's needs and options. The importance of well-coordinated care has been documented by many studies. One such study, for example, showed what one would predict—the greater utilization of laboratory studies and higher cost of care when patients were seen in emergency rooms compared to a comprehensive pediatric care program.[9]

Continuity

Continuity clearly facilitates ongoing personal care with the least fragmentation, and has important implications for acceptability, cost, quality, and even outcome of care. The use of the problem-oriented medical record and well-structured coverage systems within group practice settings allows continuity of care in instances when the individual primary care provider is not available.

Accountability

Accountability is not unique to primary care, but essential to it.[8] Accountability calls for a range of activities as shown in Table 4–1. It also requires that the primary care provider assume moral and legal responsibility for the ongoing care of the patient.

SOME ISSUES IN PRIMARY CARE

As pointed out earlier, the greatly expanded interest in primary care within medicine and in other segments of society during the last 15 years has raised a number of fundamental issues within primary care education and practice. Some of the more important issues will be discussed briefly here in an effort to round out a more complete picture of recent developments in primary care.

What Do Patients Want?

The traditional health care system has tended to reflect the interest and perceptions of health care providers more than those of patients, and until recent years comparatively little attention was paid to patient perceptions of their needs. Much of the recent interest in patient perceptions has focused on patient satisfaction studies, but some excellent work has also been done by health services researchers on health-seeking behaviors of different population groups. That this is an extremely complex area is suggested by Figure 4–1, which displays some of the factors influencing the behavioral options of patients in seeking care.[10]

Much more needs to be learned about patients' desires and expectations concerning any part of the health care system. Since patients' preferences are known to vary greatly according to socioeconomic factors, cultural, and other demographic characteristics, only fragmentary information is available with respect to patients' preferences vis-a-vis primary care. Some of the following examples, however, point to the priorities expressed by patients from various population groups in some recent studies:

1. In a large national study involving more than 5400 respondents conducted by the Center for Health Administration Studies and the National Opinion Research Center at the University of Chicago, greater patient satisfaction was observed for people who have a regular source of care instead of no regular physician and for those who visit a private physician's office or group practice compared to those visiting outpatient clinics or emergency rooms; the three most highly valued criteria for satisfaction were amount of concern the physician expressed, quality of care provided, and information from the physician, respectively.[11]

2. In a recent study by Fletcher and colleagues, a representative sample of patients attending the medical clinics of a university teaching hospital in North Carolina were asked to rate their relative priorities for eight different attributes of medical care: continuity, coordination, comprehensiveness, availability, convenience, cost, expertise, and compassion. The sampled group included a balanced distribution by age, sex, source of payment, problem duration, and severity. Continuity of care was rated highest by the overall group, with cost and convenience lowest. Older patients valued continuity and comprehensiveness most highly, while patients less

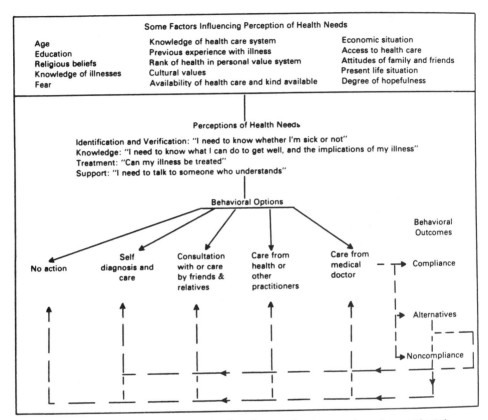

Figure 4-1. Flow chart of behavioral options and outcomes based on patients' perceptions of health care. *(From Bruhn JG, Trevino FM: A method of determining patients' perceptions of their health needs. J Fam Pract 8(4):809, 1979, with permission.)*

than 30 years old valued coordination most. Patients with acute problems rated coordination and expertise most highly while patients with chronic problems ranked continuity highest.[12]

3. Starr and colleagues, studied patient expectations for comprehensive health care among 563 patients representing consecutive visits to 4 family practice centers in urban and suburban communities in Nebraska; the population sampled was representative of the practices in terms of age, sex, and sources of payment. High expectations were found for office visits, emergency services, yearly physical examination, eye examination, and performance of proctoscopy, blood tests and chest x-ray; a majority of respondents did not feel that psychiatric services, marital counseling, youth counseling, nursing home care, and health education were necessary parts of comprehensive health care.[13]

4. A recent study by Romm examined patient expectations of the periodic health examination in terms of expected content and frequency. The study group attended a family practice center in North Carolina, was well balanced by age for adults over 20 years old, was 80 percent female, 71 per-

cent white, and 25 percent black. Over 90 percent of respondents desired an annual checkup, and their preferences generally exceeded those recommended by an expert group as being helpful in early diagnosis or prevention of disease (e.g., women in their twenties and thirties expected mammograms to be part of their checkup at least as often as did older women, although the efficacy of this procedure has not been demonstrated for women less than 50 years of age).[14]

5. Karaly and colleagues studied the perceptions of patients attending an urban family practice center in Ohio with respect to their utilization of mental health services. The study group was 80 percent female, 78 percent black, 22 percent white, and well balanced by age over 18 years of age. The family physician was preferred mainly for personal problems associated with physical manifestations, while other providers (e.g., social worker, psychiatrist, psychologist) were preferred for predominantly social or emotional problems.[15]

6. In a study involving more than 80,000 patient visits to the Department of Family Practice at the Kaiser-Permanente Medical Care Program in San Diego, California, Kelly found that female patients were about 1.5 times more likely than males to select a female physician, whereas male patients were 1.14 times as likely as females to select a male physician. In this program about 25 percent of family physicians are female; these women physicians were found to have panels comprising two-thirds female patients, compared to male physicians with just over one-half female patients.[16]

The findings of these studies help to point out the diversity of patient perceptions and expectations of primary health care, and in some cases are at variance with the customary views of physicians. Patients' views need to be considered as an important element of health planning and policy development but available information in this area is still incomplete at best.

How Important Is Continuity of Primary Care?

Although continuity of care has been adopted as a highly valued goal by all of the primary care specialties, its effects on the process and outcomes of health care have been subject to considerable debate for some years. The major difficulty prompting confusion has been the lack of consensus for a single definition of continuity so that the many studies of continuity have examined different measures in various settings without a common conceptual base. Continuity of care may exist between a patient and individual provider and/or an institution (e.g., an HMO, a clinic), and can also be related to various elements of the process of care. In primary care, most agree that continuity of care requires an ongoing personal relationship involving the patient and his/her physician that exists over time regardless of the patient's health status.[17] Hennen has identified the following basic dimensions of continuity of care:[18]

- Chronologic (i.e., longitudinal continuity, care provided over time to a defined population)
- Geographic (i.e., site continuity, constancy of physician availability whether in office, home, or hospital)
- Interdisciplinary (i.e., including coordination by primary care physician when consultative services are involved)
- Interpersonal (i.e., involving the personal physician-patient relationship)

- Informational (i.e., the medical record and other forms of communication between patient and provider, together comprising a cumulative knowledge base of the patient's problems and needs)

Two excellent recent reviews have appeared which have analyzed in some depth what is known and not known about the value of continuity of care. Wall has proposed a useful conceptual model integrating the determinants of continuity of care into a dynamic, multidimensional model illustrated in Figure 4–2.[19] The complexity of continuity is apparent from the diversity of variables involving the provider, the patient, and their encounters.

In the most rigorous assessment of past studies of continuity of care yet performed, Dietrich and Marton analyzed the methods and results of all such studies reported in the English literature between 1964 and 1980. They reviewed only those papers which met the following criteria:[17]

- Primary data reported
- At least one measure of quality of care applied whereby the effect of an ongoing physician–patient relationship could be separated from other concurrent interventions
- Studies with internal validity and general applicability

In order to determine whether each study reached reasonable conclusions from its findings, four additional questions were asked:

- Was longitudinal care studied and different between groups?
- Were the clinical and demographic characteristics of the patient groups comparable before the interventions?
- Are the conclusions statistically justified by the results?
- Are the conclusions logically justified by the results?

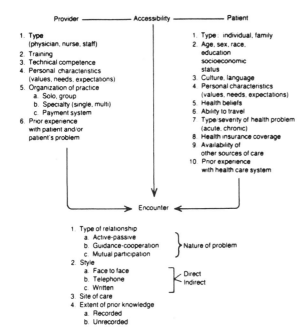

Figure 4–2. Determinants of continuity. (*From Wall EM: Continuity of care and family medicine: Definition, determinants, and relationship to outcome. J Fam Pract 13:655, 1981, with permission.*)

Table 4-2 summarizes the effects of 16 studies which were analyzed by these criteria. Dietrich and Marton were able to conclude that longitudinal care has been found to lead to increased patient and physician/staff satisfaction in a variety of settings, greater compliance with medication and appointments, and increased readiness to disclose confidential information by mothers of child patients. No studies were found which met their criteria addressing morbidity, mortality, preventive services, costs, or speed of referral.[17]

TABLE 4-2. SUMMARY OF STUDIES THAT EVALUATED CONTINUOUS OR LONGITUDINAL CARE WITH A PROVIDER

| Reference | Reported Effect[a] | | |
	Increased Quality	No Difference	Decreased Quality
Alpert	Appointment compliance		
Caplan and Sussman	Staff satisfaction		
Charney et al.	Medication compliance		
Gordis and Markowitz		Medication compliance	
Becker et al.	Medication and appointment compliance		
Miller			Later referral for specialty care
Becker et al.	Patient satisfaction and confidence, staff satisfaction, appointment compliance	Preventive care	
Morehead and Donaldson			Conformance with standards of care
Poland	Appointment compliance		
Shortell	Patient satisfaction		
Boethius	Medication compliance		
Starfield et al.	Recognition of identified problems		
Shortell et al.	Patient satisfaction		
Woolley et al.	Patient satisfaction		
Hennelly and Boxerman		More illness visits with less continuity[b]	
Roos et al.			Conformance with standards of care

[a]Direction of reported effect is given, if not obvious. If study author did not characterize an effect as increasing or decreasing quality, it is listed under No Difference and designated as such.
[b]Author did not characterize this change as increasing or decreasing quality.
(From Dietrich AJ, Marton KI: Does continuous care from a physician make any difference? J Fam Pract 15(5):929, 1982, with permission.)

One must conclude that further studies of the effects of continuity of care are needed, particularly with respect to costs and health status outcomes. One very recent study provides an excellent model of the kind of studies needed. In a double-blind randomized trial of almost 800 men aged 55 years and older, it was found that the continuity group had fewer emergent hospital admissions (20 percent versus 39 percent) and a shorter average length of stay (15.5 versus 25.5 days) over the 30-month study period than the discontinuity group.[20]

How Comprehensive Should Primary Care Be?

Most agree that comprehensiveness of care is an essential part of primary care. A number of attempts have been made to define this comprehensiveness, such as by the James' stages outlined earlier in Chapter 1. While there may be widespread support for this concept today, this support starts to break down into controversy when the real content and scope of comprehensive care are viewed in practical terms.

One basic issue involves the distinction between "medical care" and "health care." In his excellent book, *Ferment in Medicine,* Magraw suggested that: "From the standpoint of the doctor's role in society as constituted now and in the future, the prevention of disease must be regarded as an extension of his primary function, the care of the sick."[21] But most definitions of comprehensive health care tend to raise more questions than they resolve. The major points of most definitions are reflected in that of Lee, who views comprehensive medicine as:

> . . . the mobilization of all appropriate resources for the care of the patient. It implies a primary concern for the patient (rather than the disease) and a consideration of all significant factors that affect his health. It implies the application of preventive measures to individuals and the employment of all practical means for the early detection of disease.[22]

From the above, comprehensive health care still seems somewhat intangible in practical terms. But it certainly involves expansion of medicine's scope beyond care of the sick to care of the presumably well. Whereas most of our current clinical efforts involve the management of symptomatic disease and are classified as "medical care," the concept of "health care" is enlarged to also include health education and preventive, rehabilitative, and restorative services.

Many difficult practical questions arise which complicate implementation of comprehensive care: Does our health care system have the capability to render comprehensive medicine to all? Can comprehensive care be afforded (by the patient and his/her family, private insurance carriers, and government health programs)? What specific programs of preventive medicine are essential? Does the "cost–benefit" justify heavy emphasis on Stage I (Foundations of Disease) and Stage II (Preclinical Disease) medicine? How, and by whom, can comprehensive care best be rendered? These questions, and others, are difficult or impossible to answer at this time, but must be kept in mind by the medical profession and health planners as future systems of medical practice are developed.

Health maintenance, for example, has already become accepted in many quarters as an unassailable advance in modern medicine, but the research base in this important area is still inadequate. Felcher has called for identification of "criteria by which selection of the scope of testing can be made on an individual rather than a mass basis."[23] Sackett has urged that randomized clinical trials of screening and other diagnostic procedures be rapidly expanded in order to ascertain and document their validity.[24]

We are on more solid ground in looking at the comprehensiveness of what are generally accepted as "medical services." Table 4–3 compares the range of services provided by four specialties in group and nongroup practice with respect to several selected common problems.[25] The comprehensiveness of general/family physicians is demonstrated in these data, as well as the relative gaps in comprehensiveness by primary care physicians limiting their practice by age or sex.

Another important dimension of comprehensiveness is by setting (i.e., ambulatory and hospital). Some have suggested that the future primary care physician restrict his/her practice to ambulatory care as is often the case abroad.[26,27] There are persuasive arguments, however, on the other side of this question, well expressed by Alpert:[7]

> Some would suggest that primary care ought to end when the patient is hospitalized, and that ambulatory care could then be said to equal primary care. Many medical problems that require secondary services are largely treated on an ambulatory basis, however, with only occasional hospitalization. Conversely, the decision to hospitalize a patient may sometimes be based on psychosocial factors in management rather than medical complexity. There is, in addition, strong support for the view that the physician who practices ambulatory and hospital machine is a better physician than the one who practices only ambulatory medicine. For these reasons, the site of care alone, whether hospital, home, or office, is an insufficient base for a definition of primary care.

In my judgment, the sharp separation of medical careers into community-oriented ambulatory care and hospital-based intensive care of acutely ill patients would involve serious problems both for medical practice and medical education. The creation of a system with built-in discontinuity between ambulatory and hospital patient care could be expected to jeopardize the quality of care, increase its cost, decrease patient compliance, and further depersonalize care. Although it is theoretically possible that the ambulatory care physician could transmit all necessary medical information to the hospital-based physician regarding each hospitalized patient, this would not be likely to happen in everyday practice. It is more probable that hospital care would be further overutilized, significant medical problems would be overlooked, unnecessary studies and procedures performed, and patient further confused by relating to an unknown physician at the time of major personal crisis. The well-trained primary care physician is equipped to manage many common health problems requiring hospitalization. When consultation is needed, team care by the primary care physician and consultant(s) offers the patient the advantages of comprehensive and coordinated care by a known physician and advocate, while simultaneously benefiting from the care of one or more consultants.

Who Provides Primary Care?

This question has been controversial during the past decade as many disciplines have claimed major interests in primary care. Cynics have been quick to suggest a correlation between these newly discovered interests with changing priorities for federal and state funding of primary care.

The Millis Commission in 1966 defined the primary care physician as one who:

TABLE 4-3. COMPARATIVE RANGE OF SERVICES AMONG PRIMARY CARE PHYSICIANS IN UNITED STATES

Service	General Practitioners		Internists		Pediatricians		Obstetricians	
	Nongroup N = 599 (%)	Group N = 111 (%)	Nongroup N = 231 (%)	Group N = 91 (%)	Nongroup N = 136 (%)	Group N = 43 (%)	Nongroup N = 150 (%)	Group N = 58 (%)
Tape (strap) sprains	86	88	56	42	78	71	16	12
Excise simple cysts	94	90	20	11	28	19	87	93
Suture lacerations	98	95	37	31	85	80	62	65
Do proctoscopic or sigmoidoscopic exam	83	86	89	91	40	39	43	33
Do uncomplicated obstetrics	59	58	—	—	3	—	97	100
Do well-baby care	91	83	7	1	97	100	14	11
Set simple fractures	80	77	6	3	50	32	5	2

(From Mechanic D: General medical practice: Some comparisons between the work of primary care physicians in the United States and England and Wales. Medical Care 10:5, 410–411, 1972, with permission.)

. . . should usually be primary in the first contact sense. He will serve as the primary medical resource and counselor to an individual or a family. When a patient needs hospitalization, the service of other medical specialists, or other medical or paramedical assistance, the primary physician will see that the necessary arrangements are made, giving such responsibiity to others as is appropriate and retaining his own continuing and comprehensive responsibility.

Few hospitals and few existing specialists consider comprehensive and continuing medical care to be their responsibility and within their range of competence.[3]

The definitions of primary care presented earlier, together with the range of indicator activities listed in Table 4–1, demonstrate the wide range of concern and function subsumed by the primary care physician. There is broad agreement that the general/family physician, general internist, and general pediatrician indeed act as primary care physicians, and these are the only primary care specialties recognized by the Bureau of Health Manpower for funding purposes. Some believe that obstetrics–gynecology should be considered a primary care specialty. Although this specialty is viewed as a primary care field by the American Medical Association, the relative lack of comprehensiveness of services, combined with a predominantly surgical orientation of the specialty greatly weaken this argument, [28,29] and the field is not considered primary care by the Bureau of Health Manpower. Claims by other specialties of major involvement in primary care clearly fall far short of the mark. Some fields may be heavily involved in first-contact care of limited scope, such as dermatology, emergency medicine, and psychiatry, but lack of breadth and continuity to function as primary care physicians.

It must be recognized that a number of specialties may devote some proportion of their efforts to incomplete and desultory primary care. In 1975, for example, a survey of physicians by *Medical Economics* showed that 60 percent of physicians surveyed in ten specialties provided some primary care, usually for economic reasons.[30] As Beck and colleagues point out, however, "although these specialists may be meeting some primary care needs, this informal system of primary care does not provide the patient with either the most appropriate or effective care.[29]

More recently, the argument has been raised by some that a substantial and expanding number of subspecialists make such contributions to primary care through a "hidden system" that the nation's deficit of primary care providers is no longer a problem. The major work which has propelled this thesis is a national study conducted by a group at the University of Southern California involving a survey of the content and patterns of practice of more than 10,000 physicians in 24 specialties and in a variety of settings between 1973 and 1976. These physicians were asked whether they considered their patients as "regular patients" for whom they provided the "majority of care." The physicians were also asked to maintain log diaries for 3-day periods for the purpose of reporting their encounters with patients. These encounters were subsequently classified in terms of the following categories: first encounter, principal care, consultative care, and specialized care. Physicians were considered to be providing principal care if they had seen the patient before and believed him or her to be a regular patient; there were no specific requirements for comprehensiveness or continuity of services within this definition. This study collected information on the nature of over 400,000 patient encounters taking place in the office, in the hospital, or by telephone.[31]

On the basis of the results of the USC study and of other national studies on practice patterns and access to medical care, Aiken and her colleagues in 1979 drew conclusions which far exceeded the limits of the results available. Among their major conclusions were the following:

1. "Specialists" (i.e., nonprimary care physicians) currently serve as "primary physicians" for almost one out of every five Americans.
2. In view of the significant amount of generalist services provided within the "hidden system" of primary care, the nation's needs for primary care services will be adequately met within another 6 to 10 years without much further change in the distribution of physicians by specialty.[31])

There are many holes in these observations, as reflected by the following points:

1. "Principal care" is by no means equivalent to, and falls far short of, "primary care" as defined by such groups as the Millis Commission,[3] the Institute of Medicine,[9] and even the Care Classification Research Advisory Committee for the USC study.[32] As pointed out by Peterson,[33] comprehensiveness of care cannot be assumed unless the physician has recognized all of his/her "principal care" patients' health problems and copes with most of them. The data collection instrument used by the USC study did not address this issue.
2. The relatively small numbers of "principal care" patients served by the limited specialties falls far short of corresponding levels for primary care physicians.
3. In speculating on the future needs for primary care physicians, inadequate attention was paid to the well-documented "leakage" of physicians to subspecialty practice in internal medicine, pediatrics, and obstetrics–gynecology.
4. Questions of cost, quality, and distribution of primary care services were not addressed.

A further point against placing much confidence in the "hidden system" of primary care arises from a recent large study involving the experience over 1 year of more than 2700 people enrolled in the Rand Health Insurance Experiment. Spiegel and her colleagues reported in 1983 that use of a "majority of care" criterion for primary care resulted in overestimation by threefold the contribution of nonprimary care physicians to primary care. They urged that definitions of primary care should include the tasks usually associated with primary care (e.g., care of common problems) as well as patients' perceptions of the role of their physicians.[34]

The central role played by general/family physicians in primary care in the United States is demonstrated in terms of the comparative proportions of office visits to the various specialties as shown in Table 4–4 and Figure 4–3.[35]

What is the Role of Middle-Level Practitioners in Primary Care?

The last 15 years have seen a proliferation of educational programs designed to train "middle-level practitioners" to participate in the delivery of primary care as assistants to the primary care physician. These health professionals, including physicians' assistants and nurse practitioners, have been viewed by the medical profession as "physician extenders" working under the direct supervision of physicians in order to extend the range and quality of services provided. Considerable emphasis has been placed on the concept of "team practice," and many positive experiences with this approach have been reported across the country.

TABLE 4-4. DISTRIBUTION OF AMBULATORY VISITS TO OFFICE-BASED U.S. PHYSICIANS ACCORDING TO PATIENT AGE AND PHYSICIAN SPECIALTY

Physician Specialty	Patient Age (%)				
	< 17	17–44	45–64	≥ 65	All Ages
General and family practice	32.6	38.0	39.1	40.0	37.4
General internal medicine	1.5	8.6	17.9	22.1	11.6
Pediatrics	44.5	0.7	0.1	0.0	9.6
Obstetrics and gynecology	1.0	18.8	4.4	1.3	8.7
General surgery	2.8	6.0	7.9	7.7	6.1
Psychiatry	0.6	4.6	2.6	0.6	2.6
Other specialties	17.3	23.3	28.0	28.3	24.0
Totals	100.0	100.0	100.0	100.0	100.0

(From Rosenblatt RA, Cherkin DC, Schneeweiss R, et al.: The content of ambulatory care in the United States: An interspecialty comparison. N Engl J Med 309:892, 1983, with permission.)

The American Medical Association defines these health professionals as follows:[36]

The assistant to the primary care physician is a person qualified by academic and clinical training to provide patient care services under the supervision of a licensed physician in a wide variety of medical care settings which are involved in the delivery of primary care. The functions of a primary care physician are interdisciplinary in nature involving medicine, pediatrics, obstetrics and psychiatry. . . .

The assistant, therefore, is involved in helping the primary care physician provide a variety of personal health services, including but not limited to:

- receiving patients, obtaining case histories, performing an appropriate physical examination, and presenting meaningful resulting data to the physician;
- performing or assisting in laboratory procedures and related studies in the practice setting;
- giving injections and immunizations;
- suturing and caring for wounds;
- providing patient counseling services; referring patients to other health care resources;
- responding to emergency situations which might arise in the physician's absence within the assistant's range of skills and experience; and
- assisting the employing physician in all settings such as the office, hospitals, extended care facilities, nursing home, and the patient's home.

The ultimate role of the assistant and his functions vary with his individual capabilities and the specific needs of the employing physician, the practice setting in which he works, and the community in which he lives.

Many of the initial issues involved in the delivery of primary care by teams of primary care physicians and these middle-level practitioners have been effectively

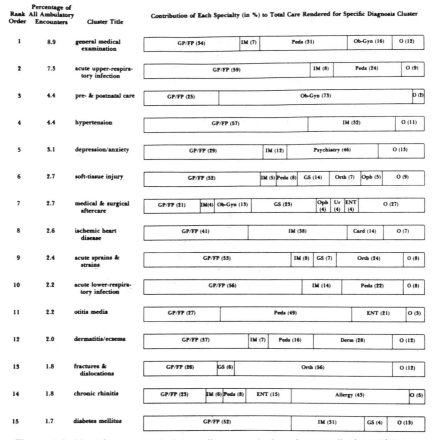

Figure 4–3. Most frequent ambulatory diagnoses in American medical practice according to physician specialty (National Ambulatory Medical Care Survey, 1977 and 1978). *(From Rosenblatt RA, Cherkin DC, Schneeweiss R, et al.: The content of ambulatory care in the United States: An interspecialty comparison. N Engl J Med 309:892, 1983, with permission.)*

resolved. Numerous studies have demonstrated that middle-level practitioners provide care of comparable quality to that of the physician, that acceptance by patients has been good, and that physician acceptance of their role has been forthcoming in many settings. Except in some remote and underserved areas, most middle-level practitioners have worked collaboratively with physicians in the same physical locations. Indeed, physicians assistant programs are designed to train graduates for this role instead of an independent practice role with less direct supervision by the physician.

A different stance has been taken by organized nursing. The nurse practitioner is not viewed by nursing as a physician extender but as a primary care provider capable of practice in a "joint" relationship with the physician. A National Joint Practice Commission was established in the mid-1970s, and adopted a definition and guidelines for joint practice in primary care. This group views joint practice in these terms:[37]

Neither the nurse nor the physician alone is prepared to address adequately the broad range of health, medical and nursing concerns of patients encountered in a primary care setting: each professional has a clear identity, each is licensed in his and her own right, and each is in command of a separate body of knowledge, although there is a shared scientific base of preparation and considerable overlap in many functions. Thus, each professional brings a different approach and additional information and expertise to the setting that the other professional recognizes, values and is unable to provide alone.

The nurse practitioner's role has been defined in broad and rather vague terms, and a variety of working relationships with physicians have evolved. In many settings nurse practitioners are heavily involved, under some physician supervision, with diagnosis and management of relatively uncomplicated common illnesses, while in other settings they emphasize social support and patient education roles. One recent study examining the extent of role agreement among physicians and nurse practitioners practicing together revealed that the nurse practitioners who were surveyed tend to prefer patient care involving psychosocial problems or requiring patient education to the traditional care of biomedical problems.[38]

There continues to be considerable confusion and controversy concerning the distinction between expanded "nursing practice" and "medical practice."[39-42] Levinson views the development of markedly expanded clinical roles of nonphysician practitioners as raising:

> . . . fundamental questions of education, certification, responsibility, organization and remuneration, not only for the new clinicians, but for all practitioners, and for the health-care system. . . . Independent practice is a contemporary not a future issue. The practice acts of many states are so vague about supervision as to be an endorsement of independent practice. The issue is pivotal and should not be decided without serious debate based on extended evaluation studies.[43]

Present health policy represents a "holding pattern" vis-a-vis the roles of middle-level practitioners in the U.S. health care system. Federal expenditures for training programs for middle-level practitioners have been plateaued for some years. GMENAC recommended no increase in these programs, and recommended that their roles in a physician surplus era should be determined soon.[43] The relationship between nursing practice and medical practice varies greatly by state based upon different legislative approaches to state nurse practice acts, prescriptive authority, and third-party reimbursement.[44] As the physician supply has increased, attempts to broaden nurse practice acts have encountered growing resistance in many states. Largely because of increasing physician resistance to independent practice by middle-level practitioners and the projected cost increase if this trend were to substantially expand (since their services are usually additive instead of substitutive for physicians' services), a major shift in this direction is not likely. At the same time, there will probably be a continued need for middle-level practitioners, usually working in a collaborative relationship with physicians, particularly caring for underserved areas and groups.[45]

How Should Primary Care Be Organized?

Recent years have seen an increasing diversity of approaches to primary care arise under the influence of various changes in medical education, federal legislation, and riembursement patterns. Brief discussion of some of the major alternative organizational approaches to the delivery of primary care services illustrates some of the issues involved. Although there are other possible approaches, five basic approaches are considered here.

1. Solo Practice. While this approach offers the primary care physician maximal autonomy and freedom to practice according to his/her individual style, this approach presents problems of coverage, comparative isolation from colleagues, and difficulty in acquiring the equipment, staff, and resources which facilitate optimal primary care. Although coverage problems can often be resolved effectively through call-sharing associations of solo physicians, solo practice is not as attractive to today's young physicians as it was in the past. Only 15 to 20 percent of graduates of family practice residency programs, for example, opt for solo practice, whereas about three-quarters choose partnership or group practice.

2. Single-specialty Group Practice. Single-specialty groups of family physicians, internists or pediatricians have been, and should continue to be, an important and effective approach to providing primary care to families, adults or children, respectively. Such groups usually include three to five physicians, and trade off some of the autonomy of solo practice for a number of advantages of group practice. These advantages include an effective on-call schedule, affording time off for continuing education and vacations, the capability to support the needed resources (physical facilities, equipment, personnel, and methods) for a comprehensive range of primary care services, and the ongoing stimulation of everyday interaction with colleagues through informal consultation and periodic audit of patient care problems.

3. Multispecialty Group Practice. Most multispecialty groups which are organized for the purpose of primary care inevitably involve much larger groups of physicians. For example, five or more internists are usually found in such groups, as well as four or more pediatricians, several obstetrician–gynecologists, and several surgeons. This is unavoidable since each specialty is neither qualified nor willing to see patients for problems outside of that specialty or to cover for colleagues in another specialty during nights and weekends. These groups tend to become quite large since the natural tendency is to add some medical and surgical subspecialists to the group. Although multispecialty groups can provide excellent medical care, an individual patient's and family's care is more fragmented than would be the case in a single-specialty primary care group. Multispecialty groups are often better suited to referral practice than to primary care.

   A possible variant of multispecialty groups oriented to primary care is the family practice group including one or more specialists in other fields, such as an internist, pediatrician, obstetrician–gynecologist, and/or general surgeon. Such groups have the advantage of extending the range of services available within the group, but often present coverage problems which may or may not be soluble within the group itself.

4. Health Maintenance Organizations (HMOs). As noted in the last chapter, prepaid group practices (HMOs) represent an expanding approach to the delivery of health services with considerable potential for effective organization of a broad range of health care services, particularly in metropolitan areas. A large HMO with a long experience is represented by the Kaiser

system on the West Coast, which utilizes a combination of family physicians, internists, and pediatricians for primary care. A somewhat smaller and extremely effective HMO developed during the last 25 years in the Pacific Northwest is the Group Health Cooperative of Puget Sound, which bases primary care more solidly on the family physician (goal of 45 percent of the group's physicians in family practice). HMOs represent well-planned, institutional approaches to providing integrated health care, particularly at primary and secondary care levels, with considerable potential for efficiency and cost containment. A recent variant in the HMO field is the development by Blue Cross and Blue Shield of a large national network presently including 38 HMOs in 21 stages. The Blues have been moving steadily toward prepaid medical practice, as evidenced by their HMO network for federal employees established in 1978 and a similar network for employees of United Airlines initiated in 1982.[46]

5. Hospital-sponsored Primary Care Group Practice. The last few years have witnessed an increasing involvement of hospitals in the United States with developing networks of primary care practices under various forms of hospital sponsorship. These satellite practices often receive assistance with startup costs from the sponsoring hospital, and their subsequent operations range from full autonomy to variable amounts of administrative controls by the hospitals. The major stimulus for this trend, of course, is the increased competition among hospitals facing reimbursement constraints through DRGs in a time of growing physician supply. Many hospitals, including teaching institutions as well as community hospitals, are trying to increase their referral base through a larger primary care base in the surrounding community served by the parent hospital.

At the same time, a strong countetrend is apparent favoring a shift of some hospital-based care to ambulatory care in the community under physician control with a more distant relationship to hospitals. Examples here include the emergence of physician group practices as HMOs with reduced utilization of hospitals; emergi-centers/urgent-care centers, and surgi-centers. Starr sees these two opposing trends as placing physicians and hospitals in increasing conflict during the 1980s and beyond. He points out that hospitals and physicians each have particular advantages in this conflict:[47] Hospitals are likely to have a stronger bargaining position in negotiations over compensation of staff physicians; the growing number of physicians may lead to increased competition among physicans for hospital staff positions and privileges. Physicians, on the other hand, have established relations with patients, can provide a large proportion of needed health care services on an ambulatory basis, have less overhead, and have fewer operational and reimbursement constraints than hospitals.

What New Issues Are Raised by the Gatekeeper Role?

As described in the previous chapter, various forms of prepaid medical practice are becoming common, especially involving HMOs and IPAs. These plans are generally based upon an established relationship between the patient and the primary care physician serving in a gatekeeping or case management capacity. Prepaid capitation plans at once create new incentives and disincentives for patients, health care professionals, and hospitals compared with the traditional fee-for-service and cost-based reimbursement systems. The inevitable result will be the forging of new expectations and relationships among patients, providers, and hospitals.

The following everyday example illustrates some of the issues involved in these plans. A patient recently enrolled in a Blue Cross Health Plus prepaid plan asks her primary care physician to approve ongoing routine consultant services which she has maintained for some years (e.g., periodic visits with ophthalmologist for vision testing and glaucoma screening, and with obstetrician–gynecologist for pelvic examination and Pap smear). The primary care physician sees these services as basic primary care which he is fully qualified to provide. By not authorizing such consultant services, both the patient and the consultants may be disturbed, but these kinds of restraints are necessary in order to contain costs within available capitation limits. Similar examples apply to discretionary services provided by other consultants, ancillary services (especially laboratory and x-ray), and hospitals.

Based upon their recent study of more than 100 HMOs in the United States, Catlin and colleagues observe that the gatekeeper/case management role can have an impact on the cost of health care in two major ways—by the primary care physician's own style of practice, and by control over utilization of other services.[48] The task of the primary care physician is to assure acceptable outcomes of care for all of the patient's health problems while limiting total expenditures for such care.

The disastrous experience of one large HMO in the Northwest sharpens some of the issues involved in the gatekeeper/case management role. United Healthcare was an HMO created in 1974 by the SAFECO Insurance Company in northern California, Washington, and Utah. Under this plan, fee-for-service reimbursement was preserved, and the risk sharing for cumulative costs was limited to 10 percent of primary care fees. Initially, there was an open-door policy for participating physicians in both primary care and other specialties, no disruption of referral patterns, and no mechanism for utilization review of office and hospital practices. By 1980, enrollment had grown to 41,000 patients and 905 participating primary care physicians, but the plan was in financial difficulty. At that point, several major changes were instituted including reduction of the physician panel in primary care as well as consulting specialties; institution of protocols for length of stay, requirements for outpatient surgery, and maximum fee schedules; preauthorization of hospital admission; increase in risk sharing to 20 percent for primary care physicians; and reduction of the benefit package with introduction of cost-sharing copayments by enrollees. These changes were too late, however, and the plan was terminated in 1982 with sizable financial losses.[49]

Several lessons emerge from the experience to date of primary care physicians serving as gatekeepers in prepaid health care plans:[50]

1. New areas of knowledge and skills will be required to effectively serve the gatekeeper/case management role, including an information system monitoring the ongoing experience of the individual patient and aggregate practice with the plan.
2. The gatekeeping role, to be effective, must be supported by needed system changes (e.g., copayment provisions for patients, utilization controls, defined practice style expectations for consultants, protocols for ambulatory and hospital care).
3. Prepaid medical practice will ultimately require renegotiation and reallocation of limited funds for the primary versus tertiary care sections; it will

be essential to preserve solid funding for primary care services by preventing a small number of tertiary care services to expend a disproportionate share of total health care dollars without reasonable limits.

COMMENT

This chapter has demonstrated considerable activity and interest in the primary care sector of a rapidly changing health care system. A variety of organizational forms of primary care are evolving which meet the five basic criteria for good primary care—accessibility, comprehensiveness, coordination, continuity, and accountability to a greater or lesser extent. Some tradeoffs of these optimal elements are probably appropriate if they appear to be more realistic in terms of meeting patients' needs in certain settings. For example, in settings where the population has demonstrated preference for convenience and ready access to episodic care over continuity or comprehensiveness of care, as is true in many underserved urban areas, emergi-centers may be more highly utilized than group practices of primary care physicians offering a full range of primary care services. As a matter of health policy, however, it would seem that the overriding goal should be to develop wherever possible a strong primary care sector with all of the elements of good primary care.

A number of current trends could lead toward strengthening the primary care base, including increased understanding of public expectations and health-seeking behaviors, growing awareness of the importance of the primary care sector, the advent of graduate training programs in the primary care specialties, the growth of group practice, and recent reimbursement changes revolving around the central role of the primary care physician as gatekeeper or case manager in prepaid health plans. Despite these promising trends, however, there are some strong countertrends toward a suboptimal delivery of fragmented, incomplete primary care services. These include the proliferation of episodic care settings (e.g., emergi-centers, urgent-care centers, excessive use of emergency rooms of hospitals for nonemergent problems) and the involvement of nonprimary care physicians "dabbling" in primary care as part of the "hidden system" of primary care without either the training or commitment to provide optimal primary care.

Urgently needed is a coherent plan for a strong primary care base of the health care system stressing all of the elements of good primary care. In viewing the problems of primary care, Sheps makes this observation:[51]

> In the industrialized nations the hospital system is today the subject of a great deal of agonized attention because of its increasing cost and its never-ending growth in size and complexity. The control measures that have been directed at hospitals in this country are notable by their general lack of success. The most important single measure that can be undertaken, which would indeed put the hospitals under appropriate control, is to develop a primary care system that is strong and pervasive, and put the primary care system on top and in control. And what we need to do is to turn that all the way over so that the hospital serves the primary care system and doesn't dominate it.

As debate and discussion of the many issues related to primary care continue, great care must be taken by all involved health care professionals to keep the welfare of the patient at the center of focus, not the special interest of any particular group of health professionals. The collective responsibility of the primary care disciplines is to provide readily accessible health care of the highest possible quality to the entire population with the least possible fragmentation at a cost which can be afforded by an increasingly burdened society.

REFERENCES

1. Fein R: Some options for the short run. In Lewis CE, Fein R, Mechanic D (eds): A Right to Health: The Problem of Access to Primary Medical Care. New York, John Wiley & Sons, 1976, p 285
2. White KL: Primary medical care for families. N Engl J Med 277:847, 1967
3. Report of the Citizens Commission on Graduate Medical Education (Millis Commission). Chicago, American Medical Association, 1966
4. Pellegrino ED: Planning for comprehensive and continuing care of patients through education. J Med Educ 43:751, 1968
5. American Academy of Family Physicians: Education for Family Practice. Kansas City, Mo., 1969
6. Magraw R: Medical education and health services—Implication for family medicine. N Engl J Med 285:1407, 1971
7. Alpert JL: New directions in medical education: Primary care. In Purcell EF (ed): Recent Trends in Medical Education. New York, Josiah Macy Jr. Foundation, 1976, p 166
8. Institute of Medicine. Primary Care in Medicine: A definition. Washington, D.C., National Academy of Sciences, 1977, p 8
9. Heagarty MC, Robertson LS, Kosa J, Alpert JL: Some comparative costs in comprehensive versus fragmented pediatric care. Pediatrics 46(4):596, 1970
10. Bruhn JG, Trevino FM: A method of determining patients' perceptions of their health needs. J Fam Pract 8:809, 1979
11. On patient satisfaction: Study points out medical manpower needs. Am Medical News, November 20/27, 1981, p 19
12. Fletcher RH, O'Malley MS, Earp JA, et al.: Patients' priorities for medical care. Med Care 21(2):234, 1983
13. Starr GC, Norris R, Patil KD, et al.: Patient expectations. What is comprehensive health care? J Fam Pract 8:161, 1979
14. Romm FJ: Patients' expectations of periodic health examinations. J Fam Pract 19:191, 1984
15. Karaly DA, Coulton CJ, Graham A: How family practice patients view their utilization of mental health services. J Fam Pract 15:317, 1982
16. Kelly JM: Sex preference in patient selection of a family physician. J Fam Pract 11:427, 1980
17. Dietrich AJ, Marton KI: Does continuous care from a physician make any difference? J Fam Pract 15:929, 1982
18. Hennen BK: Continuity of care in family practice: Part 1. Dimensions of continuity. J Fam Pract 2:371, 1975
19. Wall EM: Continuity of care and family medicine: Definition, determinants, and relationship to outcome. J Fam Pract 13:655, 1981
20. Wasson JH, Sauvigne AE, Mogielnicki P, et al.: Continuity of outpatient medical care in elderly men: A randomized trial. JAMA 252:2413, 1984
21. Magraw RM: Ferment in Medicine. Philadelphia, W.B. Saunders, 1966, p 61
22. Lee PV: Medical schools and the changing times. J Med Educ 36:72, 1961
23. Felcher WC: Does preventive medicine really work? Prism 1(7):26, 1973
24. Bombardier C, McClaran J, Sackett DC: Medical care policy rounds: Periodic health examinations and multiphasic screening. Can Med Assoc J 109:1123, 1973

25. Mechanic D: General medical practice: Some comparisons between the work of primary care physicians in the United States and England and Wales. Medical Care 10(5):410, 1972

26. Proger S: A career in ambulatory medicine. N Engl J Med 292:1318, 1975

27. Petersdorf RG: Internal medicine and family practice: Controversies, conflict and compromise. N Engl J Med 293:331, 1975

28. Lee PR: Graduate medical education 1976. Will internal medicine meet the challenge? Ann Int Med 85:2, 251, 1976

29. Beck JC, Lee PR, LeRoy L, Stalcup J: The primary care problem. Clin Research 24:258, 1976

30. Rosenberg CL: How much general practice by specialists? Med Econ (Sept 15):131, 1975

31. Aiken LH, Lewis CE, Craig J, et al.: The contributions of specialists to the delivery of primary care: A new perspective. N Engl J Med 300:1363, 1979

32. Phillips TJ: The delivery of "primary care" by specialists. Letter to the editor. N Engl J Med, 301:893, 1979

33. Peterson ML: The place of the general internist in primary care. Ann Intern Med 91:305, 1979

34. Spiegel JS, Rubenstein LV, Scott B, et al.: Who is the primary physician? N Engl J Med 308:1208, 1983

35. Rosenblatt RA, Cherkin DC, Schneeweiss R, et al.: The content of ambulatory care in the United States: An interspecialty comparison. N Engl J Med 309:892, 1983

36. Educational Programs for the Physician's Assistant. Chicago, American Medical Association, Department of Allied Medical Professions and Services, Summer 1974, p 3

37. Joint Practice in Primary Care: Definition and Guidelines. Evanston, Ill., National Joint Practice Commission, July 1977

38. Davidson RA, Fletcher RH, Earp JA: Role disagreement in primary care practice. J Comm Health 7(2):93, 1981

39. Breslau N: The role of the nurse-practitioner in a pediatric team: Patient definitions. Med Care 15(12):1014, 1977

40. Schoen EJ, Erickson RJ, Barr G, Allen H: The role of pediatric nurse practitioners as viewed by California pediatricians. West J Med 118(1):62, 1973

41. Levinson D: Roles, tasks and practitioners. N Engl J Med 296(22):1291, 1977

42. Geyman JP: Is there a difference between nursing practice and medical practice? J Fam Pract 5:935, 1977

43. Jacoby I: Physician manpower: GMENAC and afterwards. Pub Health Rpts 96(4):295, 1981

44. Trandel-Korenchuk DM, Trandel-Korenchuk KM: Current legal issues facing nursing practice. Nursing Admin Quart 5(1):37, Fall 1980

45. Ginzberg E, Brann E, Hiestand D, et al.: Milbank Mem Fund Quart/Health Soc 59(4):508, 1981

46. Blues create national HMO network. Am Med News, Dec. 23/30, 1983, p 12

47. Starr P: The Social Transformation of American Medicine. New York, Basic Books, 1982, p 426

48. Catlin RF, Bradbury RC, Catlin RJO: Primary care gatekeepers in HMOs. J Fam Pract 17:673, 1983

49. Moore SH, Martin DP, Richardson WC: Does the primary-care gatekeeper control the costs of health care? Lessons from the SAFECO experience. N Engl J Med 309:1400, 1983

50. Geyman JP: Family practice and the gatekeeper role. J Fam Pract 17:587, 1983

51. Sheps CG: Primary care: The problem and the prospect. Ann NY Acad Sciences 310:273, 1978

5 Changing Trends in Medical Education

In 1910, Flexner dealt with the gap between what was then known and what was taught in medical schools. Today, we have a different gap: between what is taught and what is needed for health care to meet public and individual need.

Cecil Sheps[1]

The last three chapters have examined some of the major problems and trends in health manpower, the health care system, and primary care. In shifting the focus to medical education itself, we find an equally dynamic state of affairs, and can be sure that changing trends in medical education will have an important infuence on future medical practice.

The purpose of this chapter is threefold: (1) to summarize briefly some of the important developments in American medical education since 1900; (2) to present an overview of some basic problems in medical education today; and (3) to outline some current trends in medical education in this country, with comment as to how these relate to primary care. An understanding of these changing directions is useful in appreciating the milieu in which family practice is developing as a major specialty in American medicine.

HISTORIC PERSPECTIVE

Evolution of the Medical School

The report prepared by Abraham Flexner in 1910 is widely regarded as a milestone in American medical education. Reviewing the standards of medical schools in the United States at that time, and comparing them against the high standards of German medical education, he called for adoption of improved standards and goals by all our medical schools.[2] There was great variation among schools as to quality, and many were substandard. He recommended a basic formula whereby medical schools structured the first 2 years for preclinical basic science and the last 2 years for clinical science with each department responsible for teaching in its own area of knowledge.[3]

This pattern was held to in a somewhat rigid way until well after World War II. Medical schools became more standardized and of more uniformly high quality. They became university centers for science and learning and escaped the older mold of trade schools.

In the years before World War II, medical schools had limited influence outside of their teaching hospitals, which were oriented primarily toward care of indigent patients. In a book published in 1930 entitled *Universities—American, English, and German,* Flexner stressed that the university's main purposes were teaching and research, and that large responsibilities for patient care as a service function within the community were to be avoided.[4] During this period, the principle province of medical education was on the undergraduate level, and there were relatively few residencies. A substantial degree of separatism often existed between the practicing physician and the academic physician, resulting commonly in a "town-gown" rivalry. The clinician in the style of Osler was the model around which teaching revolved. Basic sciences were taught in pragmatic terms as required for diagnosis and treatment of patients.[5]

The 25 years since World War II saw a rapid increase in biomedical research. The new academic physician became more the "scientist–physician" than the clinician, and often spent more time in research than on patient care.[5] This period witnessed a proliferation of teaching hospitals and residencies, with a new stress on graduate medical education. At the same time, there were increasing expectations by the public and surrounding hospitals and medical communities for support and consultation. Innovative curriculum changes became common since the experiment in interdisciplinary teaching initiated by Western Reserve University School of Medicine in 1952. Medical schools during the 1960s became highly variable in terms of philosophy, goals, and teaching methods.

The complexity of the modern medical school is well illustrated by the following statement made by Anlyan in 1969:[6]

> Today the dean finds himself at the helm of an academic medical center comprising a complex of undergraduate medical education programs; graduate PhD programs in the basic sciences; graduate medical education with interns, residents, and fellows equal in number to the number of medical students; continuing education for physicians in the region; a multimillion dollar research program (which in many instances is multidisciplinary and multidepartmental); one or more teaching hospitals which hover on the brink of financial insolvency; a fast-changing and expanding interest of federal and state government in health affairs; expanding needs of society in health care; and, not the least of all, a health manpower shortage combined with a maldistribution of physicians and health personnel. Within the academic medical center, many of the major departments have operational complexities larger than the total medical school of two decades ago.

It has become popular, perhaps to an unfair extent, to hold university medical schools largely responsible for the many deficiencies in our health care system. Medical schools are being looked to for leadership in areas of patient care and methods of health delivery. This creates a difficult dilemma for the medical school: How can it respond to such demands without compromising its primary functions of research, teaching, and advancement of scientific medicine?

Growth of Teaching Programs

In viewing medical education in the United States since 1940, one is immediately struck by the rapid growth in the size and number of teaching programs at all levels. The number of medical schools has increased by over 60 percent during this period, with a threefold increase in the enrollment.

At the graduate level, there has been a fivefold increase in the number of internship and residency positions offered in the United States since 1940. There are presently more than 4500 accredited residency programs sponsored by more than 1500 hospitals and agencies in 39 specialties and subspecialties.[7]

The dramatic growth of residency positions in the United States since 1940 reflects widespread recognition that graduate medical education has become an essential requisite for competent medical practice in all fields. Before 1940 many physicians were adequately prepared for practice by their medical school training and subsequent internship. Today well over 90 percent of the graduates of U.S. medical schools enter, and most complete, residency training.

Specialization

The process of specialization in this country over the past 50 years has already been considered in some detail in earlier chapters. There is no need to recount these developments here, but it is important to recognize this process as a major feature of medical education in this century.

The specialty boards were established by the medical profession as a voluntary credentialing mechanism in their respective fields, and have become active parties in the patterns and policies of medical education in this country. By setting standards of graduate medical education in each specialty, these boards exert a major influence on specialty practice. The 23 specialty boards today confer general and special certificates in approximately 60 areas of medical practice. The inevitable cycle involved in the process of certification in medicine has been described by Chase as follows:[8]

1. As a result of advances in a field or development of new technology, a new group develops special expertise in this area.
2. An organization or society is formed for an exchange of ideas and to display advances to one another.
3. Membership in the organization becomes a mark of distinction in the field and, in an effort to externalize that recognition, certification of excellence in the field becomes established.
4. Institutions with responsibility for quality of health care soon accept certification as evidence of competence and limit care within the field to those certified.

SOME BASIC PROBLEMS IN MEDICAL EDUCATION

Although it is beyond the scope of this chapter to examine in any depth the many problems in medical education, it is useful to briefly consider five fundamental problems which plague medical education today.

Imbalance Between Product and Public Need

There is good reason to credit medical schools with the strengths of American medical education as well as to hold them accountable in large part for the deficiencies of the system. Medical schools today represent a constituency of 127 schools and 415 major teaching hospitals whose beds comprise about one-quarter of all the hospital beds for acute care in the United States. Their teaching and patient care programs therefore greatly affect the operation of the country's health care system.

Heavy emphasis on biomedical research during the last 30 years has led to a remarkable increase in biomedical knowledge and extensive subspecialization

TABLE 5-1. NUMBER OF POSITIONS OFFERED, BY SPECIALTY

Specialty	1974–1975	1980–1981	1981–1982	1982–1983	1983–1984	1984–1985
Allergy and immunology	—	207	228	248	273	282
Anesthesiology	2,260	2,813	3,116	3,465	3,562	3,683
Colon and rectal surgery	34	42	44	46	44	46
Dermatology	778	781	818	785	767	692
Dermatopathology	—	36	35	41	42	43
Emergency medicine	—	—	—	878	988	1,028
Family practice	3,342	7,004	7,669	7,477	7,670	7,652
Internal medicine	11,353	16,576	18,113	17,503	17,703	17,948
Neurologic surgery	645	547	631	639	657	674
Neurology	1,124	1,216	1,348	1,331	1,398	1,412
Nuclear medicine	129	226	240	247	256	250
Obstetrics-gynecology	3,652	4,361	4,851	4,744	4,731	4,613
Ophthalmology	1,579	1,518	1,563	1,540	1,555	1,565
Orthopedic surgery	2,454	2,492	2,702	2,747	2,759	2,732
Otolaryngology	1,049	981	1,028	1,033	1,067	1,087
Pathology	3,404	2,522	2,700	2,656	2,777	2,775
Blood banking	—	39	40	42	54	49
Forensic pathology	60	31	46	44	53	48
Neuropathology	66	74	72	69	83	95
Pediatrics	4,988	5,505	6,292	5,912	6,031	6,364
Pediatric allergy	135	2	—	—	—	—
Pediatric cardiology	142	145	139	130	145	151
Physical medicine and rehabilitation	507	562	649	662	694	706
Plastic surgery	422	391	416	384	390	417
Preventive medicine General	246	179	188	203	208	271
Aerospace medicine	111	43	54	53	57	49
Occupational medicine	48	85	100	95	128	162
Public health	104	35	39	37	39	51
Psychiatry	5,012	4,563	4,859	4, 596	4,804	4,921
Child psychiatry	744	555	634	636	649	669
Radiology, diagnostic	3,200	2,882	3,231	3,185	3,243	3,291

TABLE 5-1. (cont)

Specialty	1974–1975	1980–1981	1981–1982	1982–1983	1983–1984	1984–1985
Radiology, diagnostic (nuclear)	—	61	64	73	129	149
Radiology, therapeutic	484	420	462	452	487	499
Surgery	7,802	7,846	8,433	8,156	8,278	7,924
Pediatric surgery	—	30	27	27	27	26
Thoracic surgery	318	260	296	282	284	299
Urology	1,156	1,036	1,136	1,067	1,062	1,046
Total	57,681	66,066	72,263	71,485	73,094	73,668

(From Graduate Medical Education. JAMA 236(26):2977, 1976; Graduate Medical Education in the United States. JAMA 250(12):1543, 1983; Summary Statistics on Graduate Medical Education in the United States. JAMA 252(12):1547, 1984, with permission. Copyright 1984, American Medical Association)

within medical schools. These gains, however, have tended to divert medical schools from other responsibilities, particularly those related to providing leadership toward improving the nation's capacity to apply biomedical advances through a more effective health care delivery system. Wilbur Cohen, as Secretary of the Department of Health, Education, and Welfare, in 1969 posed these fundamental questions to medical schools, all of which remain pertinent today:

- Does your responsibility rest only in educating the physician with no obligation to develop new patterns of patient care?
- What action do you plan to take in response to the Millis Commission's recommendations dealing with the need for family physicians?
- Are you contributing toward analyzing and meeting the health manpower make the wisest use of the physician's time?
- Are you contributing toward analyzing the meeting the health manpower needs of your community, your state, and your region?
- Should you extend your efforts to assist the medical education programs of the community hospitals of your region?

Medical schools have shown some concern for some of these larger issues in recent years but have been relatively ineffective in planning and implementing some of the fundamental changes needed. Change of the specialty distribution within graduate medical education is a good example of a chronic and pressing issue which still has not yet been effectively addressed. The "mix" within today's graduate medical education by specialty clearly is the single most important factor in determining future specialty distribution to and beyond the year 2000. As noted in Chapter 2, there is ample evidence that many specialties are already in surplus, with others projected for surplus numbers in the next several years. Yet the numbers of residency positions offered in surplus specialties, such as most of the surgical specialties, have usually not been reduced and in many instances have actually increased over the last 10 years as shown in Table 5–1.

Limited Relevance of Medical Education to Medical Practice

There is growing awareness that predoctoral and graduate medical education could be made more relevant to the needs of society and improved patterns of medical practice. Some feel that medical education is too incomplete. Millis, for instance, has observed that though medical education prepares students well for the care of the 10 percent of patients who are critically ill, teaching of common health care of most of the population is largely neglected.[10]

Jason views the issue of relevance in medical education in these terms:[11]

> Clearly, my assumption is that medical education should be relevant to medical practice. This presumes that medical school is, in fact, a preparation for medical practice. It is no secret that there are a significant number of schools that adopt the posture that they are not actually preparing students for medical practice but, rather, for careers as instructors and investigators. The facts are, however, that there is no school which has more than 13 percent of its graduates in faculty positions, and only four schools have more than 10 percent of their graduates in academic work. On the other hand, fully 90 percent of all graduates of this country's medical schools are in clinical practice. Indeed, there is no school from which less than 74 percent of the graduates are primarily involved in a career of patient care. Our schools obviously have an obligation to provide preparation for the careers their students will in fact pursue. To do otherwise is nothing less than educational malpractice.

Much of the problem of relevance in medical education has been due to the setting in which most predoctoral and graduate teaching is carried out—the hospital, which often is heavily oriented to tertiary care. That the student's (resident's) clinical exposure is severely limited by this kind of setting is clearly demonstrated by the classic work of Kerr White which showed that only 1 patient out of every 250 adults consulting a physician each month is sent to a university medical center (Figure 5–1).[12] The extent of this problem is suggested by the fact that as recently as 1981 more than one-third of U.S. medical schools did not require ambulatory care experiences for medical students.[7]

Traditional medical education has neglected, and frequently denigrated, primary medical care as either a productive educational setting or as a worthy career option for medical students and residents. As pointed out by Sheps:[1]

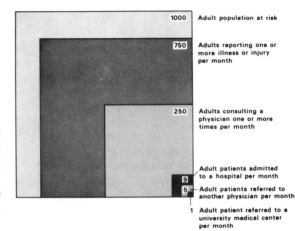

Figure 5-1. Prevalence of illness and utilization of medical care resources among 1000 adults in the United States and Great Britain. *(From White KL, Williams TF, Greenberg BG: The ecology of medical care. N Engl J Med 265:890, 1961, with permission.)*

1000 Adult population at risk

750 Adults reporting one or more illness or injury per month

250 Adults consulting a physician one or more times per month

9 Adult patients admitted to a hospital per month

5 Adult patients referred to another physician per month

1 Adult patient referred to a university medical center per month

The overemphasis on tertiary care in the university medical centers distorts their education programs. The fixation on the disease concept of illness in biological terms only is an inadequate, inappropriate, and skewed preparation for the care of most patients in the community.

Lack of a Coordinated Health Manpower Plan

Ineffective past and current efforts to address the problem of specialty maldistribution of physicians by specialty provides clear evidence for the present lack of a coordinated health manpower plan. This is by no means due to lack of previous attempts to resolve this issue.

Rosemary Stevens, a leading expert on the subject of specialization and physician manpower supply in this country, had this to say about the lack of follow-up to a recommendation by the AMA Council of Medical Education 35 years ago to control the number of residency positions and reduce the number of internship positions by 20 to 30 percent:[13]

> There was no incentive for any group to limit the supply of house staff; it was quite the reverse. Attending physicians liked both to teach and to have house staff available; hospitals wanted house staff; specialty boards were, on the whole, interested in expanding the number of diplomates; and medical schools were still reluctant to intervene. There was thus continuing avoidance of the effects of increasing numbers of house staff on the underlying questions of graduate medical education.

Today, faced with an increasingly severe problem of maldistribution of physicians by specialty, there is still no accepted national plan for redistribution of physician manpower which is endorsed by the various organizations and parties needed to implement needed changes. The structure of graduate medical education in the nation's medical schools and teaching hospitals remains a nonsystem featured by uncoordinated local control on a departmental basis. More than two-thirds of residents in training in the United States are based in medical schools and their major teaching hospitals.[7] Nevertheless, individual institutions have been unable or unwilling to consider future national, state, or regional needs for physicians by specialty as an important factor in the planning and operation of their residency programs. In the mid-1970s the federal government attempted to shift the balance toward primary care by tying capitation grants to the percentage of residents in the primary care specialties. This initiative has now phased out with the termination of capitation funding. Meanwhile, the boards, colleges, and specialty societies which could have substantial influence on specialty maldistribution, have failed to address the problem. As Petersdorf observes:[14]

> (These organizations) are charter members of an academic "right to life movement." They need to justify their existence and that of their specialties. However, in feeding the system an excess of their products, they have made these products all but indigestable.

Constraints of Funding

The costs of medical education have increased exponentially during the past 25 years. The number of full-time faculty in U.S. medical schools increased more than fourfold between 1960 and 1980 as the enrollment tripled in these schools. These faculty members were supported by combinations of state and private support, research and training grants, and patient care revenue. Recent years have seen erosion of state and private support, termination of federal capitation and special projects grants, increased difficulty in securing research funding, continued inflation of available dollars, and an increased pressure for medical faculty to support the costs of medical education through patient care activities. In addition to seeing patients, medical faculty is expected to teach, generate grants, conduct research, and in many cases, administer programs. Allocation of more time in patient care is often at the expense of teaching.

The proportion of federal support to medical education fell by almost one-half between 1965 and 1979, while the contribution in constant dollars from medical school and university sources (largely patient care revenue) increased almost 15-fold from $91 million in 1960–1961 to $1347 million in 1978–1979.[15] Meanwhile, as NIH funding became increasingly competitive, federal research grants were awarded to a smaller proportion of medical schools. For example, in 1978–1979, three-quarters of these funds were received by 40 of the nation's 127 medical schools with one-half of the funds received by 20 medical schools.[7]

The question of who will pay the costs of medical education has become a critical issue. Reimbursement procedures by third parties for patient care services provided within teaching programs have become more restrictive. Teaching hospitals are faced with growing operational costs and increasing regulation limiting their capacity to recover costs. Governmental agencies at all levels are increasingly hard pressed to maintain past levels of support of medical education programs.

The Carnegie Council on Policy Studies in Higher Education in 1976 completed in excellent, indepth report of current problems in medical and dental education in the United States. Two of its five "urgent recommendations" are even more pertinent today as they were almost a decade ago:[16]

> The nation has a vital stake in maintaining high standards of health among its residents. In recognition of the social benefits flowing from medical and dental education, the federal government should pursue a stable policy of financial support of university health science centers. It should provide a basic floor of support for these centers which can be supplemented by support from state governments and private sources. . . .
>
> The federal government should pursue a stable and consistent policy of support of research in the health sciences, increasing its allocations for this purpose along with the rise in real GNP. Federal allocations should cover full research costs and should encourage increased emphasis on ways of achieving greater efficiency in the training of health manpower and in the delivery of health care.

Competition in a Physician-Surplus Era

An earlier chapter clearly demonstrated that a surplus of most subspecialties has already occurred and that no substantial correction of this problem has yet evolved. The impact of this situation is severe and threatens the very survival of the medical education system as it is presently constituted. The typical scenario starts with the young graduate in cardiology, cardiovascular surgery, or another surplus medical or surgical subspecialty looking for a place to practice. Because of the increasing concentration of subspecialties in urban, suburban, and more peripheral communities of smaller size, the subspecialist just out of training often migrates to yet another community hospital whose administrator and medical staff welcomes the opportunity to add new technology to the community. The reimbursement system has favored the expansion of such highly specialized services beyond the need of the population to an increasing number of hospitals and communities. Medical schools have thereby found themselves surrounded by a tightening "golden noose" of competing community hospitals providing larger amounts of what has been their traditional responsibility for tertiary care. The dilemma of medical schools is graphically described by Schroeder as follows:[17]

> Historically, at least for the past 30 years or so, the academic medical center has responded to a national mandate to train physicians with specialized skills, to expand the national biomedical research capability, and to care for patients with increasingly specialized problems. In order to do so, the academic medical center has created increasingly specialized clinical facilities for undergraduate and graduate medical education. It now appears that, at least in most urban areas, academic medical centers are becoming victims of their own success. They find themselves competing for patients with their own graduates in areas that are saturated with recently trained, highly qualified subspecialists. In order to retain their share of the patient care market, they must indulge in a technologic "arms race" and emphasize tertiary, highly specialized care in order to attract referred patients.

As the competition increases with community hospitals, academic medical centers find themselves especially at risk because of several inherent problems:

- They are not known for their primary care base.
- They are dependent on referrals which are diminishing in many areas.
- They have multiple missions beyond patient care, including teaching at many levels and research.
- They often have a larger share of public sector patients with lesser reimbursement than private sector patients.
- They must maintain costly facilities for the highest intensity of services as institutions of "last resort."
- Increasing uncertainties surround present mechanisms for funding the costs of medical education, and the physician faculties of medical schools are already stressed with multiple responsibilities, including growing commitments in patient care.

SOME MAJOR TRENDS IN MEDICAL EDUCATION

Stabilization of Growth

An important change which has received wide acceptance since the close of the 1970s is the need for stabilization of growth of medical education programs at both undergraduate and graduate levels. The previously mentioned Carnegie Council on Policy Studies in Higher Education issued this warning:[16]

> We are in serious danger of developing too many new medical schools, and decisive steps need to be taken by both federal and state governments to stop this trend.

This group went further in questioning the desirability of continuing to develop a number of beginning medical schools.

Other national groups have called for limitation of growth of enrollment levels. The Institute of Medicine of the National Academy of Sciences, for example, recommended in 1978 that the number of entrants to medical schools remain at current levels.[18]

In 1976, federal legislation recognized for the first time the trend toward surplus in the country's physician supply. In the declaration of policy in the Health Professional Educational Assistance Act of 1976, Congress stated that "there is no longer an insufficient number of physicians and surgeons in the United States such that there is no further need for affording preference to alien physicians and surgeons in admissions to the United States under the Immigration and Nationality Act."[19] That Act sharply restricted the entry of foreign medical graduates and shifted the focus from increasing the total number of physicians to specialty and geographic redistribution of physicians.[20]

Almost 10 years after these several initiatives to stabilize the growth of medical education programs in the United States, it is clear that brakes on previous growth are beginning to take effect. The number of entrants to U.S. medical schools showed a slight decrease for the first time in 1982, and declined by another 0.5 percent in the fall of 1983 to 16,480. At this writing, however, only 7 medical schools have actually reduced the size of their entering classes, whereas 24 schools are projecting a decrease in class size.[21] At the graduate level, the number of first-year graduate positions has plateaued at approximately 21,000. Even though the total number of foreign medical graduates applying for U.S. graduate medical education positions has declined since the mid-1970s, the number of U.S. citizen foreign medical graduates has increased. The result is the current shortfall of graduate medical education positions vis-a-vis the entire applicant pool, which totalled about 24,000 medical graduates in 1984 (including 16,500 U.S. graduates and 2500 U.S. citizen foreign medical graduates). There are presently 1.3 positions available for every U.S. medical graduate.[22]

This represents a major change over the last 30 years—in 1983 more than four times as many applicants competed for less than one-half the number of positions in comparison with 1952.[23] In 1983, only one-half of U.S. citizens graduating from foreign medical schools gained positions in U.S. graduate training programs through the NRMP.[24] Figure 5–2 shows a recent decline in the total number of positions per active applicant, an increasing percentage of unmatched foreign medical graduates, and a small comparatively stable percentage for unmatched U.S. graduates (8 percent in 1983).[25]

Emphasis on Primary Care

The increased emphasis on primary care in recent years must certainly be included among the important trends in American medical education today. It involves a redirection in curriculum content, teaching methods, teaching settings, and philosophy and style of practice.

Family practice teaching programs have enjoyed considerable flexibility in their organizational and curriculum development because of their lack of dependence on past traditions and structures of education. It has been more difficult for residency programs in general internal medicine and general pediatrics to develop in medical schools and teaching hospitals with long-standing commitments to subspecialty training. In an excellent paper dealing with residency training in these two fields, Charney has pointed out that these disciplines have traditionally "focused on the complex rather than the routine, the diagnosis rather than the management, the acute rather than the chronic, the cure rather than the prevention."[26] Fundamental changes of existing residency programs in these fields are therefore required in order to train internists and pediatricians for primary care.

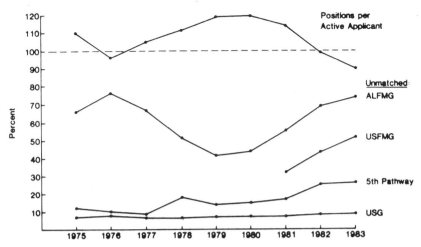

Figure 5-2. Relation between positions per active applicant and the success of groups of applicants in the National Residency Matching Program. ALFMG = alien foreign medical graduates, USFMG = U.S. foreign medical graduates, and USG = U.S. graduates. *(From Stimmel B, Graetting JS: Medical students trained abroad and medical manpower: Recent trends and predictions. N Engl J Med 310:234, 1984, with permission.)*

As previously noted, the federal government has recognized three primary care disciplines—family practice, general internal medicine, and general pediatrics. Federal health manpower policy of the late 1970s required that the percentage of graduates entering primary care residencies in these fields exceed 50 percent in 1980 in order for medical schools to be eligible for capitation grants. This requirement was easily met, since the requirement had no effective means of distinguishing between residents training in internal medicine and pediatrics with primary care or subspecialty goals and interests.

Fifteen years after the formation of the American Board of Family Practice and multiple efforts at various levels to increase the numbers of physicians entering the primary care specialties, there is incontrovertible evidence that this surge has fallen well short of the mark. Table 5–2 displays the trends among U.S. medical graduates entering primary care and other specialties between 1970 and 1980.[27] Although various groups (e.g., the Willard Committee on Education for Family Practice) and health manpower experts have called for a national goal of 25 percent of U.S. medical graduates entering family practice residencies,[28,29] this number has plateaued at about one-half of that level. Steinwachs and colleagues have developed a model to estimate the "leakage" of residents in internal medicine and pediatrics into subspecialty training and other nonprimary care specialties. The result is a projection for primary care specialties well below the 50 percent goal, as shown in Table 5–3.[27] In view of the pervasive influence of subspecialization, Petersdorf has questioned the 50 percent goal for primary care specialties and calls for only 10 to 20 percent of medical graduates entering the nonprimary care specialties.[14]

Decentralization and Community Involvement

The trend toward growing numbers of university affiliations with community hospitals represents a major change in medical education. There was more than a two-fold increase in the number of university affiliations with community hospitals during

TABLE 5-2. TRENDS AMONG U.S. PHYSICIANS ENTERING GRADUATE MEDICAL EDUCATION FROM 1970 TO 1980

Category	1970[a]		1974[a]		1975[a]		1976[b]		1980[b]	
	%	No.	%	No.	%	No.	%	No.	%	No.
Rotating internship	44.1	3558	21.1	2306	—	—	—	—	—	—
Flex year	—	—	—	—	—	—	—	—	—	—
Primary care	38.0	3068	52.4	5725	57.7	6845	59.1	7622	57.5	8592
Internal medicine	27.1	2189	33.7	3686	36.3	4307	36.4	4695	34.4	5142
Pediatrics	9.4	762	9.7	1064	9.9	1171	10.0	1284	9.6	1428
Family practice	1.4	117	8.9	975	11.5	1367	12.7	1643	13.5	2022
Obstetrics/gynecology	1.3	104	4.3	469	5.4	646	5.5	704	6.3	937
General surgery	12.6	1013	14.6	1603	14.4	1708	12.9	1667	14.0	2086
Surgical specialties	0.1	9	0.7	76	0.7	84	1.9	242	2.9	426
Hospital-based specialties	1.9	157	3.3	362	2.9	339	5.8	746	6.8	1009
Other specialties	2.0	161	3.6	392	4.4	526	5.1	659	4.4	663
Total	100.0	8070	100.0	10,933	100.0	11,869	100.0	12,904	100.0	14,930

[a]*(From American Medical Association Physician Masterfile, with permission.)*
[b]*(From National Residency Matching Program data on first-year positions, with permission.)*

TABLE 5-3. PROJECTED SPECIALTY OF U.S. MEDICAL-SCHOOL GRADUATES, ACCORDING TO YEAR OF STARTING GRADUATE MEDICAL EDUCATION[a]

Category	1970		1974		1976		1980	
	%	No.	%	No.	%	No.	%	No.
Internship or flex year only	6.8	551	3.3	360	2.0	253	1.6	243
Primary care	21.3	1721	29.5	3229	32.2	4157	31.8	4747
Internal medicine	11.2	904	13.4	1465	14.0	1801	13.2	1975
Pediatrics	7.0	568	7.1	779	6.6	855	6.3	948
Family practice	3.1	249	9.0	985	11.6	1501	12.2	1824
Medical specialties	14.3	1156	17.0	1861	17.6	2277	16.7	2489
Pediatric specialties	2.0	163	2.3	251	2.2	289	2.2	321
Surgical specialties	29.3	2361	27.0	2952	25.1	3233	27.0	4041
General surgery	5.9	480	5.4	592	4.2	541	4.4	664
Obstetrics/gynecology	5.4	436	6.5	716	6.5	838	7.2	1073
Other specialties	17.9	1445	15.0	1644	14.4	1854	15.4	2304
Hospital-based specialties	13.3	1072	10.4	1136	10.8	1392	11.4	1700
Anesthesiology	3.2	255	2.2	243	2.8	367	3.4	514
Pathology	2.9	236	3.2	349	2.9	380	2.7	402
Radiology	7.2	582	5.0	544	5.0	645	5.3	784
Other specialties	13.0	1046	10.5	1143	10.1	1303	9.3	1389
Psychiatry	7.6	610	6.8	740	5.9	761	5.1	758
Neurology	2.0	165	1.5	169	1.6	206	1.4	214
Other	3.4	271	2.1	234	2.6	388	2.8	418
Total	100.0	8070	100.0	10,933	100.0	12,904	100.0	14,930

[a]Percentages and numbers do not total exactly because of rounding off.
(From Steinwachs DM, Levine DM, Elzinga DJ, et al.; Changing patterns of graduate medical education: Analyzing recent trends and projecting their impact. N Engl J Med 306(1): 10, 1982, with permission.)

the period from 1966 to 1976, while the number of unaffiliated hospitals declined by over 40 percent in that same period.

This trend does not reflect a "university takeover" of teaching programs in community hospitals, but a genuine interdependence between medical schools and community hospitals with benefits to both parties. The university gains much needed clinical and teaching resources for its medical students and residents, as well as a desirable shift in clinical teaching to less highly selected patients more representative of health problems to be encountered commonly by its graduates later in practice. The involved communities also have much to gain from such affiliations, including enhanced opportunities for continuing medical education for community physicians and a tendency toward improved quality of patient care in their teaching hospitals.

Closely related to the trend of increasing university affiliations with community hospitals is the development of new regional linkages between medical schools and their surrounding areas. There are numerous examples of excellent medical education programs which have been developed on a regional basis by medical schools for both undergraduate and graduate medical education. The University of Washington and Michigan State University are two such examples. The WAMI program is a well-established and viable program with an emphasis on decentralized medical student teaching involving four states in the Pacific Northwest— Washington, Alaska, Montana, and Idaho—in affiliation with the University of Washington.[30] Michigan State University has likewise developed teaching programs linking a substantial area of Michigan with the medical school, and has even demonstrated that experimental undergraduate tracks can be conducted in distant rural communities with teaching effectiveness and learning outcomes comparable to those of teaching programs based in metropolitan communities.[31]

Coordination of Undergraduate, Graduate, and Continuing Medical Education

The last 15 years have seen vigorous efforts to achieve some degree of coordination across the continuum of medical education encompassing the needs of medical students, residents, and practicing physicians. Traditionally, undergraduate, graduate, and continuing medical education have been disconnected functionally and conceptually, and the concept of a "continuum of medical education" has until recently been merely a hollow phrase without content.

In 1972 the Coordinating Council on Medical Education (CCME) was organized under the auspices of five parent bodies: the Association of American Medical Colleges (AAMC), the American Board of Medical Specialties (ABMS), the American Hospital Association (AHA), the American Medical Association (AMA), and the Council of Medical Specialty Societies (CMSS). The CCME was established to "coordinate the activities of the various liaison committees that serve as accrediting bodies and to review and recommend policy decisions relating to medical education to the five parent organizations."[32] Initially the CCME addressed its efforts to the coordination of the activities of the Liaison Committee on Medical Education (LCME), responsible since 1942 for the accreditation of medical schools, and the Liaison Committee for Graduate Medical Education (LCGME), which in 1975 became the official accrediting body for residency training. In 1977 the Liaison Committee for Continuing Medical Education (LCCME) was established as the third group under the LCME.

The termination of the free-standing internship during the early 1970s and its integration as the first year of residency training by 1975 represents an example of more effective coordination within the continuum of medical education. The net result of this change today is to regard residency training as the final phase of the young physician's basic medical education.

By the late 1970s, however, the precise roles and authority of the CCME remained both uncertain and controversial. Some viewed CCME as a coordinating organization without authority, while others proposed that it become an independent, free-standing commission with authority to regulate all levels of medical education.[32] The CCME was asked by the federal government to enter into a contract with the Department of Health, Education, and Welfare to develop and implement a system designed to assure the training of the optimal number and mix of specialists, but declined to accept a regulatory function.[33]

From the beginning, the CCME was plagued by differences vis-a-vis the respective responsibilities of the various groups, together with issues of authority, autonomy, financing, and staffing. It was apparent, for example, that CCME could not act in a coordinating or supervisory role over LCME, which is recognized as the official accrediting body for U.S. medical schools by the U.S. Office of Education. After considerable debate and negotiation, the CCME was disbanded in 1980 and replaced by the Council for Medical Affairs (CFMA). The CFMA was intended to serve as a forum for representatives of the five parent organizations to consider issues related to medical education and other issues of mutual concern. It has no authority over policy decisions of the various liaison committees.[34]

After similar difficulties, some reorganization was also required for the liaison committees themselves. Most of the differences in LCGME were resolved by 1981, when this body was continued under a new name, the Accreditations Council for Graduate Medical Education (ACGME). The Liaison Committee for Continuing Medical Education (LCCME) encountered severe conflict leading to temporary withdrawal by the American Medical Association, but was reorganized in 1981 as the Accreditation Council for Continuing Medical Education (ACCME).[34]

It remains to be seen whether voluntary efforts by these organizations can be effective in addressing the major problems within their purview. Certainly the track record of voluntary efforts by the medical profession to rebalance medical education in response to public need have been unimpressive to date. Beck and colleagues seem to be on solid ground in this view.[35]

> Voluntary efforts have stressed quality in individual training programs and the needs of the individual medical specialties. This has not been adequate to address the broader problems of specialty and geographic maldistribution. We do not believe that voluntary action by the medical profession alone will be adequate. We support expanding the federal-academic medicine partnership to certifying and accrediting bodies. Only when the medical profession takes actions which require professional expertise and the federal government assures enforcement of these actions through programs such as capitation payments to medical schools and reimbursement for services will graduate medical education be effectively regulated in the public interest.

Changes in Licensure

Trends in graduate and continuing medical education are closely related to some fundamental changes being developed and studied in the licensure of physicians. Traditionally, medical school graduates have received unlimited licensure for life following satisfactory completion of an internship and passage of one of several licensure examinations. A report in 1973 of the Committee on Goals and Priorities of the National Board of Medical Examiners (the G.A.P. Report) recommended that unlimited licensure be withheld until completion of residency training. Periodic recertification during later practice years was also proposed as shown in Figure 5–3.[36]

Although the G.A.P. Report has generated continuing debate in terms of the applicability of its full recommendations, it represents a direction which is gaining momentum, and may be even more influential in future years. Brief mention of some emerging developments in medical licensure illustrates the complexity of the issues involved.

Medical licensure in the United States is the sole prerogative and authority of state medical boards. These agencies have the responsibility to assure the public that the physicians they license have the education and training to practice in a satisfactory manner. The state medical boards in all states have three basic requirements for licensure: (1) the candidate is of sound moral and ethical character, (2) hold an M.D. degree from an acceptable school, and (3) has passed a recognized extramural examination. Currently, graduates of LCME-accredited U.S. and Canadian medical schools are eligible for licensure in most states after completion of 1 year of graduate medical education, although in a few states medical graduates gain this eligibility immediately upon graduation.

Two principal pathways are available in order to qualify for licensure on the basis of extramural examination—the Parts I, II, and III sequence of the National Board of Medical Examiners (NBME), and the FLEX I–FLEX II sequence of the Federation of State Medical Boards (FSMB). Presently, 48 states accept NBME Parts I, II, and III as qualification for licensure, and over three-quarters of U.S. medical graduates are licensed through this pathway.[37] The Federation Licensing Examination (FLEX) complements the National Boards, is derived from the same ques-

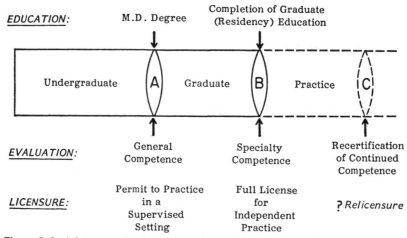

Figure 5-3. A future evaluation system for certification and licensure. The chart depicts the proposed interrelationships of education, evaluation, and licensure in the projected educational continuum. *(From National Board of Medical Examiners: Committee on Goals and Priorities. Evaluation in the Continuum of Medical Education. Philadelphia, National Board of Medical Examiners, June 1973, p 51, with permission.)*

tion pool as the National Boards, and is administered by all state licensing agencies.[38] The NBME is an independent private agency established in 1915 for the purpose of preparing and conducting examinations for physician licensure; it thereby stands at the interface between the educational and licensing systems.[37] The FSMB was founded in 1912 as a voluntary, nonprofit agency composed of 62 licensing authorities, including the medical boards of the 50 states.[38]

One issue which has challenged the licensure system is the problem of foreign medical training of variable quality, in many cases substandard (e.g., some proprietary medical schools in the Caribbean without any accreditation standards whatsoever). Some states (e.g., New York State) are considering methods to assess the quality of foreign medical schools using a self-evaluation questionnaire patterned after that used by the LCME in the United States. The FSMB has called for a single national approach to this problem, together with a uniform national licensure process through the FLEX I–FLEX II pathway. FLEX I would be a qualifying examination for the limited practice of medicine under supervision in a graduate training program while FLEX II would qualify one for the unrestricted general practice of medicine. The FSMB believes that such a single licensure system would bring equity to the process for graduates of U.S., Canadian, and foreign medical schools alike.[38]

Meanwhile, the NBME is developing a new examination, the Comprehensive Qualifying Examination (CQE) as a single qualifying examination with a clinical emphasis to be given to medical students before graduation from medical schools. The CQE would replace Part II of the National Boards, and the Part I–II–III sequence would no longer be required. Some medical educators have expressed concern that the CQE could lead to demise of the present NBME sequence and weaken basic science in U.S. medical education.[37,39]

The present climate continues as one of controversy over the basic issues raised by the G.A.P. Report over 10 years ago. Despite the views of organized medicine and the medical education community, it will be the state medical boards who will decide what changes in present licensing methods will be adopted. There are already eight state boards which grant licensure on the basis of specialty-board certification (Maryland, Massachusetts, Nevada, New Hampshire, Oregon, Pennsylvania, Virginia, and West Virginia), with five restricting practice to the respective specialties and three involving unlimited general licensure.[38] In addition, an increasing number of states require some form of relicensure. Table 5–4 lists those states which have adopted requirements for continuing medical education for reregistration of the medical licenses.[40]

Looking to the future, the predictions offered by Ruhe in 1978 vis-a-vis medical licensure still have currency:[41]

1. Within the next decade there will be pressures from within and from outside the profession for limited licensure of physicians, i.e., restriction of the type of practice to the specific fields in which the individuals have had residency training or have been board certified. This will inevitably lead to restrictive definitions of the boundaries of permissible practice in the various specialties.
2. Completion of residency training will become a requirement for licensure in most states.
3. Regular participation in continuing medical education will become a de facto requirement for all physicians to continue to practice medicine.

TABLE 5-4. STATES WITH LEGISLATION REQUIRING CONTINUING MEDICAL EDUCATION (CME) FOR REREGISTRATION OF LICENSE TO PRACTICE MEDICINE

State	Legislation Requiring CME, Date	CME Requirement Operational	Physician's Recognition Award Accepted for CME Requirement
Alaska	1976	No	No
Arizona	1976	Yes	Yes
Arkansas	1977	No	No
California	1977	Yes	Yes
Hawaii	1976	Yes	Yes
Iowa	1979	Yes	Yes
Kansas	1978	Yes	Yes
Kentucky	1972	No	No
Maine	1979	Yes	No
Maryland	1978	Yes	No
Massachusetts	1977	Yes	Yes
Michigan	1977	Yes	No
Minnesota	1977	Yes	No
Nebraska	1976	No	No
Nevada	1979	No	No
New Hampshire	1978	Yes	Yes
New Mexico	1972	Yes	Yes
Ohio	1977	Yes	No
Pennsylvania	1978	No	Yes
Puerto Rico	1976	No	No
Rhode Island	1977	Yes	No
Utah	1976	Yes	Yes
Washington	1976	Yes	Yes
Wisconsin	1977	Yes	No

(From Continuing medical education. JAMA 252:1561, 1984, with permission. Copyright 1984, American Medical Association.)

4. With residency training compulsory, or nearly so, the significance of the M.D. degree will increasingly be called in question. Eventually the M.D. degree may be granted only at the successful completion of residency training and, like the Ph.D. today, may be granted in a specific discipline, e.g., M.D. in Surgery, M.D. in Family Practice, M.D. in Radiology. This in turn will increase the pressures for limited licensure of physicians according to specialty area of practice.

5. Specialty board certification will inevitably change in nature and may even be supplanted by "specialized" M.D. degrees. Specialty boards will come under increasing pressure from the Federal Trade Commission and others as alleged elitist groups in restraint of competition. Board certification may become a prerequisite for licensure limited to a specialty field.

The Changing Medical Student

Recent years have seen strong efforts by admissions committees in U.S. medical schools to select medical students better representing a cross-section of the general population. Medical students today represent more diverse cultural, social, and economic groups within our society than at any time in the past, which should increase the capability of medical graduates to meet the diverse health care needs of the nation. Particular progress has taken place in the increasing enrollment of women and minorities in medical schools. The proportion of women enrolled in U.S. medical schools increased by sixfold over the last 30 years from 5 percent in 1959 to 30 percent in 1983. By 1977 the proportion of students from underrepresented racial minorities (black, American Indian, Mexican American, and mainland Puerto Rico) totalled 8.3 percent in U.S. medical schools.[21]

The present generation of medical students is quite different in many respects from previous generations. Many medical students today are more interested than their predecessors in the human and social aspects of medicine. Medical students today are claiming, and being accorded, a more active role in the planning and evaluation of curricula, teaching methods, and other functions within the medical schools. Medical students frequently participate in course planning and review and often serve on admissions committees and other committees. Many are more aware and less accepting of social injustices and the deficiencies in our health care system. Many are better informed about the world and its problems, and better prepared for graduate education.[42]

Another interesting difference between today's medical students and those of past generations is the changing pattern of specialty choice among women medical graduates. In 1971, for example, women represented 21 percent of pediatricians, 19 percent of public health physicians, 14 percent of anesthesiologists, and 13 percent of psychiatrists; at the same time, they tended to avoid some fields (e.g., they represented only 4 percent of general/family physicians, 1 percent of general surgeons, and 0.5 percent of orthopedists.[43] By contrast, the proportion of women among residents in training in 1983 for various specialties showed much wider diversity: internal medicine, 24 percent; pediatrics, 47 percent; obstetrics–gynecology, 37 percent; psychiatry, 36 percent; family practice, 23 percent; surgery, 10 percent; anesthesiology, 20 percent; diagnostic radiology, 22 percent; and orthopedic surgery, 4 percent. Among the 16,341 women residents in training in the United States in 1982, their leading seven choices of specialty were as follows: internal medicine, 24 percent; pediatrics, 16 percent; obstetrics–gynecology, 10 percent; psychiatry and family practice, 9 percent each; pathology and surgery, about 5 percent each.[44]

COMMENT

Perhaps the single most important issue facing medical education and the nation's health care system is the need to restore an appropriate balance between the primary care and nonprimary care specialties. There is overwhelming evidence that the balance has shifted much too far toward the subspecialties with resultant distortion of the medical education and health care delivery systems. Despite the importance of this issue, however, the progress of the 1970s toward strengthening the primary care specialties has now slowed markedly, and inertia in the system stands in the way of resolving the issue.

As noted previously, today's problems in medicine have become sufficiently large as to require fundamental changes in both medical education and medical practice. Two overall approaches could be taken to the current problem of maldistribution of physicians by specialty—accommodative or revisionary. An accommodative approach would involve relatively minor changes of the existing system through whatever political accommodations may be required to satisfy the principal conflicting interests. A revisionary approach would involve fundamental changes to strengthen the primary base of medicine, probably including concerted efforts to redistribute graduate medical education portions by specialty, implementation of a case management/gatekeeper role for primary care physicians, and providing new incentives to attract physicians into primary care practice. Based upon trends described in this and earlier chapters, two divergent future outcomes could be expected to result from following each of these approaches, as summarized in Table 5–5.[45]

An accommodative approach would place inappropriate reliance on the hidden system of primary care (i.e., that provided by nonprimary care physicians). This falls far short of most current definitions of primary care because of its episodic nature, fragmentation, and narrow range of services within each specialist's interest, training, and experience. For a variety of reasons, the problems inherent in the "hidden system" approach to primary care are not yet widely appreciated. First of all, there is a perception among many medical educators and others in the more limited specialties that primary care is readily mastered, and that any specialist can provide good general medical care regardless of the limits of his specialty. This perception may be supported by a belief that predoctoral education in medical school, together with a year or so of some graduate training, provides adequate preparation for general medical care. Traditional licensing practices have also fostered this belief, based as they are on an unrestricted license in most instances.

There is considerable evidence refuting these perceptions. In terms of predoctoral education, for example, the fourth year in medical school is for many students an unstructured potpourri of electives, often with a narrow focus to better prepare the graduate for a contemplated residency in a given specialty. For example, only two-fifths of fourth-year students in the 1981 class in U.S. medical schools took an emergency medicine clerkship, while only 22.4 and 15.8 percent took clerkships in ophthalmology and otolaryngology, respectively.[7] Moreover, only a minority of medical graduates today can be said to take a broad first graduate year. Gonnella has shown that residents in the nonprimary care specialties without a broad first graduate year score considerably lower than residents in the primary care specialties on Part III of the National Boards.[46] As one examines the broad spectrum of graduate training required over 3 years for today's practice of family medicine,

TABLE 5–5. DIVERGENT OUTCOMES BASED ON ADEQUACY OF PRIMARY CARE

Weak Primary Care Base	Strong Primary Care Base
Fragmented access to care	Improved access to care
More episodic care	More continuity of care
Care less personal	Care more person oriented
Uncontrolled costs	Effective cost containment
Inconsistent quality of care	Improved overall quality of care
Persistent geographic maldistribution of physicians	Improved geographic distribution of physicians
Increased duplication and waste	Reduced duplication and waste

(From Geyman JP: Future medical practice in the United States: A choice of scenarios. JAMA 245:1140, 1981, with permission. Copyright 1981, American Medical Association.)

together with the clinical content of family practice to be described in future chapters, it becomes clear that "general medical care" has become a specialty per se. Thus, the primary care system is best based on residency-trained physicians in the three primary care specialties.

There are no simple answers to the complex and interrelated problems that have collectively produced an overspecialized medical profession without an adequate generalist base. Many parties and interests will need to join in an enlightened and positive strategy to strengthen the primary care base. A coherent health care policy for physician manpower is yet to be devised. Some of the elements that could well be part of such a policy, however, include the following:

1. Continue, and expand, federal and state funding for residencies in primary care.
2. Expand the number of family practice residency positions as the most effective approach to training physicians for primary care, since this is the only specialty without appreciable "leakage" to subspecialty practice.[47]
3. By means of both national and local institutional approaches, contract the number of residency positions in surplus specialties, with full-time staff physicians and/or faculty replacing many of the functions previously carried by these residents in clinics and on the ward services of teaching hospitals.
4. Within each medical school, provide increased administrative support and resources to the primary care specialties for enlargement of their faculties and expansion of their activities in patient care, teaching, and research.
5. Expand the primary care base of medical schools and teaching hospitals through the development of satellite primary care practices as a means to provide increased teaching and research opportunities in primary care together with an expanded referral base for these institutions.
6. Further develop reimbursement systems which provide incentives for the full range of primary care services and disincentives to excessive application of technology and procedures.

With regard to future health policy initiatives to redress the generalist–specialist imbalance in American medicine, Steinwachs and his colleagues view the problem in these terms:[27]

Recommendations by GMENAC to reduce the total number of physicians trained while increasing the number in primary care will involve changes for graduate medical education and for the hospitals providing the training experience. Federal and state policies directed at achieving these recommendations will have to consider the combined effects of educational initiatives and other health-care initiatives, including cost containment, improving the geographic distribution of physicians, and stimulating the growth of health-maintenance organizations. To ensure that manpower goals are directed at achieving a proper balance between the production of different kinds of physicians and the demand for services in such a complex environment, it will be necessary to monitor closely the trends in medical-school admissions, the special preferences of medical-school graduates, and the residency offerings of hospitals during the 1980s, as well as changes in the demand and need for specific services by the population. This will provide policy makers and planners with an aggregate assessment of the impact of their efforts to tailor the future supply of physicians to the country's anticipated needs.

REFERENCES

1. Sheps CG: Education for what? A decalogue for change. JAMA 238(3):234, 1977
2. Editorial. A new Flexner report? JAMA 290:930, 1969
3. Strassman HD, Taylor DD, Scoles J: A new concept for a core medical curriculum. J Med Educ 44:170, 1969
4. Glaser RJ: The university medical center and its responsibility to the community. J Med Educ 43:793, 1968
5. Funkenstein DH: Implications of the rapid social changes in universities and medical schools for the education of future physicians. J Med Educ 43:443, 1968
6. Anlyan WG: What has happened to the AAMC since the Coggeshall Report of 1965. JAMA 210:1897, 1969
7. An Overview of the General Professional Education of the Physician and College Preparation of Medicine and Questions that Should be Addressed. Washington, D.C., Association of American Medical Colleges, 1982, p 7
8. Chase RA: Proliferation of certification in medical specialties; productive or counterproductive. N Engl J Med 294:497, 1976
9. Cohen WJ: Medical education and physicians manpower from the national level. J Med Educ 44:15, 1969
10. Editorial. What's wrong with medical education? JAMA 211:1849, 1970
11. Jason H: The relevance of medical education to medical practice. JAMA 212:2093, 1970
12. White KL, Williams TF, Greenberg BG: The ecology of medical care. N Engl J Med 265:890, 1961
13. Stevens RA: Graduate medical education: A continuing history. J Med Educ 53:13, 1978
14. Petersdorf RG: Is the establishment defensible? N Engl J Med 309:1055, 1983
15. Ebert RH, Brown SS: Academic health centers. N Engl J Med 308:1200, 1983
16. Progress and Problems in Medical and Dental Education: Federal Support versus Federal Control. Report of the Carnegie Council on Policy Studies in Higher Education. San Francisco, Jossey-Bass, 1976, pp 1–15
17. Schroeder SA: Medical technology and academic medicine: The doctor-producers' dilemma. J Med Educ 56:638, 1981
18. A Manpower Policy for Primary Health Care. Washington, D.C., National Academy of Sciences, Institute of Medicine, 1978, p 6
19. 94th Congress: Health Professions Educational Assistance Act of 1976 (Public Law 94–484). Washington, D.C., U.S. Government Printing Office, 1976
20. Whiteside DF: Training the nation's health manpower—the next 4 years. Public Health Rep 92(2):99, 1977
21. Weekly Report No. 83–39, Washington, D.C., Association of American Medical Colleges, Nov. 3, 1983, p 2
22. For U.S. graduates, enough residencies, study says. Am Med News, Oct. 19, 1984, p 8
23. Section on Medical Schools Report. Chicago, American Medical Association, Feb. 1983, p 2
24. Women, minorities make gains. Am Med News, Dec. 2, 1983, p 8
25. Stimmel B, Graettinger JS: Medical students trained abroad and medical manpower: Recent trends and predictions. N Engl J Med 310:234, 1984
26. Charney E: Internal medicine and pediatric residency education for primary care. Supplement to J Med Educ 130, December 1975
27. Steinwachs DM, Levine DM, Elzinga DJ, et al.: Changing patterns of graduate medical education: Analyzing recent trends and projecting their impact. N Engl J Med 306(1):10, 1982

28. Willard WA, Ruhe CHW: The challenge of family practice reconsidered. JAMA 240:454, 1978
29. Morrow JH, Edwards AB: U.S. health manpower policy: Will the benefits justify the costs? J Med Educ 51:803, 1976
30. Schwarz MR: WAMI—An experiment in regional medical education. West J Med 121(4):333, 1974
31. Werner PT, Richards RW, Fogle BJ: Ambulatory family practice experience as the primary and integrating clinical concept in a four-year undergraduate curriculum. J Fam Pract 7:325, 1978
32. Medical education in the United States, 1976–1977. JAMA 238(26):2762, 1977
33. Editorial: Specialty distribution and the CCME. J Med Educ 52(10):861, 1977
34. Future Directions for Medical Education. Chicago, American Medical Association, Council on Medical Education, 1982, p 87
35. Beck JC, Lee PR, LeRoy L, Stalcup J: The primary care problem. Clin Research 24:266, 1976
36. National Board of Medical Examiners; Committee on Goals and Priorities: Evaluation in the Continuum of Medical Education. Philadelphia, National Board of Medical Examiners, June 1973, p 51
37. Holden WD, Levit EJ: Medical education, licensure, and the National Board of Medical Examiners. N Engl J Med 303:1357, 1980
38. Cramblett HG: National policies for medical licensure through the Federation of State Medical Boards. N Engl J Med 303:1360, 1980
39. Barrett-Connor E: Whither National Boards? N Engl J Med 303: 1356, 1980
40. Continuing medical education. JAMA 250:1558, 1983
41. Ruhe CHW: Looking ahead in medical education. AHME J 26, Spring 1978
42. Davidson CS: Student revolt and our medical schools. In Popper, H (Ed): Trends in New Medical Schools. New York, Grune & Stratton, 1967, p 124
43. Pennell MY, Renshaw JE: Distribution of women physicians, 1971. J Am Med Wom Assoc 28:181, 1973
44. Summary statistics on Graduate Medical Education in the United States. JAMA 252:1549, 1984
45. Geyman JP: Future medical practice in the United States: A choice of scenarios. JAMA 245:1140, 1981
46. Gonnella JS: The impact of early specialization on the clinical competence of residents. N Engl J Med 306:275, 1982.
47. Jacoby I: Graduate medical education: Its impact on specialty distribution. JAMA 245:1046, 1981

6 Predoctoral Education for Family Practice

Family medicine has an opportunity to focus on those things that make life worth-while—for yourselves, for your students, for your colleagues, and for your patients. The orientation of family medicine has from the outset been a natural for this approach. The greatest contribution an ideal department of family medicine can make to a medical school is to be the conscience of the school, and to see that these qualities are recognized as paramount in the goals and objectives of the institution and all of the departments of the school.

Marvin R. Dunn[1]

Shifting the focus now to education for family practice, this is the first of three chapters which will deal with the continuum of education in the specialty. The first phase in this continuum—the undergraduate or predoctoral phase—has been an area of remarkable development during the last 15 years. In 1970, there were just a handful of organized teaching programs in family practice in U.S. medical schools. Today, over 85 percent of medical schools have organized teaching programs in family practice, which already have made considerable impact on the milieu of predoctoral medical education and on the growth of student interest in family practice as a career.

The purpose of this chapter is threefold: (1) to discuss some basic issues which underlie the development of predoctoral teaching programs in family practice; (2) to outline the major requisites for these programs; and (3) to comment on some of the lessons which have been learned from these efforts over the last 15 years.

SOME BASIC ISSUES

At the initial stages of planning for any teaching program in family practice for medical students, a number of fundamental issues present themselves. Five of these merit consideration as a means of better understanding the content, style, and problems of those programs which have developed to date.

Content of Teaching

Two legitimate questions inevitably asked by medical educators and academicians in other disciplines are: (1) What is the definition of family medicine? (2) What can family practice contribute to the medical student's education that is not already being presented by the other departments? The first question has been dealt with in the first chapter, and will not be recounted here. The second question can be answered partly in terms of the content and process of family practice as a delivery mode, and partly in terms of gaps in existing predoctoral medical curricula.

The content of predoctoral teaching in family practice can logically be based on the functions of the family physician which have already been described. Thus, as Leaman suggests, the medical student needs exposure and active involvement with the following functional content areas of family practice:[2]

1. First contact care of clinical problems seen in primary care
2. Comprehensive health care for over 90 percent of the health problems of patients of either sex or any age
3. Health maintenance
4. Intrafamily psychodynamics
5. Community medicine
6. Home care
7. Continuity of care
8. Close physician–patient relationship

The dimensions of predoctoral teaching in family medicine include the knowledge, skills, and attitudes derived from the role of the family physician. As pointed out by Pellegrino:

> Any such curriculum must teach a set of skills—intellectual and practical—that are specific to the clinical function of the generalist and the family practitioner. Defining these skills more precisely; illustrating their use, and demonstrating them clinically in the domain of the family are the special educational assignments of a department of family medicine.[3]

The Task Force on Predoctoral Education of the Society of Teachers of Family Medicine have developed a comprehensive and extremely useful monograph describing current and recommended approaches to predoctoral teaching in family medicine, including curriculum development and evaluation.[4] This Task Force has identified three groups of curricular goals for family medicine as shown in Table 6–1. A central element of clinical teaching in family medicine involves the teaching and learning of the family physician's approach to problem solving of undifferentiated problems as presented by the whole patient as a person (Figure 6–1).

In addition to teaching involving the content and process of family practice per se, departments of family medicine have contributed to a number of gap areas in the existing curricula of their medical schools. Whether on a departmental or interdisciplinary basis, family medicine in many medical schools has participated in teaching programs involving a wide range of courses, including gerontology, human sexuality, medical ethics, nutrition, preventive medicine, sports medicine, and other areas.

Parkerson and colleagues recently reported the results of a study comparing the clinical experience of medical students at Duke University on the five traditional required clerkships (internal medicine, surgery, pediatrics, obstetrics–gynecology, and psychiatry) with that gained during the family medicine clerkship. Although all six clerkships were 2 months in duration, major differences were found in the setting and type of clinical problems encountered. On the traditional clerkships, medical students saw mostly hospitalized patients (88 percent); on the family medicine clerkship, they saw mostly ambulatory patients (80 percent). The total number of patients seen over the 2 months' clerkships averaged five times greater

TABLE 6-1. FAMILY MEDICINE GOALS IN THE PREDOCTORAL CURRICULUM

Goal Group I:

Teach, demonstrate and facilitate practice of the knowledge, skills and attitudes of family medicine

    1. Diagnosis and management of common, undifferentiated problems in ambulatory and community settings

    2. Approach to the patient as a whole person, with emphasis on wellness and health promotion

    3. Primary care problem-solving approaches

    4. Communication skills

    5. Data collection and record-keeping as tools of patient care

    6. Care of the family as a unit

    7. Consultation, referral, and continuity of care

    8. Special diagnostic and therapeutic modalities of family medicine

    9. Community-oriented skills and attitudes

Goal Group II:

Foster student self-understanding and development

    10. Life-long learning

    11. Self-understanding and personal growth

Goal Group III:

Other aspects of family medicine

    12. Family medicine as a career choice

    13. Organizational and management issues involved in practice and cost-effective medical care

    14. Family medicine research

    15. Health care teams

(From Predoctoral Education in Family Medicine. The Task Force on Predoctoral Education. Kansas City, Mo., Society of Teachers of Family Medicine, 1981, with permission.)

for the family medicine clerkship compared with the other required clerkships. Table 6–2 shows important differences in clinical content between the family medicine and traditional required clerkships. This study therefore provides solid evidence that the family medicine clerkship contributes a substantive and different dimension to the overall clinical curriculum beyond that offered by any one or the collective group of the five traditional required clerkships.[5]

Site of Teaching

Several basic issues are important with respect to the location of predoctoral teaching in family medicine, such as: (1) What should be the relative emphasis between ambulatory and hospital-based teaching? (2) To what extent should teaching programs be based in the University, in the community, or in a combination of both settings?

Since the predominant focus of family practice, together with the other primary care specialties, is on ambulatory care, it is quite appropriate that the family practice office serve as the principal base of predoctoral teaching in family medicine. Since the family physician, however, is involved in continuity of care based on the needs of the patient, other ambulatory settings will be involved to a lesser

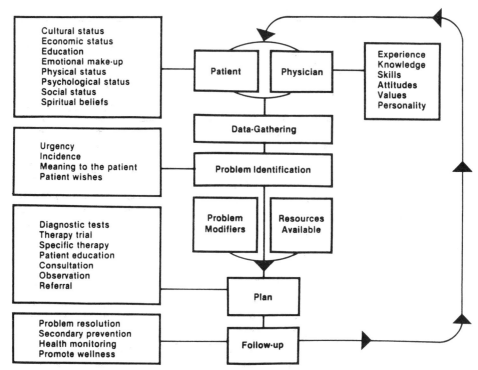

Figure 6-1. Family medicine problem-solving process. *(From Predoctoral Education in Family Medicine. The Task Force on Predoctoral Education. Kansas City, Mo., Society of Teachers of Family Medicine, 1981, with permission.)*

extent (i.e., the emergency room, the nursing home, and the patient's home), and the hospital will likewise be involved for inpatient care provided by the family physician.

There is ample evidence that house staff in the various specialties have provided a substantial part of medical education for many years, and that students often learn best from students and residents just 2 or 3 years ahead of them in their training. Medical students need to form some impression of the nature of residency training in family practice and to see role models of young physicians in graduate training in this field. For these reasons, it is advantageous that some portion of predoctoral teaching in family medicine be provided in the context of the family practice residency program. In addition, medical students gain additional valuable exposure to family practice residents while working with them on their various hospital rotations in the other specialties.

Since family practice is based in the community as a primary care delivery mode, it is logical that community settings, whether urban, suburban or rural, be emphasized in the predoctoral teaching of family medicine. There is an important need, however, for university-based teaching of family medicine which affords medical students ready access to family practice faculty and residents as visible role models. There are special problems in developing a teaching practice by family physicians in the university setting. Nevertheless, this has been effectively accomplished

TABLE 6-2. COMPARISON OF THE 15 MOST FREQUENT PROBLEM CONTACTS PER STUDENT PER 2-MONTH CLINICAL CLERKSHIP IN THE TRADITIONAL CLERKSHIPS WITH THOSE IN THE FAMILY MEDICINE CLERKSHIP FOR 40 DUKE UNIVERSITY MEDICAL STUDENTS, 1978–1982

Clerkship/Problem	Traditional Clerkships[a] (n = 300 Problems)		Family Medicine Clerkshipe (n = 416 Problems)	
	%	Rank	%	Rank
Traditional and family medicine				
Depressive neurosis	4.1	1	1.9	7
Chronic ischemic heart disease	2.1	7	2.1	6
Medical examination	2.1	8	5.4	2
Diabetes mellitus	1.8	11	3.6	4
Traditional only				
Medical or surgical procedure	3.7	2	—[b]	
Alcohol abuse	2.7	3	—	
Malignant neoplasm, female	2.5	4	—	
Schizophrenia	2.4	5	—	
Other nervous system diseases	2.3	6	—	
Other endocrine, nutritional, metabolic disorders	1.9	9	—	
Other malignant neoplasms	1.9	10	—	
Other urinary system diseases	1.7	12	—	
Normal delivery	1.6	13	—	
Complicated delivery	1.5	14	—	
Congenital anomaly, heart and circulatory system	1.5	15	—	
Family medicine only				
Hypertension, uncomplicated	—[b]		7.5	1
Acute upper respiratory tract infection	—		4.4	3
Cystitis and urinary tract infection	—		2.2	5
Abdominal pain	—		1.7	8
Prenatal care	—		1.6	9
Acute otitis media	—		1.6	10
Low back pain	—		1.5	11
Heart failure	—		1.5	12
Other cerebrovascular disease[c]	—		1.4	13
Chronic obstructive pulmonary disease	—		1.4	14
Obesity	—		1.4	15
All Other Problems	66.2		60.8	
Total	100.0		100.0	

[a]Mean values for the five traditional clerkships: internal medicine, surgery, pediatrics, obstetrics-gynecology, and psychiatry.
[b]Dashes indicate that rank order of this problem is not in the top 15 reported in this type of clerkship.
[c]Includes mostly cerebrovascular accidents.
(From Parkerson GR, Muhlbaier LH, Falcone JC: A comparison of students' clinical experience in family medicine and traditional clerkships. J Med Educ 59:124, 1984, with permission.)

by family practice programs in many medical schools, and the maintenance of these teaching practices poses no major obstacles as long as the concepts of family practice remain their orienting focus and excessive involvement in the total needs of the institution for undifferentiated primary care are avoided.

A national study by Walbroehl and colleagues conducted in 1979 provides an overall picture vis-a-vis the settings used by departments of family medicine for predoctoral teaching of medical students. Based on responses from 87 departments of family medicine, they found that family practice clerkships have been based mainly in the ambulatory setting in both family practice clinics and private physicians' offices.[6]

Organization of Curriculum

Another basic issue which immediately surfaces whenever an undergraduate teaching program in family medicine is being considered in any institution is the question of how its curriculum should be organized and integrated within the medical school. This larger question subsumes a number of related questions, such as:

1. To what extent is there consensus within the medical school faculty concerning the desired goals and product of predoctoral medical education?
2. How much of the medical school class should receive exposure to family medicine?
3. Should a family physician "track" or "pathway" be organized within the curriculum?
4. What should be required and/or elective in the family medicine curriculum?
5. To what extent can curriculum time be made available for new courses in another discipline in an already crowded undergraduate curriculum?
6. What is the present and projected capability of the family practice faculty to develop and maintain new predoctoral courses in family medicine?
7. What lead time is needed to implement each increment of family medicine teaching to the overall curriculum?

Assuming that sufficient resources are available to the family practice department and that the institution is committed to the education of future family physicians in substantial numbers, the ideal responses to these questions would clearly involve meaningful exposure of all medical students to family medicine and sufficient flexibility of the overall curriculum to accomplish this aim. But this option is often not available to a department of family medicine early in its development when other commitments are great (e.g., patient care, resident training, and developing research programs) and the faculty size is often limited. In 1979, 60 of 87 reporting medical schools had required courses in family medicine for all medical students.[6]

Coordination With Graduate Education in Family Practice

Another fundamental question in family practice, as in other clinical disciplines, concerns what should be offered at the predoctoral level as opposed to later residency training in the field. Although there will inevitably be some overlap at each level, the resolution of this issue can be aided by making a distinction between "education" and "training."

In Britain the Royal Commission on Medical Education has addressed this question in the following terms, which seem equally applicable in the United States.[7]

> We cannot emphasize too strongly that the undergraduate course in medicine should be primarily educational. Its object is not to produce a fully qualified doctor, but an educated man who becomes fully qualified in the course of postgraduate training.

Wright elaborates on this point in this way:[8]

> . . . while the hallmark of training is its particularity, the hallmark of education is its universality. Training is predominantly concerned with the preparation of an individual for specific tasks, i.e., with skills (and with knowledge insofar as it is relevant to those skills). Education, by contrast, is not confined to specific tasks, nor to skills and their related knowledge, but is also much concerned with ways of thinking and attitudes. It aims to develop a capacity for "transfer"—the ability to apply the insights of any one discipline to the problems of another and a capacity for intellectual integration and synthesis.

Logistic Problems

It is one matter to identify the needs and develop a plan for a predoctoral teaching program in family medicine, but quite another to implement such a program. One critical dimension in the implementation phase relates to logistic problems, particularly those concerned with the limited resources of most family practice departments in their beginning years.

As relative newcomers in academic medicine, family practice departments are charged with broad responsibilities simultaneously, including the need to develop their clinical base, organize residency training programs, recruit and develop faculty, initiate research and other scholarly activities in the discipline, and acquire the necessary funding to permit all of these activities. Since these departments usually have limited funding and numbers of faculty to meet all of these goals, priorities need to be established as to what is possible to accomplish within the limits of available resources. Perhaps the most challenging dilemma in this respect is the relative emphasis to be directed to graduate versus predoctoral teaching, since both are essential and interrelated needs.

REQUISITES FOR PREDOCTORAL TEACHING PROGRAM

With this background, it is useful to outline briefly some basic requisites for any developing or projected predoctoral teaching program in family medicine.

Department of Family Practice

Given the scope of the mission of the developing family practice program in the medical school, an academic and administrative unit is clearly needed which can best mobilize and support this effort. A free-standing department is required, and is the principal approach being taken in U.S. medical schools, which by 1983 had organized 103 such departments. As a division of another department, or as a free-standing division responsible to the dean, the capability of the family practice program to develop and flourish in the competitive academic environment is compromised.

The Department of Family Practice (or Family Medicine) should have its own clinical and teaching service (both ambulatory and inpatient), adequate budget, and full representation as a major clinical department within the medical school.

The department should preferably be headed by a family physician with both teaching and practice experience.

Exemplary Clinical Settings

The clinical sites for medical student teaching in family medicine should effectively illustrate the full dimensions of family practice as defined earlier. These sites will usually include the department's clinical base at the university, but should include an emphasis on community-based practices, whether associated with affiliated family practice residency programs or exemplary group practices of family physicians in the community. The full spectrum of clinical problems seen in the primary care of a diverse patient population should be represented, and ready access to consultants and other community resources should be available.

These clinical settings should be actively involved in the monitoring of quality of care through audit, and in the maintenance of modern medical record and data retrieval systems. An atmosphere of critical inquiry is essential to the learning climate for all involved in the teaching program.

Coordinated 4-Year Curriculum

In order to make available to medical students appropriate exposure to the knowledge, skills and attitudes of the family physician, as well as to provide sufficient experience to allow an informed career decision for their future specialties, family medicine must be offered in each year of the overall curriculum, usually over a 4-year period. The curriculum in family medicine should be planned carefully to assure coordination of learning objectives and content, and provisions for progressive levels of responsibility should be made.[9] It is also desirable to maximize continuity of care for medical students as much as possible within the time constraints of each particular course. In some cases long-term continuity can be provided for excellent learning opportunities with "longitudinal patients."[10]

Alfred North Whitehead has divided the process of learning into three phases: (1) *romance*, (2) *precision*, and (3) *generalization*, or *synthesis*.[11] This concept can serve as a useful framework for progression from a largely passive observational learning experience for first-year medical students (romance), to a more focused, content-based third-year clerkship experience (precision), to a fourth-year advanced clerkship at a subinternship level (synthesis).

In addition to intradepartmental coordination of the predoctoral curriculum in family medicine, further coordination is needed in order to integrate the program within the medical school curriculum. An example is the integration of preclinical family medicine electives with required Introduction to Clinical Medicine courses.[9]

Table 6–3 provides a summary of family medicine course offering and requirements in 87 U.S. medical schools in 1979. About two-thirds of these schools had required courses in family medicine at that time, generally in the form of a continuous block clerkship.[6]

Family Practice Role Models

Perhaps the single most important element in the quality and effectiveness of the predoctoral teaching program in family medicine is the caliber of the family physicians themselves as teachers and role models. Teachers must be carefully selected who best demonstrate the attributes of the excellent family physician. As noted by Scherger when a medical student: "The clinical student interested in an alternative

TABLE 6-3. CURRICULUM YEARS IN WHICH FAMILY PRACTICE COURSES ARE OFFERED AND REQUIRED (n = 87)

	% of Schools Offering Courses[a]	% of Schools Requiring Courses[a]
Year 1	49	23
Year 2	51	18
Year 3	53	32
Year 4	75	28
No. courses offered	3	—
No. courses required	—	31

[a]Sum of percentages greater that 100, as several institutions offer courses in more than 1 year.
(From Walbroehl GS, Painter AF, Gillen JC: Family practice undergraduate education. JAMA 245(15):1552–1553, 1981, with permission. Copyright 1981, American Medical Association.)

to the secondary and tertiary care of the academic center will be taking a very close look at the family physician, his life style, and his practice."[12]

Beyond a high level of clinical competency in dealing with the wide range of clinical problems in family practice, the family physician teacher needs to display a genuine concern for the well-being of his/her patients and their families, together with a blending of the art and science of medicine. In addition, the family physician teacher should be comfortable in sharing with students his personal philosophy of practice, including his views of the challenges and satisfactions of everyday practice.

Family medicine faculty involved in predoctoral teaching include full-time faculty, family physicians in community practice (both paid and voluntary), and family practice residents.[6] That residents are heavily involved in medical student teaching is well documented by Plumb's 1977 survey of U.S. family practice residencies. Based upon a response rate of 84 percent of programs, Plumb found that three-quarters of these programs were engaged in predoctoral teaching, with more than 90 percent of their residents so involved and carrying a substantial share of medical student teaching.[13]

Advising Program

Today's medical student is confronted by a curriculum of increasing complexity and the need to select a field for further training and practice from among a growing number of specialties and subspecialties. This is made more difficult by the elimination in recent years of the internship year, which forces medical students to make what are usually lifetime decisions by the end of the third year or the first part of the fourth year in medical school. The pressure of early career decisions represents a difficult dilemma for many medical students. This can be partly alleviated by an active counseling and advising program by faculty. Family practice faculty members need to be fully involved as advisors for students interested in this field, both as role models and for help with selection of courses and options for residency training.

Evaluation System

All parts of the predoctoral teaching program in family medicine require periodic evaluation and revision as needed. The evaluation process includes students and faculty performance, student assessment of courses and faculty, and the content of students' actual learning experiences. Evaluation of educational programs may be of two basic kinds: (1) formative (e.g., assessment of the teaching/learning experience as it proceeds so that feedback can change the process); and (2) summative (e.g., a final examination after the learning experience has been completed).

A variety of techniques have been applied in the evaluation of family medicine teaching programs around the country. Daily student logs have been found useful, for example, in the evaluation of decentralized family medicine clerkships by recording frequency, level of responsibility and site of experience for diagnoses and procedures.[14] Other evaluation techniques in common use include videotaping with feedback, the use of simulated patients, oral and written examinations, chart audits, and self-assessment.[15-19]

COMMENT

It is of interest now to comment briefly on some of the lessons which can be derived from family medicine's efforts over the past 10 to 15 years in predoctoral medical education in the United States. Several useful findings were revealed by a national survey in 1975 of U.S. and Canadian predoctoral teaching programs in family medicine. The purpose of the study was to examine the relationship between administrative structure, size of program, faculty size, and type of predoctoral curriculum to the number of graduates selecting graduate training in family practice. This study involved a response rate of 90 percent, and demonstrated a clear relationship between the commitment of the medical school to family practice, the size of the program, and the presence of required courses in the curriculum to the success of the program as reflected by the proportion of graduates choosing family practice residencies.[20] Positive correlations were established between increased numbers of graduates opting for family practice and the presence of a Department of Family Practice (Table 6–4), a larger number of full-time family physicians on the faculty (Table 6–5), and required family practice clerkships and preceptorships (Table 6–6). An organized Department of Family Practice was also found to influence the extent to which preclinical courses, clerkships, and preceptorships in family practice were required in the medical school's curriculum (Table 6–7).

TABLE 6-4. TYPE OF ADMINISTRATIVE UNIT AND PROPORTION OF STUDENTS CHOOSING FAMILY PRACTICE RESIDENCIES

Administrative Unit	Proportion Choosing Family Practice				
	0–10%	11–20%	21–30%	31–40%	n
Department	10.6	51.1	27.7	10.6	47
Division	66.7	22.2	11.1	0.0	9
Other	50.0	50.0	0.0	0.0	6
n	14	29	14	5	62

(From Beck JD, Stewart WL, Graham R, Stern TL: The effect of the organization and status of family practice undergraduate programs on residency selection. J Fam Pract 4:663, 1977, with permission.)

TABLE 6-5. NUMBER OF FULL-TIME SALARIED FAMILY PHYSICIANS AND PROPORTION OF STUDENTS CHOOSING FAMILY PRACTICE RESIDENCIES

Number of Full-Time Family Physicians	Proportion Choosing Family Practice				
	0-10%	*11-20%*	*21-30%*	*31-40%*	*n*
0-2	35.0	40.0	25.0	0.0	20
3-5	20.8	58.3	20.8	0.0	24
6-9	0.0	53.8	15.4	30.8	13
10+	40.0	0.0	40.0	20.0	5
n	14	29	14	5	62

(From Beck JD, Stewart WL, Graham R, Stern TL: The effect of the organization and status of family practice undergraduate programs on residency selection. J Fam Pract 4:663, 1977, with permission.)

If one looks at one outcome measure—the proportion of medical graduates attracted to careers in family practice—a wide range in career choice patterns is apparent. The proportion of graduates from public medical schools who opt for family practice is almost double that of graduates from private medical schools (Table 6–8). That private medical schools have been slower than the public medical schools to establish departments of family practice is undoubtedly a major factor. In addition, substantial regional differences in career choice of family practice have been identified, ranging from a low of 7.5 percent of graduates in New England to a high of 18.6 percent in the West North Central region. Table 6–9 shows that number and percentage of graduates from each U.S. medical school who were family practice residents during the 1981–1982 year.[21]

In appraising the first 10 years of predoctoral programs in family medicine, Leaman has observed a shift of emphasis as the new programs started to mature:[22]

The educational goals chosen by teachers of family medicine for predoctoral students a decade ago differ substantially from the present goals. The original goals were to increase the number of family physicians, provide them with the basic knowledge and skills to practice, integrate the concepts of family medicine

TABLE 6-6. ASPECTS OF CURRICULUM AND PROPORTION OF STUDENTS CHOOSING FAMILY PRACTICE RESIDENCIES

		Proportion Choosing Family Practice				
		0-10%	*11-20%*	*21-30%*	*31-40%*	*n*
Clerkship Required	% Yes	20.0	40.0	13.3	26.7	15
	% No	22.7	47.7	27.3	2.3	44
	n	13	27	14	5	49
Preceptorship Required	% Yes	11.1	44.4	33.3	11.1	9
	% No	23.5	47.1	21.6	7.8	51
	n	13	28	14	5	60

(From Beck JD, Stewart WL, Graham R, Stern TL: The effect of the organization and status of family practice undergraduate programs on residency selection. J Fam Pract 4:663, 1977, with permission.)

TABLE 6-7. RELATIONSHIPS BETWEEN TYPE OF ADMINISTRATIVE UNIT AND CURRICULUM

		% Yes	% No	n
		Required Preclinical Courses		
Department		82.0	18.0	50
Division		44.4	55.6	9
Other		20.0	80.0	5
	n	46	18	64
		Required Clerkships		
Department		35.8	64.2	53
Division		23.1	76.9	13
Other		0.0	100.0	6
	n	22	50	72
		Required Preceptorships		
Department		22.2	77.8	54
Division		15.4	84.6	13
Other		16.7	83.5	6
	n	15	58	73

(From Beck JD, Stewart WL, Graham R, Stern TL: The effect of the organization and status of family practice undergraduate programs on residency selection. J Fam Pract 4:663, 1977, with permission.)

into the total medical school curriculum, and develop the "attitudes and ideals" of the good family physician. . . .The present curriculum has an increased emphasis on clinical skills in family practice and on integration of behavioral science; there is a new emphasis on the role of the physician in the community and a better understanding of health care systems. Future directions for family medicine include increasing the emphasis on interpersonal communications, clinical synthesis, and clinical assessment.

TABLE 6-8. NUMBER OF PERCENTAGE OF GRADUATES FROM MEDICAL SCHOOLS WHO WERE FIRST-YEAR RESIDENTS IN FAMILY PRACTICE BY TYPE OF MEDICAL SCHOOL, DECEMBER 1981

Type of Funding of Medical School	Graduates July 1980 to June 1981 Number	Graduates Entering as First-Year Residents in FP Programs	
		Number	%
Public (74)	9,250	1,437	15.5
Private (48)	6,417	564	8.8
Total	15,667	2,001	12.8

(From Schmittling G, Clinton C, Brunton S: Entry of U.S. medical school graduates into family practice residencies: A national study. J Fam Pract 17:283, 1983, with permission.)

TABLE 6-9. NUMBER AND PERCENTAGE OF MEDICAL SCHOOL GRADUATES, BY MEDICAL SCHOOL, WHO WERE FIRST-YEAR RESIDENTS IN FAMILY PRACTICE, DECEMBER 1981

State by Medical School	Medical School Graduates July 1980 to June 1981 Number	Graduates Entering as First-Year Residents in Family Practice Programs	
		Number	%
Alabama			
Alabama, Univ. of	164	20	12.2
South Alabama	67	8	11.9
Arizona			
Arizona, Univ. of	86	9	10.5
Arkansas			
Arkansas, Univ. of	136	28	20.6
California			
California, Davis	91	14	15.4
California, Irvine	89	15	16.9
California, Los Angeles	164	20	12.2
California, San Diego	90	8	8.9
California, San Francisco	161	25	15.5
Loma Linda	166	31	18.7
Southern California	150	21	14.0
Stanford	83	6	7.2
Colorado			
Colorado, Univ. of	133	20	15.0
Connecticut			
Connecticut, Univ. of	83	5	6.0
Yale	112	0	0.0
District of Columbia			
Georgetown	206	22	10.7
George Washington	147	20	13.6
Howard	113	8	7.1
Florida			
Florida, Univ. of	119	17	14.3
Miami	175	13	7.4
South Florida	93	12	12.9
Georgia			
Emory	118	3	2.5
Georgia, Med. Coll. of	189	10	5.3
Hawaii			
Hawaii, Univ. of	80	8	10.0
Illinois			
Chicago Medical	128	16	12.5
Chicago, Pritzker	108	5	4.6
Illinois, Univ. of	320	25	7.8
Loyola, Stritch	167	14	8.4
Northwestern	175	4	2.3
Rush	126	23	18.3
Southern Illinois	72	12	16.7

(continued)

TABLE 6-9. (cont.)

State by Medical School	Medical School Graduates July 1980 to June 1981 Number	Graduates Entering as First-Year Residents in Family Practice Programs	
		Number	%
Indiana			
Indiana, Univ. of	301	64	21.3
Iowa			
Iowa, Univ. of	178	38	21.3
Kansas			
Kansas, Univ. of	111	14	12.6
Kentucky			
Kentucky, Univ. of	96	19	19.8
Louisville	142	28	19.7
Louisiana			
Louisiana, New Orleans	178	20	11.2
Louisiana, Shreveport	86	12	14.0
Tulane	152	4	2.6
Maryland			
Johns Hopkins	111	2	1.8
Maryland, Univ. of	182	37	20.3
Uniformed Services Univ.	67	8	11.9
Massachusetts			
Boston	145	9	6.2
Harvard	171	2	1.2
Massachusetts, Univ. of	101	12	11.9
Tufts	166	14	8.4
Michigan			
Michigan, Univ. of	237	28	11.8
Michigan State	95	18	18.9
Wayne State	248	35	14.1
Minnesota			
Mayo	39	8	20.5
Minnesota, Minneapolis	295	86	29.2
Mississippi			
Mississippi, Univ. of	145	39	26.9
Missouri			
Missouri, Columbia	112	21	18.8
Missouri, Kansas City	60	11	18.3
St. Louis	148	14	9.5
Washington, St. Louis	141	6	4.3
Nebraska			
Creighton	112	18	16.1
Nebraska, Univ. of	82	13	15.9
Nevada			
Nevada, Univ. of	48	5	10.4
New Hampshire			
Dartmouth	62	8	12.9

TABLE 6-9. (cont.)

State by Medical School	Medical School Graduates July 1980 to June 1981 Number	Graduates Entering as First-Year Residents in Family Practice Programs	
		Number	%
New Jersey			
CMDNJ–New Jersey	136	10	7.4
CMDNJ–Rutgers	93	8	8.6
New Mexico			
New Mexico, Univ. of	75	15	20.0
New York			
Albany	126	4	3.2
Columbia	146	6	4.1
Cornell	107	4	3.7
Einstein	172	16	9.3
Mount Sinai	126	2	1.6
New York Medical	197	11	5.6
New York Univ.	178	4	2.2
Rochester	106	6	5.7
SUNY, Buffalo	145	14	9.7
SUNY, Downstate	216	14	6.5
SUNY, Stony Brook	57	9	15.8
SUNY, Upstate	141	25	17.7
North Carolina			
Bowman Gray	107	20	18.7
Duke	119	14	11.8
East Carolina	28	12	42.9
North Carolina, Univ. of	160	18	11.3
North Dakota			
North Dakota	39	5	12.8
Ohio			
Case Western Reserve	149	15	10.1
Cincinnati	196	20	10.2
Northeastern Ohio	42	6	14.3
Ohio State	224	35	15.6
Ohio, Toledo	129	23	17.8
Wright State	44	13	29.5
Oklahoma			
Oklahoma, Univ. of	173	20	11.6
Oral Roberts	0	0	0.0
Oregon			
Oregon, Univ. of	114	11	9.6
Pennsylvania			
Hahnemann	177	23	13.0
Jefferson	224	31	13.8
Pennsylvania, Med. Coll. of	121	18	14.9
Pennsylvania, Univ. of	156	10	6.4
Pennsylvania State, Hershey	95	12	12.6
Pittsburgh	132	16	12.1
Temple	179	21	11.7

(continued)

TABLE 6-9. (cont.)

State by Medical School	Medical School Graduates July 1980 to June 1981 Number	Graduates Entering as First-Year Residents in Family Practice Programs	
		Number	%
Puerto Rico			
Puerto Rico, Univ. of	148	5	3.4
Rhode Island			
Brown	67	9	13.4
South Carolina			
South Carolina, Medical Univ. of	166	44	26.5
South Carolina, Columbia	22	5	22.7
South Dakota			
South Dakota, Univ. of	46	19	41.3
Tennessee			
East Tennessee State	0	0	0.0
Meharry	112	7	6.3
Tennessee, Univ. of	181	25	13.8
Vanderbilt	102	3	2.9
Texas			
Baylor	181	22	12.2
Texas, Galveston	199	31	15.6
Texas, Houston	149	30	20.1
Texas, San Antonio	137	26	19.0
Texas, Southwestern	198	17	8.6
Texas, A & M	32	5	15.6
Texas Tech	42	11	26.2
Utah			
Utah, Univ. of	97	14	14.4
Vermont			
Vermont, Univ. of	84	15	17.9
Virginia			
Eastern Virginia	76	17	22.4
Virginia, Med. Coll. of	168	32	19.0
Virginia, Univ. of	132	24	18.2
Washington			
Washington, Univ. of	173	57	32.9
West Virginia			
Marshall	18	2	11.1
West Virginia, Univ. of	85	11	12.9
Wisconsin			
Wisconsin, Med. Coll. of	149	18	12.1
Wisconsin, Univ. of	152	26	17.1
Total	15,667	2,001	12.8

(From Schmittling G, Clinton C, Brunton S: Entry of U.S. medical school graduates into family practice residencies: A national study. J Fam Pract 17:283, 1983, with permission.)

Phillips has noted another dimension of change in predoctoral programs over their first 10 years.[23]

> A decade or more ago, many of us entered enthusiastically upon our new roles as medical educators bent on finding, recruiting, and proselyting students for family practice and teaching them how to be family doctors. Some faculty concerned themselves with improving the education of all students as their primary goal, but that wasn't the dominant attitude. The dominant attitude worked all right in an era which valued differentiation of students at the pre-M.D. level. It works less well today. In an era which values a standard, basic medical education for all students to produce an undifferentiated, basic M.D., the family medicine teacher must be clear about his or her role in that basic medical education. He or she must teach from a solid base of knowledge generated through scholarship and experience. We must be prepared to make that knowledge relevant, exciting, and useful for all medical students—not just those we're trying to attract into family practice. We as faculty members must change along with our schools and departments as we enter the new era.

It is inevitable that considerable variability exists among predoctoral family medicine programs around the country. Programs naturally differ in the extent to which family medicine teaching is decentralized, and in the way the family medicine curriculum is integrated within the overall medical school curriculum. These differences illustrate one point which has been learned from the early years—that the organization and conduct of predoctoral teaching in family medicine need to be adapted to the goals, needs, and settings of each individual institution, and further depend upon what is possible within resource constraints of each department at its particular stage of development. Despite these differences, however, excellent progress has been made during the last 10 to 15 years in the predoctoral teaching of family medicine in U.S. medical schools. These efforts to date have emphasized the romance and synthesis phases of Whitehead's trilogy. Further growth and development of Departments of Family Practice in coming years, particularly as the research base expands in the discipline, can be expected to lead to refinement of these predoctoral teaching programs and to an increased degree of precision in their courses.

REFERENCES

1. Dunn MR: Contributions of an ideal Department of Family Medicine to a medical school. Fam Med 13(4):15, 1981
2. Leaman TL: A predoctoral curriculum in family medicine. J Fam Pract 2:107, 1975
3. Pellegrino ED: The academic viability of family medicine: A triad of challenges. JAMA 240(2):133, 1978
4. Predoctoral Education in Family Medicine. Kansas City, Mo., Society of Teachers of Family Medicine, 1981
5. Parkerson GR, Muhlbaier LH, Falcone JC: A comparison of students' clinical experience in family medicine and traditional clerkships. J Med Educ 59:124, 1984
6. Walbroehl GS, Painter AF, Gillen JC: Family practice undergraduate education. JAMA 245(15):1552, 1981

7. Royal Commission on Medical Education (1968). Report. Cmnd. 3569, London, H.M.S.O.

8. Wright HJ: The logic of medicine—the contribution of general practice to the understanding of clinical method. J Royal Coll Gen Pract 25:531, 1975

9. Smith CK, Gordon MJ, Leversee JH, Hadac RR: Early ambulatory experience in the undergraduate education of family physicians. J Fam Pract 5:227, 1977

10. Geyman C, Smith L, Clayton J, et al.: Benefits of early predoctoral experiences in longitudinal patient care. J Fam Pract 18:911, 1984

11. Miller G: Teaching and Learning in Medical School. Cambridge, Mass., Harvard University Press, 1961, p 67

12. Scherger JE: A medical student's perspective on preceptors in family practice. J Fam Pract 2:201, 1975

13. Plumb JD: The family medicine resident and medical student teaching. J Fam Pract 7:1171, 1978

14. Zinser EA, Wiegert HT: Describing learning experiences of undergraduate medical students in rural settings. J Fam Pract 3:287, 1976

15. Kauss DR, Robbins AS, Abrass I: The long-term effectiveness of interpersonal skills training in medical schools. J Med Educ 55:595, 1980

16. Coggan PG, Knight P, Davis P: Evaluating students in family medicine using simulated patients. J Fam Pract 10:259, 1980

17. Norman GR, Feightner JW: A comparison of behavior on simulated patients and patient management problems. J Med Educ 15:26, 1981

18. Smith SR, MacLeod NM: An innovative family medicine clerkship. J Fam Pract 13:687, 1981

19. Harris DL, Bluhm HP: An evaluation of primary care preceptorships. J Fam Pract 5:577, 1977

20. Beck JD, Stewart WL, Graham R, Stern TL: The effect of the organization and status of family practice undergraduate programs on residency selection. J Fam Pract 4:663, 1977

21. Schmittling G, Clinton C, Brunton S: Entry of U.S. medical school graduates into family practice residencies: A national study. J Fam Pract 17:283, 1983

22. Leaman TL: Predoctoral education in family medicine: A ten-year perspective. J Fam Pract 9:846, 1979

23. Phillips TJ: Medical school curricula and family medicine in the 1980's. Fam Med 13(3):12, 1981

7 Graduate Education for Family Practice

Perhaps the single most impressive feature of the progress demonstrated by the new specialty of family practice over the last 15 years is the remarkable growth and development of graduate education in the field. At this writing, there are 384 approved family practice residency programs in operation in the United States with over 7400 residents in training. Residencies in family practice are carefully designed as coordinated 3-year programs, with the first year taking the place of the older rotating internship. Residency development has been based upon the *Essentials for Graduate Training in Family Practice,* a document first prepared through the joint efforts of the American Academy of Family Physicians, the American Board of Family Practice, the Section on General/Family Practice of the American Medical Association, and the AMA Council on Medical Education. This document has been periodically revised and updated since then, and the current revision was adopted in 1983.

Family practice residency training represents several important shifts of direction when compared to other kinds of residency programs: from episodic to continuous and comprehensive care; from a disease-oriented emphasis to a focus on the whole patient; from an individual to a family focus; and from the solo physician to the physician as a member of a group.

This chapter will examine the nature of family practice residency training in this country with three purposes in mind: (1) to present some common features of family practice residencies; (2) to provide an overview of the goals, content, and current directions of family practice residency training in the United States; and (3) to comment briefly on some of the lessons which have been learned to date concerning graduate education in this field.

COMMON FEATURES OF FAMILY PRACTICE RESIDENCIES

Family Practice Center

The Family Practice Center is the clinical and teaching base of the family practice residency program. It is designed and located so as to maintain the identity and functions of a group practice of family physicians. It may be located within its related hospital or at some distance from its related hospital(s) (usually not over 2 or 3 miles away). The Family Practice Center serves as the resident's base for the continuing care of his/her growing practice over a 3-year period, and is the site for much of the resident's training in ambulatory care. To the maximal possible extent, the functions of a family practice group in the community are replicated in the Family Practice Center, including its own separate medical record and practice management systems. In some programs, especially larger ones, a second satellite Family Practice Center is also used; in this case, the additional center must satisfy the same accreditation criteria as the primary center.

The Family Practice Center, even in the smallest residency program, is usually at least 3600 to 5000 square feet in size. It invariably includes a waiting room, business and medical record office, examination rooms, minor surgery room, office laboratory, conference room/library, and faculty/resident offices. X-ray facilities may also be located in the Family Practice Center, although many programs utilize the x-ray facilities of a nearby hospital. There is generally a sufficient number of examination rooms to provide each resident working in the Family Practice Center with two such rooms at any given time.

The patient population served by the Family Practice Center should represent a broad socioeconomic spectrum from the surrounding community with all age groups included. Individuals and families should be included in the practice who desire continuity and comprehensiveness of care, not just episodic care for acute medical problems. In most programs, the first-year family practice resident is assigned about 25 families for ongoing care, and spends 1 (sometimes 2) half-days each week in the Family Practice Center. In the second and third years, the resident becomes responsible for 100 to 150 families, and spends more time in the Family Practice Center (usually 2 to 4 half-days per week) as the emphasis on hospital training during the first year shifts more toward ambulatory care by the third year. As residents progress through the family practice residency, they are expected to become more proficient in seeing patients expeditiously as will be needed in their future practices. Under normal circumstances, residents see an average of 5, 10, and 10 to 12 patients each half-day in the Family Practice Center during their first, second, and third residency years, respectively.

Beyond the usual clerical and clinical support staff required in most family practice offices, many of the residency programs employ other allied health professionals in the Family Practice Center on either a part-time or full-time basis. Thus, medical social workers, clinical psychologists, clinical pharmacists, physician extenders (Medex, physician assistant, and/or nurse practitioner), and others may be involved in the teaching programs. In addition, residency programs are often able to arrange for consultants in other specialties to teach and consult in the Family Practice Center, so that rather extensive teaching resources can be made available to the resident at the program's home base.

Hospital Training

The family practice residency program requires a close linkage to one or more hospitals for the dual purpose of hospital-based teaching services and hospitalization of patients from the Family Practice Center. Geographic settings vary from large teaching hospitals in metropolitan areas to 150- or 200-bed general hospitals in communities as small as 40,000 in population. Under some circumstances the residency program relates to one hospital (usually at least 200 beds), but often 2 (and occasionally 3) hospitals are needed to accommodate all of the required services. If multiple hospitals are involved, care must be taken to avoid undue fractionation of the program's clinical and teaching efforts, but this is often unavoidable in a community where some hospitals' services have been consolidated. Figure 7–1 shows the current breakdown of family practice residency programs by type and setting in the United States. It can be noted that more than one-half of these are university-affiliated community hospitals, and this proportion has been increasing.

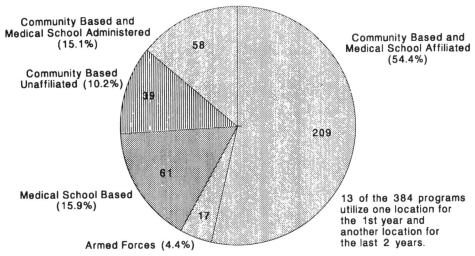

Figure 7-1. Breakdown of 384 accredited family practice residency programs by type and setting. July 1984. *(From Division of Education. American Academy of Family Physicians. Kansas City, Mo., with permission.)*

Almost all family practice residency programs involve a fixed base over the full 3-year period of residency training. A small number of programs, however, are organized on a "one-and-two" basis, with the first year in a larger metropolitan community with its Family Practice Center and large teaching hospital, and the final 2 years of training in a smaller community with the principal Family Practice Center there linked to one or more smaller community hospitals.[1]

Most programs maintain an active Family Practice Service in a nearby hospital(s) for the care of patients from the teaching practice who require hospitalization. This assures continuity of care of family practice patients, with consultation requested as needed. Medley and Halstead have reviewed their experience in one family practice residency program, where the Family Practice Service provided care for 631 patients over a 1-year period. Consultation was requested in one-third of patients, and in these instances the family physicians continued to share responsibility for patient care with the consultants. Table 7-1 lists the most common discharge diagnoses encountered during the study.[2]

Hospital teaching rotations are required on all of the major clinical services, including internal medicine, pediatrics, obstetrics–gynecology, and general surgery. The family practice resident also needs inpatient teaching rotations in cardiology and neurology, and often takes electives on other services. Emergency room experience and various specialty clinics, when available, add further to the resident's training.

Size of Program
The majority of family practice residency programs range from 4 residents in each year of the 3-year program to 12 residents per year, with a typical program having 18 residents (6-6-6). Since the family practice residency is a complex entity requiring continuity of patient care and teaching in the Family Practice Center and its related hospital(s), there must be a sufficient number of residents to meet the program's commitment to patient care, teaching, and related activities. In addition,

TABLE 7-1. MOST COMMON DIAGNOSES ON ONE FAMILY PRACTICE RESIDENCY INPATIENT SERVICE

Diagnoses	No. of Cases	Diagnoses	No. of Cases
Intrauterine pregnancy (uncomplicated)	96	Urinary tract infection	8
Newborns (uncomplicated)	90	Herniated nucleus pulposus	7
Newborns (complicated)[a]	26	Chronic obstructive pulmonary disease	6
Chest pain, possible MI	26	Bronchitis, acute	6
Gastroenteritis	17	Pelvic inflammatory disease, tuboovarian abscess	6
Arteriosclerotic heart disease, acute MI	16	Bony trauma	6
Asthma	15	Leg pain	4
Arteriosclerotic heart disease, not specified	14	Cellulitis	4
		Supraventricular tachycardia	4
Arteriosclerotic heart disease, congestive failure	13	Seizures	4
Diabetes mellitus	13	Croup	4
		Viral illnesses	4
Intrauterine pregnancy (complicated)	13	Spontaneous abortion	4
		Reflux esophagitis	3
Low back pain other than herniated nucleus pulposus	13	Depression	3
		Ureteral colic	3
Pneumonia	12	Excessive weight gain	2
Overdose	11	Pyelonephritis	2
Concussion	10	Conversion reaction	2
Soft tissue trauma	10	Situational stress reaction	2
Abdominal pain	9	Epididymitis	2
Thrombophlebitis	8	Other	126
Hypertension	8	Total	631

[a]Includes all newborns with jaundice requiring photo therapy, as well as respiratory distress syndrome, congenital defects, etc.
(Modifed from Medley ES, Halstead ML: A family practice residency inpatient service: A review of 631 admissions. J Fam Pract 6:4, 817–822, 1978, with permission.)

it is well known that a substantial amount of everyday teaching and learning takes place on a housestaff level between residents 1 or 2 years apart in their levels of training. There is now a general consensus that the minimal number or "critical mass" of residents in a family practice residency program should be 12 residents (4-4-4). The optimal size of any one program depends on a number of practical considerations, such as: (1) the extent of educational resources; (2) the need for family physicians in the area served by the program; (3) the availability of funding and other kinds of support for the program; (4) the logistics of inpatient teaching rotations; (5) the logistics of night and weekend coverage; and (6) the size of the teaching practice.[3]

The Faculty

The faculty of the typical family practice residency program generally includes at least three or four full-time family physicians, with the number depending on the size of the program. Accreditation requirements call for one full-time equivalent family physician teacher for every six residents in the program, in addition to the program director, who also is preferably a family physician with a background in practice and teaching. The full-time family physician faculty members are actively involved in the teaching practice in the Family Practice Center, and participate actively in other parts of the teaching program, such as conferences and didactic sessions. On a rotational basis, one of them makes daily rounds on the Family Practice Service in the hospital(s), and is available to the residents on call during nights and weekends.

Other specialties are also involved actively in the teaching program, sometimes on a full-time basis and more often on a part-time basis. The specialties most commonly represented in this capacity include internal medicine, pediatrics, obstetrics–gynecology, and psychiatry. University-based and community hospital programs differ considerably in their arrangements for teaching involvement by other specialties. The larger teaching hospitals tend to have existing full-time and part-time teaching staffs involved in the conduct of their respective teaching services. Family practice residencies in smaller community hospitals often employ part-time consultants in the major specialties to teach in the program as well as to arrange and coordinate the teaching efforts by other consultants in their specialty on a voluntary basis.

Most family practice residencies include a full-time or part-time behavioral science teacher on the regular faculty. Jones and colleagues recently studied the patterns of mental health training in U.S. family practice residency programs, and found that more than 1600 individuals are involved in behavioral science teaching in 246 programs, most often on a part-time basis. Of this total, 42 percent are psychiatrists, 21 percent psychologists, and 18 percent social workers.[4]

Clinical pharmacists have taken an increasingly active role in teaching in family practice residencies in recent years. A recent study by Thies and colleagues showed a wide range of teaching and service roles for clinical pharmacists in more than three-fifths of responding programs.[5]

In addition to the above faculty, the typical family practice residency involves a substantial number of volunteer physicians, in family practice and all of the other specialties. They may participate as attending physicians in the Family Practice Center or on hospital teaching services, present didactic sessions, or contribute to periodic teaching conferences. Thus the family practice residency, regardless of its setting or size, invariably involves the active participation of a large number of physicians in all of the specialties as well as nonphysicians in other health professions.

Educational Goals

Goals and objectives for any educational program cannot be developed without understanding the needs for the program, its graduates, and individual residents within the program. Some of the issues requiring consideration in formulating the goals of a family practice residency program are these: (1) What are the needs of the community? (2) What is the "community" being served (socioeconomic, cultural, and geographic)? (3) What kinds of practice settings are likely for program graduates? (4) How are patterns of health care changing, and how do they influence future needs? Resolution of these issues for any given program clearly relates closely to curriculum, resident selection, design and function of the Family Practice Center, and many other elements of the program.

Two overall goals of a family practice residency program might therefore be formulated as follows:

1. To train family physicians able to respond to changing health care needs of the area/region served by the program
2. To produce well-trained clinicians capable of providing definitive care of about 95 percent of the health problems of individuals and their families for which medical care is sought

More specific goal statements for family practice residents have been developed and endorsed by the Society of Teachers of Family Medicine:[6]

The family practice resident shall, after completion of a residency:

1. Demonstrate clinical excellence, utilizing current biomedical knowledge in identifying and managing the medical problems presented by his/her patients
2. Provide continuing and comprehensive care to individuals and families
3. Demonstrate the ability to integrate the behavioral/emotional/social/environmental factors of families in promoting health and managing disease
4. Recognize the importance of maintaining and developing the knowledge, skills, and attitudes required for the best in modern medical practice in a rapidly changing world and pursue a regular and systematic program of life-long learning.
5. Recognize the need and demonstrate the ability to utilize consultation with other medical specialists while maintaining continuity of care
6. Share tasks and responsibility with other health professionals
7. Be aware of the findings of relevant research; understand and critically evaluate this body of research; and apply the results of the research to medical practice
8. Manage his/her practice in a business-like, cost-effective manner which will provide professional satisfaction and time for a rewarding personal life
9. Serve as an advocate for the patient within the health care system
10. Assess the quality of care that he/she provides and actively pursue measures to correct deficiencies
11. Recognize community resources as an integral part of the health care system; participate in improving the health of the community
12. Inform and counsel patients concerning their health problems, recognizing patient and physician backgrounds, beliefs, and expectations
13. Develop mutually satisfying physician–patient relationships to promote comprehensive problem identification and problem solving
14. Use current medical knowledge to identify, evaluate, and minimize risks for patient and family
15. Balance potential benefits, costs, and resources in determining appropriate interventions

Curriculum

The curricular content of a family practice residency program is described in general terms in the recently revised *Essentials for Graduate Training in Family Practice*. The curriculum is directed toward three distinct capability levels:[7]

1. Definitive capability (including, for example, the management of most common clinical and behavioral problems of families and life-threatening emergencies)
2. Partial capability (including the initiation of appropriate diagnostic and/or therapeutic measures for more complex clinical problems requiring consultation and/or referral)
3. Limited capability (including the recognition or suspicion of rare or complex problems for referral)

The curriculum is likewise focused on the various stages of comprehensive care—prevention, early diagnosis of asymptomatic disease, care of symptomatic disease, rehabilitation, and care of terminal illness.

Although there are some individual program and regional differences in the curricula of family practice residencies in various parts of the country, a basic curriculum has emerged in recent years which meets the current criteria of the Residency Review Committee for Family Practice as well as the recommended guidelines of the Residency Assistance Program,[8] a national program jointly sponsored by the American Board of Family Practice, the American Academy of Family Physicians, and the Society of Teachers of Family Medicine.

The resident's experience and training are derived from the care of patients in the Family Practice Center, in the hospital on the Family Practice Service, on inpatient rotations on other services, and in other specialty clinics or community settings. Over a 3-year period, the family practice residency program usually involves teaching rotations of about 1 year in internal medicine (including such medical selectives as cardiology, neurology, and dermatology; 6 months of pediatrics, 3 to 6 months of obstetrics–gynecology, 6 months of surgery and its subspecialties (including ophthalmology, otolaryngology, orthopedics, and urology), and 2 months of emergency medicine. In addition, a strong thread of behavioral science is presented longitudinally over the 3-year program, with or without a 1-month rotation in psychiatry. Table 7–2 illustrates the curriculum in a "typical" family practice

TABLE 7-2. CURRICULUM IN "TYPICAL" FAMILY PRACTICE RESIDENCY

	Inpatient Rotations	Family Practice Center
First year		
Medicine	4 mo	
Pediatrics	3 mo	
Obstetrics–gynecology	2 mo	1–2 half-day/wk
Surgery	2 mo	
Emergency room	1 mo	
Second Year		
Medicine	4 mo	
Pediatrics	3 mo	
Obstetrics–gynecology	2 mo	2–4 half-days/wk
Cardiology	1 mo	
Psychiatry	1 mo	
Emergency room	1 mo	
Third Year		
Medical subspecialties	4 mo	
Surgical subspecialties	4 mo	3–4 half-days/wk
Electives	4 mo	

residency today, and Table 7–3 shows generally accepted minimum durations for some of the major curricular areas.

Although there are many practical reasons leading to the common use of this kind of time-based curriculum, it is important to recognize that the amount of time devoted to a specific curricular area does not fully describe the learning experience or level of competency achieved by the resident on completion of this experience. The value of a particular teaching rotation, for example, depends on such variables as the characteristics of the learning setting, clinical volume, level of resident responsibility, and the resident's motivation and capability levels.

In three instances, interspecialty agreements have been developed specifying recommended core curricular for family practice residents. The first to be developed resulted from the joint efforts of the American Academy of Family Physicians (AAFP) and the American College of Obstetricians and Gynecologists.[9] More recently similar agreements have been concluded between the AAFP and the American College of Cardiology and the American Academy of Ophthalmology. These agreements define in some detail the recommended content of cognitive knowledge and skills at both basic and more advanced competency levels in these respective areas.

Several studies in the past few years have characterized in further detail the clinical experience and training of family practice residents on the major specialty rotations. Meza and Lapsys compared the adult medicine inpatient experience on their family practice adult medicine inpatient service with that of the internal medicine service in the same multispecialty hospital. They found that the range of problems cared for by family practice residents was quite similar to that of the internal medicine resident (Table 7–4), and that the family practice service included a rich and broad experience in general medicine.[10] In pediatrics, a national survey involving an 82 percent response rate polled program directors concerning their assessment regarding level of competency of their family practice residents after their pediatric training, which totalled 9 months (including an average of 5.6 months on pediatrics rotations and 3.4 equivalent months in the Family Practice Center over 3 years). Their perceptions for inpatient and ambulatory care are displayed

TABLE 7-3. MINIMAL DURATION OF CORE CURRICULAR AREAS[a]

General medicine	8 mo
Cardiology	200 hr
Dermatology	60–120 hr
Other medical subspecialties	3 mo
Pediatrics	4 mo
Obstetrics	2 mo
Gynecology	1 mo
General surgery	2 mo
Orthopedics	160–200 hr
Ophthalmology	40–80 hr
Otolaryngology	40–80 hr
Urology	40–80 hr
Emergency medicine	1 mo

[a]Behavioral science teaching presented as longitudinal thread during program.

TABLE 7-4. COMPARATIVE RESIDENT EXPERIENCE ON TWO TEACHING SERVICES[a]

Disease Category	Family Practice Patients (%)		Internal Medicine Patients (%)		Statistical Significance[b]
Cardiovascular	284	(41.0)	166	(28.6)	$P<0.001$
Gastrointestinal	125	(18.1)	137	(23.6)	$P<0.05$
Respiratory	66	(9.5)	67	(11.5)	NS
Neurology	82	(11.8)	64	(11.0)	NS
Endocrine	23	(3.3)	34	(5.9)	$P<0.05$
Miscellaneous	112	(16.2)	112	(19.3)	NS
Total	692		580		

[a]Based on random sample of 251 patients (20 percent of hospital admissions over 1-year period).
[b]Chi-square test for significant differences between the proportion of patients in a disease category for each training program.
(From Meyer F, Lapsys FX: Adult medicine inpatient experience: A comparison of family practice and internal medicine residency services. J Fam Pract 13:701, 1981, with permission.)

in Figures 7–2 A and B, respectively.[11] In obstetrics and gynecology a survey of 190 U.S. family practice residencies in 1975 revealed the level of experience being obtained in normal and abnormal obstetrics by family practice residents in training (Table 7–5).[12] In surgery, a 1981 study (57 percent response rate) identified the range of general surgical procedures that are included in the training of family practice residents (Table 7–6).[13] In psychiatry, a 1981 study with a 64 percent response rate revealed that almost all programs offered psychiatry and behavioral science on a longitudinal basis over 3 years, together with a block rotation on psychiatry (usually 1-month) in 60 percent of programs.[4]

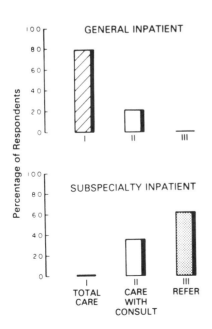

Figure 7-2A. Percentage of respondents indicating the optimal level of competency for family physicians in inpatient child health care. *(From Rabinowitz HK, Hervada AR: Pediatric training in family medicine residency programs. J Fam Pract 11:575, 1980, with permission.)*

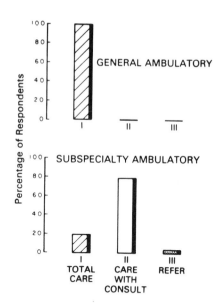

Figure 7–2B. Percentage of respondents indicating the optimal level of competency for family physicians in outpatient child health care. *(From Rabinowitz HK, Hervada AR: Pediatric training in family medicine residency programs. J Fam Pract 11:575, 1980, with permission.)*

Continuity of Care

Continuity of care is an important element in the design, operation, and accreditation of all family practice residency programs. Many pressing and real conflicts arise, however, in all family practice residencies in implementing continuity of care in

TABLE 7-5. EXTENT OF OBSTETRIC EXPERIENCE

No. of Normal Deliveries	No. of Residencies	%
0–49	33	19.0
50–99	56	32.3
100–149	46	26.4
150–199	28	16.1
200–249	9	5.1
250–299	0	0.0
Total	174	100.0

No. of Complicated Deliveries	No. of Residencies	%
0	35	20.2
1–5	20	11.5
6–10	31	17.9
11–15	24	13.9
16–20	19	11.0
21–25	13	7.5
26–50	25	14.5
50	6	3.5
Total	173	100.0

(From Harris BA, Scutchfield FD: Obstetrical and gynecological teaching in family practice residency programs. J Fam Pract 4:749, 1977; data based on a survey of 190 U.S. family practice residency programs during 1975, with permission.)

TABLE 7-6. PROCEDURAL SKILLS

	Percentage of Programs
Proctoscopy	97
Suture	97
Central venous line placement	93
Curretage	93
Paracentesis, thoracentesis	91
Simple fractures	90
Endotrachial intubation	89
Closed tube thoracotomy	69
Vasectomy	68
Peritoneal lavage	65
Tracheostomy	54
Electrosurgery	52
Breast biopsy	49
Hernias	27
Appendectomy	24
Cholecystectomy	20

(From Shamblin WR, Burleson J, Moss CN: Surgical training of family practice residents. J Fam Pract 15:364, 1982, with permission.)

a complex training program, especially due to the numerous commitments of the residents and the differing expectations of the resident by other faculty members and services. Residents frequently find themselves in a double bind, torn between Family Practice Center responsibilities and inpatient responsibilities, including rounds, ward duties, and night call.

There are a number of practical and effective approaches to this dilemma.[14] One important approach is to organize the residency into resident teams, or modules, preferably involving both staff and physical space units within the residency.[15] An 18-resident program may thereby include 3 teams of 6 residents (2 in each residency year) facilitating continuity of care on a team basis and fostering the development of attitudes and skills needed by the residents in future group practice. Another useful approach to providing continuity of care in a family practice residency is by pairing of residents on certain hospital services whereby one resident of the pair covers the inpatient service while the other is in the Family Practice Center.[16,17] Other approaches involve the maintenance of a family practice service by advanced residents, the use of the problem-oriented medical record for improved communication, and the promotion of a group versus solo ethos of patient care by the faculty.[14] In a study of the level of continuity of care actually achieved in one university-based family practice residency program, it was found that third-year residents averaged 83 percent continuity with their individual patients and 70 percent continuity with their assigned families.[18]

Evaluation

Evaluation is a critical component in all educational programs, and has been viewed by Worthen and Sanders as the "most widely discussed but little used phenomena in today's educational systems."[19] The development, however, of effective and often innovative evaluation systems has received strong emphasis in U.S. family practice residency programs. Evaluation has been recognized as an essential part of a feedback loop to the resident, to the teacher, and to the program director. As Corley has pointed out: "Formative in-training evaluation enriches training programs by assessing residents' progressive mastery of professional knowledge, skills and attitudes. It can play a significant role in upgrading a residency."[20]

Evaluation is approached on three levels by most family practice residency programs: (1) at the overall program level; (2) at the level of individual parts of the program (e.g., an inpatient teaching rotation); and (3) at the level of the experience and performance of the individual resident. At the first level, external review by local or national reviewers has been found particularly useful in identifying strengths and weaknesses of programs which might not be readily apparent to those most closely associated with a program. Some departments of family medicine, such as at the University of Iowa and the University of Washington, conduct a regular process of periodic internal review within their networks of affiliated residency programs, involving site visits by faculty not directly involved with the program being reviewed. On the national level, the Residency Assistance Program provides 2-day consultation visits by experienced family practice educators to residency programs requesting assessment and consultation.[8]

The evaluation of individual rotations and individual resident's experience has been addressed in a variety of ways. The experience of family practice residents has been monitored with a problem category index;[21] by practice profiles involving the use of a diagnostic index, the E-book;[22,23] and more recently by diagnosis clusters.[24]

Various methods have been used to evaluate the clinical performance of residents, including chart review,[25] patient profiles,[26] videotape with feedback,[27] and even feedback of patient perceptions.[28] In-training examinations have also been found of value in a number of family practice residencies;[29,30] the in-training examination developed by the American Board of Family Practice is used by many programs today.

Another important dimension of evaluation involves periodic assessment by residents of faculty performance, and this too is being addressed by some programs.[31] An excellent model of evaluation as a means of faculty developed has been described by Whitman and Schwonk based upon ratings by learners, self-ratings, and consultation with an educational consultant.[32]

Costs and Funding

The costs of graduate medical education in any field are substantial. Current estimates for the cost per resident year in family practice are over $50,000, including the resident's salary (average $17,000 per year) and prorated costs for faculty, staff, teaching materials, operational costs of the Family Practice Center, and related costs. There are invariably additional start-up costs of the program before the arrival of residents, especially those costs involved by remodeling, or even new construction, of the Family Practice Center.

There are four major sources of funding to offset program costs: (1) patient care revenue; (2) the contributions of the participating hospital(s); (3) state funding, often on a capitation basis; and (4) grants from federal, foundational, or other sources. The last category must be considered "soft," since these funds are often uncertain from year to year and are intended more for start-up needs than ongoing operational needs. Patient care revenue is an important source of support for the program, but should not be expected to cover more than 50 percent of total progam costs. The contribution of the program's hospital(s) must therefore provide a solid floor of funding for the residency program. Most hospitals with residency programs include house staff costs in their daily per diem charges. Since the house staff contributes directly to the availability and quality of patient care in the hospital, it is reasonable that a small portion of the patient's daily bill be directed to medical education. State funding has been an essential source of support for many family practice residencies throughout the country, and constitutes a wise ongoing investment by the states toward the solution of their common problems of specialty and geographic maldistribution of physicians.

Experience over the years has clearly shown that strong sponsorship by the participating hospitals is vital to the successful operation and viability of any family practice residency. The association of family practice residencies and their sponsoring hospitals meets a number of needs for each party. Through this association the family practice residency acquires a site for inpatient care of its own patients, access to both inpatient teaching services and selected ambulatory services (e.g., emergency room), and a linkage to other clinical and teaching resources of the institution. In turn, the participating hospital realizes several important benefits, including (1) some increase in utilization of both inpatient and ambulatory hospital services; (2) maintenance and enhancement of quality of patient care; (3) house staff coverage of inpatients on teaching services, as well as increased capability to respond to and manage inhospital emergencies; (4) augmented opportunities for continuing education for the medical staff; and (5) positive image of the hospital in the community. Some of the benefits to sponsoring hospitals are directly measurable, others are less tangible but often more important (i.e., especially those related to an expanding primary care base for the hospital). A simple approach to estimating the contributions of a family practice residency to the utilization of hospital services is illustrated in Table 7–7.[33] A useful and more indepth framework to analyze the direct, indirect, and intangible costs and benefits of such a program in a community hospital has recently been described by Patrick and his colleagues.[34]

TABLE 7-7. CONTRIBUTIONS OF FAMILY PRACTICE RESIDENCY TO UTILIZATION OF HOSPITAL SERVICES

	FPC Patients Admitted Directly	FPC Patients Admitted by Referral	Graduates' Patients Admitted Directly	Graduates' Patients Admitted by Referral
Annual number of admissions				
Annual number of patient days				
Average cost per patient day				
Estimated hospital charges				
Laboratory charges				
X-Ray charges				
Total hospital charges				
Collection ratio				
Estimated total income to hospital				

(From Geyman JP: Family practice residencies and their sponsoring hospitals: Mutual interests and unrecognized potential. J Fam Pract 11:1019, 1980, with permission.)

COMMENT

Four major points, in my view, stand out as especially important in commenting upon the overall development of graduate training in family practice over the last 15 years.

1. Viability and Quality of Family Practice Residencies: The 1970s and early 1980s have amply demonstrated that excellent family practice residency programs can be developed and maintained with the capability to attract sustained student interest and to produce well-trained graduate family physicians to meet public needs. These programs have been very competitive in attracting residents of high caliber, and the fill rate has averaged about 97 percent. A number of extensive graduate follow-up studies have demonstrated that graduates feel generally well prepared for the needs of their practices and have a high level of professional satisfaction in their work.[35-39] A close correlation has been documented between the content of their residency training and the content of their future practice. In late 1975, for example, a large practice content study was completed representing the health care problems of about 88,000 patients presenting to 118 family physicians (including 82 family practice residents) over a 25-month period. This study revealed that the content of teaching practices was almost identical to that of nonteaching practices in Virginia.[40]

   Despite the organizational and funding difficulties of starting new programs in a time of constrained resources, there has been very little attrition among these programs. In addition, quality control mechanisms have been developed which will assure the future viability of these programs.

2. Need for Flexibility: First-rate family practice residency programs can and should be developed in varied settings ranging from university medical centers to 200-bed general hospitals in smaller outlying communities. The organizational approaches and structure, however, of programs in such diverse settings must necessarily be flexible and adapted to local and institutional needs and resources. There is no single or fixed blueprint for a successful family practice residency. The quality and value of learning experiences for residents depend on such factors as the characteristics of the learning setting, clinical volume, level of resident responsibility, availability and competence of teaching faculty, and the motivation and capability levels of individual residents.

   Beyond the importance of organizational flexibility, there remains a need for curricular flexibility to allow continued innovations in teaching strategies and appropriate revision of curricular content as the specialty evolves. Rigidity is the inevitable hazard of teaching programs in all fields as they mature, and this tendency is spurred on by the accreditation process. With regard to predoctoral medical education, Abramson has recently described several important diseases of the curriculum (Table 7–8).[41] These same diseases occur in graduate medical education, and family practice education is at full risk for these endemic problems.

3. Value of University Affiliation: The increasing trend toward university affiliation of community hospital-based family practice residencies reflects a growing awareness that more can be accomplished through the cooperative efforts of groups of programs than by isolated individual programs.

TABLE 7-8. DISEASE OF THE CURRICULUM

Disease	Underlying Problems
Curriculosclerosis	Hardening of the categories
Carcinoma of the curriculum	Uncontrollable growth of one segment of curriculum
Curriculoarthritis	Dysfunction of articulations and communications between related segments of curriculum
Iatrogenic curriculitis	Excessive tampering and meddling with curriculum
Curriculum hypertrophy	Progressive increase in didactic teaching requirements
Idiopathic curriculitis	Mask for poor teaching
Curriculum ossification	Casting in concrete; often epidemic

(From Abramson S: Diseases of the curriculum. J Med Educ 53:951, 1978, with permission.)

The partnership between medical school departments of family practice and affiliated family practice residencies within a network provides many benefits to all parties, including sharing of clinical and educational resources, joint planning and problem solving, enhanced linkages with predoctoral and continuing medical education activities, and the potential for collaborative research.[42] Table 7–9 lists the various benefits to the university and to the community hospital through an affiliation relationship.

4. Importance of Shared Funding Sources: As noted earlier, there are four major sources of funding to support family practice residency programs: (1) patient care revenue; (2) contributions from participating hospitals; (3) state funding, often on a capitation basis; and (4) other grants (e.g., federal, foundations). Many primary care services are inadequately compensated under current third-party reimbursement policies, and extensive teaching commitments necessarily limit the service capability of a program. It is, therefore, not possible for a program to generate much more than one-half of its total costs from patient care services. The continued support of participating hospitals is vital, together with ongoing supplemental funding by government.

While the principal focus of family practice residency programs is naturally upon resident training, they have much to contribute in other areas—predoctoral and postgraduate teaching as well as research. At the predoctoral level, family practice residencies provide excellent learning settings for advanced medical students in family practice clerkships. Several kinds of benefits accrue to residency programs involved in such clerkships: (1) expansion of the capacity of teams within the residency; (2) provision of opportunities to residents to teach (and learn through teaching); (3) assistance with special projects within the residency; and (4) assessment of potential future resident applicants through daily contact with medical students during their clerkships.[43]

It is inevitable that family practice residencies will become active sources of

TABLE 7-9. BENEFITS OF UNIVERSITY AFFILIATION

Benefits to Community Hospital	Benefits to University
Assistance in residency program development through the pooled experience of other affiliated programs	Increased opportunity to contribute to the training of the required number of family physicians
Assistance with the formulation of education objectives and the evaluation of resident performance	Extension of continuing medical education to a larger area beyond the medical school itself
Expansion of teaching resources through visiting professor programs and various teaching materials	Increased clinical resources and learning opportunities for medical students, residents, and allied health personnel
Augmented effectiveness of teaching through teacher development programs	Opportunities to participate in the development of new models of education and health care delivery
Enhanced potential for recruitment of residents of high caliber because of university affiliation and associated medical student clerkship programs	Enhanced potential for collaborative research in family practice
Increased opportunities for resident electives, both at the university and elsewhere within the network	Facilitation of improved linkages between primary, secondary and tertiary care on a regional basis
Potential for increased funding through the university and/or grant funds acquired for the network	Potential for increased utilization of the university for consultation and referral

continuing medical education in their areas. The residency program of itself is an educational system involving the Family Practice Center, related hospital(s), physicians, and other health professionals within the community. This system usually can accommodate more learners, and the educational needs of practicing family physicians and advanced family practice residents are similar in many aspects. Self-assessment and teaching methods which are developed for residents are equally applicable to practicing physicians, and can be made readily available to larger numbers of practicing family physicians because of the wide geographic distribution of these programs.[43]

Family practice residencies likewise have considerable opportunities to become involved in research and innovative demonstration projects whether related to teaching or clinical practice. These residency programs are directly involved in the definition and implementation of modern concepts in family medicine, and increasingly have available the necessary tools and resources for substantive research of various types.[44] Some programs have already become involved in research activities. If the teaching practices and Family Practice Centers of family practice residencies are considered "laboratories," then the faculty and residents in these programs can contribute immeasurably to research in family medicine.

Much progress has been made over the past 15 years in the development of family practice residency programs of high quality throughout the country. Their capacity, however, still falls short of the need. The challenge ahead is to maintain the standards of excellence which have been established and to develop additional programs at a rate which will allow family practice to make an impact on the delivery of health care which is so urgently needed.

REFERENCES

1. Geyman JP: The "one-and-two" program: A new direction in family practice residency training. J Med Educ 52:999, 1977
2. Medley ES, Halstead ML: A family practice residency inpatient service: A review of 631 admissions. J Fam Pract 6:817, 1978
3. Geyman JP: Prevention of complications in initial development of family practice residency programs. J Fam Pract 4:1111, 1977
4. Jones LR, Badger LW, Parlour RR, et al.: Mental health training in family practice residency programs. J Fam Pract 15:329, 1982
5. Thies PW, Helling DK, Rakel RE: Clinical pharmacy services in family practice residency programs. J Fam Pract 15:1173, 1982
6. STFM Board approves educational goal statements. Fam Med Times 10(5):11, 1978
7. Geyman JP: A competency-based curriculum as an organizing framework in family practice residencies. J Fam Pract 1:34, 1974
8. Stern TL, Chaisson GM: The Residency Assistance Program in family practice. J Fam Pract 5:379, 1977
9. Stern TL: A landmark in interspecialty cooperation. J Fam Pract 5:523, 1977
10. Meza F. Lapsys FX: Adult medicine inpatient experience: A comparison of family practice and internal medicine residency services. J Fam Pract 13:701, 1981
11. Rabinowitz HK, Hervada AR: Pediatric training in family medicine residency programs. J Fam Pract 11:575, 1980
12. Harris BA, Scutchfield FD: Obstetrical and gynecological teaching in family practice residency programs. J Fam Pract 4:749, 1977
13. Shamblin WR, Burleson J, Moss CN: Surgical training of family practice residents. J Fam Pract 15:364, 1982
14. Geyman JP: Continuity of care in family practice: Implementing continuity in a family practice residency program. J Fam Pract 2:445, 1975
15. Geyman JP: A modular basis of resident training for family practice. J Med Educ 47:292, 1972
16. Phillips TJ, Holler JW: A university family medicine program. J Med Educ 46:821, 1971
17. Lincoln JA: The three-year paired residency program: A solution to a teaching dilemma. J Fam Pract 1:31, 1974
18. Curtis P, Rogers J: Continuity of care in a family practice residency program. J Fam Pract 8:975, 1979
19. Worthen BR, Sanders JR: Educational Evaluation: Theory and Practice. Worthington, Ohio, Charles A. Jones, 1973
20. Corley JB: In-training residency evaluation. J Fam Pract 3:499, 1976
21. Tindall HL, Henderson RA, Cole AF: Evaluating family practice residents with a problem category index. J Fam Pract 2:353, 1975
22. Boisseau V, Froom J: Practice profiles in evaluating the clinical experience of family medicine trainees. J Fam Pract 6:801, 1978
23. Terrell HP: Documentation of resident exposure to disease entities. J Fam Pract 6:317, 1978
24. Schneeweiss R: Diagnosis clusters: A new approach to reporting the diagnostic content of family practice residents' ambulatory experiences. J Fam Pract 20:487, 1985
25. Kane RL, Leigh EH, Feigel DW, et al.: A method for evaluating patient care and auditing skills of family practice residents. J Fam Pract 2:205, 1975
26. Given CW, Simoni L, Gallin RS, Sprafka RJ: The use of computer generated patient profiles to evaluate resident performance in patient care. J Fam Pract 5:831, 1977

27. Zabarenko RN, Magero J, Zabarenko L: Use of videotape in teaching psychologic medicine. J Fam Pract 4:559, 1977
28. Falco D: Patient perception as a tool for evaluation and feedback in family practice resident training. J Fam Pract 10:471, 1980
29. Donnelly JE, Yankaskas B, Gjerde, C, et al.: An in-training assessment examination in family medicine: Report of a pilot project. J Fam Pract 5:987, 1977
30. Geyman JP, Brown T: An in-training examination for residents in family practice. J Fam Pract 3:409, 1976
31. Kelly J, Woiwode D: Faculty evaluation by residents in a family medicine residency program. J Fam Pract 4:693, 1977
32. Whitman N, Schwenk T: Faculty evaluation as a means of faculty development. J Fam Pract 14(6):1097, 1982
33. Geyman JP: Family practice residencies and their sponsoring hospitals: Mutual interests and unrecognized potential. J Fam Pract 11:1019, 1980
34. Patrick K, Castle CH, Danforth N: Impact of a family practice residency on a community hospital: A case study of costs and benefits. J Fam Pract 14:727, 1982
35. Ciriacy EW, Bland CJ, Stoller JE, et al.: Graduate follow-up in the University of Minnesota Affiliated Hospitals Residency Training Program in Family Practice and Community Health. J Fam Pract 11:719, 1980
36. Mayo F, Wood M, Marsland DW, et al.: Graduate follow-up in the Medical College of Virginia/Virginia Commonwealth University Family Practice Residency System. J Fam Pract 11:731, 1980
37. Geyman JP, Cherkin DC, Deisher JB, et al.: Graduate follow-up in the University of Washington Family Practice Residency Network. J Fam Pract 11:743, 1980
38. Hecht RC, Farrell JG: Graduate follow-up in the University of Wisconsin Family Practice Residency Program. J Fam Pract 14:549, 1982
39. Black RR, Schmittling G, Stern TL: Characteristics and practice patterns of family practice residency graduates in the United States. J Fam Pract 11:767, 1980
40. Marsland DW, Wood M, Mayo F: A data bank for patient care, curriculum and research in family practice: 526,196 patient problems. J. Fam Pract 3:25–28, 36–68, 1976
41. Abramson S: Diseases of the curriculum. J Med Educ 53:951, 1978
42. Geyman JP, Brown TC: A network model for decentralized family practice residency training. J Fam Pract 3:621, 1976
43. Geyman JP: Family practice residencies and the continuum of medical education. J Fam Pract 5:743, 1977
44. Geyman JP: Research in the family practice residency program. J Fam Pract 5:245, 1977

8 Continuing Education in Family Practice

Traditional continuing medical education (CME) keeps physicians aware of the state of the art. It has limitations, however, as a quality-assurance tool: it is memory based, involves a group endeavor with diffuse goals, often unrelated to practice, is an inappropriate remedy for many problems in patient care, is hampered by poor-quality evaluation, and is governed more by market factors than educational outcomes. The self-study of practice and practice-linked CME offer rich potential for development. The physician's monitoring of his work, with appropriate improvements in performance, is valuable CME. Computers provide facts and guidance at the time and place the physician is developing diagnostic plans, diminishing reliance on memory. The next step in CME is for hospitals, societies, and medical schools to perfect methods of self-study of practice and practice-linked CME.

Phil R. Manning[1]

The steady growth of medical knowledge in recent years, together with continuously changing patterns of practice and an increasing emphasis on public accountability in medicine as in other fields, have made continuing medical education an area of major concern in the United States today. Although the concept of life-long learning in medicine has been endorsed on a voluntary basis for many years, the past 15 years have seen a progressive momentum toward mandatory continuing medical education (CME) for all physicians. CME requirements have now been adopted as requisites for membership in many national and state medical societies, hospital medical staffs, and, as noted earlier, as legislated requirements in 24 states and territories for reregistration of the license to practice medicine.[2]

Continuing medical education has burgeoned to become a large industry in this country. In 1976 it was estimated by the newly formed Alliance for Continuing Medical Education that approximately $2 billion were then being spent each year for CME, including the costs of faculty remuneration, conduct of programs and accreditation.[3] According to the American Medical Association, the number of CME courses per year increased from about 1000 in 1955 to more than 8500 in 1981.[4]

As CME has become recognized as increasingly important, its goals, content, and methods have been subjected to closer scrutiny. It has become painfully obvious that this is a special kind of education which requires different approaches from those taken in predoctoral and graduate medical education.

Each physician's needs for CME represent an individual matter, even within the same field. It is difficult for busy physicians to be aware of their individual needs at any given time, and to compare their own knowledge and performance with that of their colleagues.

Since CME must be directed in so many different directions and meet such a diverse range of individualized needs, development of curricula and appropriate methods for such education becomes a formidable task. The task is made even more complex when one realizes that as many as 50 percent of practicing physicians are often said to be poorly motivated to pursue their own continuing education.

Several special features of continuing medical education illustrate the complexities of this area: (1) both students and teachers are usually part time; (2) the classroom model, or even models derived from graduate medical education, are not usually applicable to the purposes of CME; (3) the objectives of CME are more particular and specific than traditional predoctoral and graduate medical education; and (4) CME is inseparable from patient care, and ideally should lead to behavioral changes in the physician as relates to the use of new knowledge in patient management, as well as to improved outcomes of patient care.

The purpose of this chapter is to present an overview of continuing medical education as it applies to family practice. Some generic problems of CME will first be considered, together with the basic requisites for effective postgraduate learning. Some current directions of CME in family practice will then be outlined, as well as the developing roles of medical school departments of family practice and some useful approaches for individual family physicians in acquiring more meaningful continuing education.

SOME GENERIC PROBLEMS OF CONTINUING MEDICAL EDUCATION

Brief consideration of various basic problems involved in CME serves to illustrate the complexities and challenges of this subject.

Expansion of Medical Information

There is no question that the volume of medical information is expanding at an exponential rate in recent years, but the implications of this process are controversial. Some believe that we are involved in a "knowledge explosion." In a paper examining information technologies and health care, for example, Moore has projected a 10 percent annual increment of new medical knowledge and estimated that 5 percent of the physician's total medical knowledge becomes obsolescent each year.[5] That a "publication explosion" has occurred cannot be denied. There are now about 2,000.000 articles published each year in the biomedical literature.[6] A good case can be made, however, that the amount of clinically applicable medical knowledge has not increased at such a rapid rate. Weiss denies the existence of a true "knowledge explosion" in this way.[7]

> The semblance of a knowledge explosion has come from using the wrong yardstick. No doubt, there has been a data explosion, liberally equatable with an information explosion, though not all of the collected data are truly informative. Furthermore we are also faced with a publication explosion. But knowledge explosion? Not by criteria of measurement on a scale of relevance.

McWhinney suggests that medical knowledge cannot be viewed simply as information-based, but includes two additional elements: (1) clinical craftsmanship as a skill, and (2) insight and awareness as an integral part of the physician's personality.[8]

Lack of Correlation Between Knowledge and Performance

Many studies have demonstrated that CME may be effective in transmitting knowledge as measured by pre- and post-CME knowledge tests. It is well known, however, that the medical knowledge of physicians often correlates poorly with their clinical performance. Ashbaugh and McKean, for example, showed that 94 percent of deficiencies in surgical practice identified by 55 audits of 5499 patient records were in the area of performance, while only 6 percent were on the basis of lack of knowledge.[9]

There are undoubtedly many reasons why physicians' practice behaviors frequently do not change based on newly acquired medical knowledge. These include force of habit, skepticism, medical "fashion," time constraints, economic disincentives, pressures by patients, and inadequate effort (i.e., time and priority) in revising one's practice methods. In addition, Scott has pointed out the subtle and easily overlooked biases that any physician may harbor, and the need to adopt habits of more critical thought.[10]

Irrelevance of Content

It is likewise readily apparent that the content of most continuing medical education programs as traditionally offered bears little resemblance to the specific learning needs of the individual physician. The dimensions of this problem are graphically stated by Brown in this way:[11]

> The concept of continuing medical education conjures up a roomful of preoccupied but hopeful physicians at a community hospital, anticipating a learned presentation by the medical school faculty either in person or by way of educational television, two-way radio or other media. The members of the audience are caught between the demands of their practices and the hope that such an educational program will somehow be useful in the care of the patients. But such a teacher or planner-oriented approach is both limited and limiting since it may only incidentally or accidentally meet the needs of the learner and possibly less often the needs of the patient. Diagnosis of patient care needs seldom precedes educational therapy.

Logistic Barriers to CME

Physicians often find themselves practicing under circumstances which make further programmed education difficult. Time is short, and the demands of their practices, families, and communities are great. They can leave their practices only occasionally, coverage of their patients may present a problem, and traditional CME has become very expensive. In most cases, physicians must individually schedule their own time off and cease income-producing activities in order to keep up to date with current developments. The demands of solo practice particularly aggravate these kinds of problems. To this extent, therefore, medicine can be said to lack an organizational structure which facilitates the continuing education and retraining of physicians.[12]

Ineffective Teaching Methods

Much of traditional continuing medical education is conducted by the lecture method, an approach which violates classic learning theory as to how adults learn.

This method has been demonstrated to be a comparatively ineffective method of teaching, partly due to the lack of active involvement of the learner and partly due to the exclusive focus of this method on information transfer alone. As pointed out by Miller:[13]

> There is ample evidence to support the view that adult learning is not most efficiently achieved through systematic subject instruction. It is accomplished by involving learners in identifying problems and seeking ways to solve them. It does not come in categorical bundles but in a growing need to know. It may initially seem wanting in content that pleases experts, but it ultimately incorporates knowledge in a context that has meaning. It is in short a process model of education.

Lack of Clear Goals and Methods of CME

There is general agreement among those who have carefully considered the role and purpose of CME that it should address three basic goals: (1) to improve physician knowledge; (2) to improve physician performance; and (3) to improve patient outcomes.[10,14-16] Most traditional CME activities, however, have addressed the first goal without any relationship to the latter two goals. Most studies to date have shown that traditional CME in its various forms has not positively influenced either physician performance or patient outcomes.[17,18] Yet the assumption has been made by many that the transfer of more medical information will meet the needs of participating physicians and their patients. The extent of this misperception is illustrated by the rapid trend toward mandatory CME. In the short span of 7 years between 1971 and 1978, 20 states passed legislation requiring designated numbers of CME credits for relicensure.[19] Manning observes that this kind of legislation had its roots in various social and political events, such as the passage of the Medicare law in 1965, that made physician accountability a public issue.[1] The problem with mandatory CME as a quality assurance method is succinctly summarized by Wilbur:[3]

> Education cannot assure knowledge; knowledge does not insure competence; and competence does not assure good performance. My opposition is to the misuse of a valuable commodity—continuing medical education—by making it mandatory. We are attempting to make CME do things it cannot, such as assure competence, knowledge, and quality patient care.

The complexities of this issue are further described by Sanazaro in these terms:[20]

> In the absence of alternatives, CME must remain the foundation stone of professional commitment to maintaining competence. But we should face up to some of its serious limitations. Specifically, CME cannot be relied upon to remove deficiencies in performance when the physicians in question already possess the necessary knowledge and simply do not apply it. Also, it is possible that those physicians most in need of CME are not able to attend conferences designed specifically to assit them in better understanding the reasons why a change in their performance is desirable. Then there is the observation that many physicians who are not providing adequate care nonetheless believe they are keeping up with new developments and feel no need for CME.[21] And finally, it is a well documented fact that on the average, with advancing age, physicians devote less effort to CME, demonstrate less cognitive learning and perform at a lower level.[21-27] Physicians under 40 years of age do more in CME and achieve better results on tests and in practice than those past 60, on the average. Taken together,

these considerations support the conclusion that CME may well be least effective in those who most need it.

SOME REQUISITES FOR CONTINUING MEDICAL EDUCATION

Brief reference to some well-accepted principles of learning is of interest before focusing on CME in family practice. It is currently believed that five basic conditions must be met for meaingful learning by adults: (1) Students must be adequately motivated to change their behavior. (2) They must be aware of the inadequacy of their present behavior (and the superiority of the behavior they are required to adopt). (3) They must have a clear picture of the new behavior. (4) They must have opportunities to practice the new behavior with a sequence of appropriate materials. (5) They must get continuing reinforcement of the new behavior.[27]

Two additional points have an important bearing on the learning process. It is well known that there is a forgetting curve—information which is not related to one's continuing practice is easily forgotten. In addition, each of us has our own individual style of learning. Some will learn best by reading, others by small-group patient-oriented discussions, and still others by self-instructional media.

These principles can be formulated into four basic requisites for meaningful continuing medical education: (1) a need to know (preferably related to patient care); (2) an active process (preferably problem-oriented instead of subject-oriented); (3) a continuous relevance to everyday medical practice (with the educational experience designed to meet identified learning needs); and (4) a format which fits the individual physician's learning style.

That these principles can be effective in meeting all of the three basic goals of CME is well illustrated by a recent example. The Professional Competence Assurance Program (PROCAP) was developed at the University of California in San Francisco as an individualized CME program based upon patient care appraisal of physicians' performance in office practice. Criteria were developed by a broad-based, participatory basis for the "ideal" diagnosis and treatment of hypertension. A group of internists and family physicians in the Bay Area were invited to participate in the project involving baseline audit, an individualized educational program involving a seminar or small-group conference call, and reassessment 12 months later. Forty-eight physicians completed the program. The process and outcome criteria are listed in Table 8–1 together with the comparative adherence to criteria at baseline and reassessment times. Improvements were demonstrated in both physician performance and outcomes of patient care.[28]

CURRENT APPROACHES TO CONTINUING EDUCATION IN FAMILY PRACTICE

Today's approaches to continuing education in family practice are based on some of the educational principles which have been mentioned, and are directly addressing some of the generic problems of CME which were considered earlier.

Profiling and Indexing of Practice Experience
Several methods have been described in recent years whereby the practicing experience of family physicians can be readily described in profile form.[29-31] The Il-

TABLE 8-1. BASELINE ADHERENCE TO CRITERIA COMPARED WITH REASSESSMENT LEVELS IN TREATMENT OF 953 PATIENTS FROM 48 PHYSICIANS' PRACTICES

	Baseline Percent	Reassessment Percent
History		
Renal signs and symptoms	55	60[a]
Neurologic signs and symptoms	82	87[a]
Risk factors and family history	83	86
Physical examination		
Funduscopic examination	62	57[a]
Laboratory		
Urine analysis for protein	77	76
Urine analysis for casts	74	75
Creatinine or blood urea nitrogen	84	82
Therapy		
Use of medications		
Beta-blockers	25.8 (246)	30.3 (289)[a]
Vasodilators	9.6 (92)	13.7 (131)[a]
Reserpine	9.1 (87)	5.9 (56)[a]
Methyldopa	14.2 (135)	13.1 (125)
Measurement of blood pressure in multiple positions	21	46[a]
Patient education		
Concerning disease	58	70[a]
Concerning diet	61	67[a]
Outcome		
Normotensive $\leq$ 90 mm Hg	74	81[a]

[a]Significant ($P<.05$). Only criteria with less than 85 percent compliance are listed.
(From Gullion DS, Adamson E, Watts MSM: The effect of an individualized practice-based CME program on physician performance and patient outcomes. West J Med 138:582, 1983, with permission.)

linois Council on Continuing Medical Education, for example, developed a handbook for physicians describing a profiling method and outlining an approach to developing a personal learning plan based on individual needs.[29] At the University of Wisconsin a successful program has been developed based on the Individual Physician Profile, which is derived by recording over a 4-week period the age and sex of every patient encountered (in the office, hospital, home, or by telephone); presenting symptoms; significant findings; major diagnoses; tests ordered; and disposition. The physician's profile is then used as the basis for an individualized self-assessment examination and educational consultation concerning specific learning experiences needed.[30] More recently, Schneeweiss has developed a new technique of profiling a family physician's ambulatory experience by diagnosis clusters, which aggregate morbidity data in a comparatively small number of categories, retain clinical specificity, and permit comparisons with peers in a group practice.[31]

Indexing systems have also been developed whereby family physicians can record on simple index cards the names and important clinical information for patients with selected problems.[32] A sample index card is shown in Figure 8–1, and the various advantages of this kind of system are listed in Table 8–2.

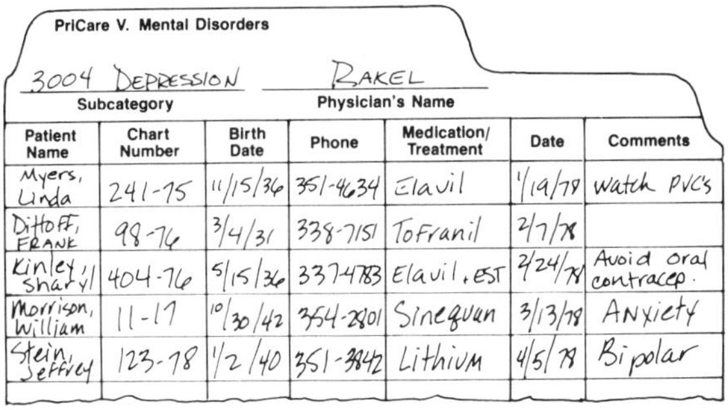

PriCare V. Mental Disorders

3004 DEPRESSION — Subcategory

RAKEL — Physician's Name

Patient Name	Chart Number	Birth Date	Phone	Medication/ Treatment	Date	Comments
Myers, Linda	241-75	11/15/36	351-4634	Elavil	1/19/78	watch PVC's
Dittoff, FRANK	98-76	3/4/31	338-7151	Tofranil	2/7/78	
Kinley, Sharyl	404-76	5/15/36	337-4783	Elavil, EST	2/24/78	Avoid oral contracep.
Morrison, William	11-17	10/30/42	354-2801	Sinequan	3/13/78	Anxiety
Stein, Jeffrey	123-78	1/2/40	351-3842	Lithium	4/5/78	Bipolar

Figure 8-1. Sample problem indexing card. *(From Rakel RE: Indexing in office practice: A system for monitoring high-risk patients and filing medical literature. Cont Educ 9:30, 1978, with permission.)*

Increasing Use of Problem-Oriented Medical Record

The problem-oriented medical record has been widely adopted by family practice teaching programs and has received growing acceptance by many practicing family physicians. The logical format of this record system not only affords improved communication among colleagues and consultants, but also facilitates assessment of quality of care through audit and data retrieval of clinical problems encountered.

Increasing Use of Medical Audit

Audit of medical records both in the office and in the hospital is increasingly emphasized in family practice, and has the potential to "close the loop" between knowledge and performance. Audit can clearly facilitate the physician's ongoing learning and the improvement of patient care through the basic steps involved in the process: (1) identification of an important problem area for audit; (2) setting of criteria by peers; (3) conduct of the audit; (4) educational response to deficits noted; and (5) reaudit of the problem at a later date to determine if improvements in patient care have actually taken place.

Most family practice residency programs stress the use of audit as a means of evaluating the quality of patient care and of learning skills which can facilitate

TABLE 8-2. ADVANTAGES OF PROBLEM INDEXING

1. Identify patients with similar problems or medications.
2. Simplify recall when updating of treatment is necessary.
3. Identify patients for whom medications must be changed to avoid newly recognized hazards.
4. Simplify recall for periodic evaluation of chronic problems.
5. Assist with self-audit by:
   a. Assessment of diagnostic accuracy
   b. Identification of areas to be stressed in continuing education
   c. Identification of conditions rarely encountered (or missed)
6. Analysis of practice content for design of teaching objectives.
7. Simplify collection of data for clinical research.
8. Identify new syndromes or unique associations between problems.
9. Retrieve cases for recertification.

(From Rakel RE: Indexing in office practice: A system for monitoring high-risk patients and filing medical literature. Cont Educ 9:30, 1978, with permission.)

the continuing education of graduates in their future practices. Some programs, such as the Family Medicine Program at the University of Rochester, have utilized audit for critical event outcome studies as a teaching tool.[33] One study of perceptions of formal in-training evaluation by residents in 20 U.S. family practice residency programs demonstrated that chart audit and regular chart review were seen by residents as having the greatest educational value of all evaluation methods used.[34]

It can be anticipated that various forms of medical audit and patient care appraisal will become commonplace in family practice as trends toward group practice, utilization review, and office applications of microcomputers continue.

Self-Assessment

The Connecticut and Ohio Academies of Family Physicians have conducted a successful self-testing and CME program since 1968 known as the Core Content Review of Family Medicine. The most comprehensive self-assessment program in family practice to date, however, is the Home Study Self-assessment Program developed by the American Academy of Family Physicians. This program consists of multimedia teaching materials, pre- and posttests, yearly examinations, and booklets providing answers, discussion, and references for each examination question. This program covers 70 subject areas essential to family practice and extends over a 6-year period, the interval established by the American Board of Family Practice as a requisite for recertification.

Increased Use of Small-Group Teaching and Self-Instruction

The traditional emphasis on the lecture as a primary teaching method has fallen into disrepute in recent years as ineffective in affecting behavioral changes in learners. Many CME programs in family practice today are giving more emphasis to other teaching methods, particularly small-group interactive teaching, multimedia teaching, and programmed learning units for self-instruction. The most recent addition to this approach is the use of microcomputers for problem solving clinical simulations which are now available on a subscription basis.[35]

Learning Through Reading

Despite the proliferation in recent years of various kinds of teaching modalities, especially involving audiovisual materials, reading remains an essential method of continuing education. A recent study based on personal interviews showed that journals are still the most used resource for continuing medical education.[36] A variety of filing systems have been developed to facilitate ready retrieval of articles. One recent study of filing systems for medical literature showed that alphabetical and numerical systems are most commonly used in U.S. family practice residency programs.[37]

Recent years have seen important advances in the types and content of literature in family practice. *The Journal of Family Practice*, for example, represents a major departure from review papers written for the family physician by consultants in the other specialties. Most of the papers in this journal represent original work in family practice settings by family physicians and others involved in the developing discipline of family medicine. The continued expansion of this literature base of original work based on careful studies of the teaching and practice of family medicine should allow family physicians to take a more critical and scholarly approach to patient care.

Learning Through Teaching

As more family practice teaching programs have developed in medical schools and community hospitals, opportunities have increased for practicing family physicians to become involved with teaching in various ways. Some serve as preceptors for medical students in their own practices, others participate in resident teaching in nearby family practice residency programs, and still others participate in collaborative research projects involving their practices and teaching programs. As family physicians are exposed to younger, more recently trained students and residents through the teaching process, the interchange is inevitably a learning experience for all involved.

Certification and Recertification by the American Board of Family Practice

The American Board of Family Practice (ABFP) was established in 1969, and was the first specialty to require recertification (at intervals of 6 years). The ABFP is independent of the American Academy of Family Physicians (AAFP). Although the great majority of board-certified family physicians are Academy members, board certification is not a requirement for AAFP membership.

The ABFP has established the following eligibility requirements to take the certifying examination: (1) completion of an approved 3-year family practice residency and (2) completion of at least 300 approved CME credit hours acceptable to the ABFP.*

The certifying examination is a 2-day examination including multiple choice, pictorial, and patient management problems. The recertification examination may involve a similar 2-day cognitive examination, but most candidates opt for a 1-day cognitive examination plus review of a total of 20 patient records representing 5 selected categories. These categories may be selected from among 20 categories, and are subject to verification and audit by the ABFP. In order to facilitate the learning process and value of office record review the ABFP has recently made available to participating family physicians an excellent series of Reference Guides for the 20 problem areas. Each provides recommended criteria for the diagnosis, management, patient education, and follow-up of each problem.

ROLES FOR DEPARTMENTS OF FAMILY PRACTICE

Departments of family practice to date have necessarily given top priority to the development of predoctoral and graduate teaching programs. They have great potential, however, to contribute to continuing medical education through the following kinds of future directions.[38]

1. Incorporate continuing education into the continuum of teaching in family practice: An active process of self-learning should be emphasized and modeled in predoctoral and graduate teaching programs in family practice. In addition, as competency-based curricula and more effective teaching methods are developed and refined in family practice residencies, there

---

*Prior to 1978, candidates could qualify for the ABFP examination by meeting the CME requirement together with practice eligibility through a minimum of 6 years of active family practice.

can be more productive overlap between graduate and postgraduate education in family practice. Departments of family practice have both the opportunity and the responsibility to relate to the surrounding area or region as their "campus," including acceptance of an active role in CME for practicing family physicians. Family practice refresher courses should be more than didactic sessions; they should provide opportunities for self-assessment and problem-oriented small-group interactive learning. Departments of family practice can also serve as an advocate for practicing family physicians in arranging for short-term learning experiences provided by other clinical departments.

2. Decentralize educational programs on a regional basis: The development of regional teaching programs, on a network basis, especially at the graduate level, allows new relationships to be established with practicing physicians over a wide area. As noted in the last chapter, such networks afford closer communication with medical school and community-based faculty, opportunities to teach in nearby residency programs, and access to clinical methods being developed in teaching programs.

3. Develop educational support methods: Several approaches are of particular value in this respect: (1) a teaching bank for multimedia self-instructional materials; (2) self-assessment materials; (3) profiling and indexing methods to analyze the practice experience of family physicians; and (4) consultation with regard to useful ways to audit or otherwise examine one's practice experience in selected areas. In addition, exchanges can be arranged between third-year family practice residents and individual family physicians in partnership or group practice. These exchanges can allow residents to gain a better perspective of anticipated practice settings (with supervision and teaching provided by the physicians' associates), while providing family physicians coverage of their practices as they pursue selective CME experiences within the residency program.

4. Involve practicing family physicians in part-time teaching: Practicing family physicians have much to offer medical students and residents in training. Students and residents greatly value "real world" role models and the teaching input for those engaged in family practice in varied settings. Departments of family practice can augment the teaching skills of part-time teachers and contribute to their satisfaction and learning derived from teaching by conducting periodic teacher development workshops for part-time faculty.

5. Carry out research and evaluation of CME methods: There has been insufficient work done to date on the effectiveness of CME in any field of medicine. It is well known that adult learning is complicated by varied individual learning styles. The practice of family medicine involves a diversity of settings, practice styles, and organizational patterns. The various approaches to CME which are being taken today in family practice require study as to their effectiveness in meeting the three basic goals of CME—increased knowledge and skills, improved clinical performance, and improved outcomes of patient care.

Practice-linked CME instead of traditional knowledge-based CME offers greater potential for enhancing physician performance and patient care outcomes. Departments of family practice can play an active role in the development and evaluation of practical methods of information management, data retrieval, and quality assurance approaches designed to examine the family physician's own individual practice. The widespread application of microcomputers in office practice will assist in this effort, as will the development of practice standards as exemplified by the audit criteria developed by the ABFP in selected areas.

6. Engage in collaborative research with practicing family physicians: Research in family practice is a wide-open field with many areas requiring study. Research efforts are now being facilitated by the establishment of departments of family practice in medical schools, the development of improved audit and record retrieval systems, and by refinements in coding for common clinical problems. Participation in collaborative research projects should be of real educational value to all physicians involved.

IMPLICATIONS FOR THE FAMILY PHYSICIAN

Based on the forgoing, several approaches can be summarized which can help the individual family physician to become involved in meaningful continuing medical education.[38]

1. Identify your needs: Several approaches have been described for this purpose, including profiling/indexing of one's practice, the use of the problem-oriented medical record, medical audit, and self-assessment materials.
2. Explore available educational resources: This involves looking at resources available within the region, including nearby family practice teaching programs, medical libraries, journals, courses offered, self-instructional materials, and the availability of consultation on patient care appraisal methods.
3. Individualize your approach to specific needs: A variety of learning options have been mentioned earlier. Family physicians should select their own approach to CME based upon their learning needs and individual learning styles.
4. Utilize consultation as a learning process: Consultation affords an important and often neglected avenue for continuing medical education. If consultants are chosen for their competence in dealing with a difficult problem as well as for their willingness and interest in teaching, each consultation can become a valuable learning experience.
5. Establish a habit for continuing medical education: This involves organizing one's practice so that time can be allocated to continuing medical education, together with reordering of personal priorities to make this happen. There are more opportunities and options available for CME in family practice than ever before, including an increased number which can be carried out locally in one's own practice without leaving town. An active interest in continuing education can lead to increased professional competence and improved patient care as well as greater satisfaction and interest in one's practice.

Many years ago Sir William Osler called attention to the importance of reviewing one's own practice experience ". . . only in this way can you gain wisdom with experience. It is a common error to think that the more a doctor sees the greater his experience and the more he knows." Today there are ample opportunities for self-renewal and productive CME for physicians everywhere who are prepared to take responsibility for their continued learning.

REFERENCES

1. Manning PR: Continuing medical education: The next step. JAMA 249:1042, 1983
2. Continuing medical education. JAMA 252:1563, 1984
3. Wilbur RS: Mandatory continuing medical education: A liability. Qual Rev Bull 4(3):12, 1978
4. Continuing medical education. JAMA 248:3287, 1982
5. Moore FJ: Information technologies and health care. Arch Intern Med 125:504, 1970
6. Bernier CL, Yerkey AN: Cogent Communication: Overcoming Reading Overload. Westport, Conn., Greenwood Press, 1979
7. Weiss PA: Living nature and the knowledge gap. Saturday Review 52(48):19, 56, 1969
8. McWhinney IR: Family medicine in perspective. N Engl J Med 293(4):176, 1975
9. Ashbaugh DG, McKean RS: Continuing medical education: The philosophy and use of audit. JAMA 236:1485, 1976
10. Scott AJ: Continuing education: More or better? N Engl J Med 295:444, 1976
11. Brown CR, Uhl HSM: Mandatory continuing education—Sense or nonsense? JAMA 213:1660, 1970
12. Lewis CE, Hassanein RS: Continuing medical education. N Engl J Med 282:258, 1970
13. Miller GE: Continuing education for what? J Med Educ 42:320, 1967
14. Haynes RB, Davis DA, McKibbon A, et al.: A critical appraisal of the efficacy of continuing medical education. JAMA 251:61, 1984
15. Berg AO: Does continuing medical education improve the quality of medical care? A look at the evidence. J Fam Pract 8:1171, 1979
16. Stein LS: The effectiveness of continuing medical education: Eight research reports. J Med Educ 56:103, 1980
17. Sibley JC, Sackett DL, Neufeld V, et al.: A randomized trial of continuing medical education. N Engl J Med 306:511, 1982
18. Lloyd JC, Abrahamson S: Effectiveness of continuing medical education: A review of the evidence. Eval Health Prof 2:251, 1979
19. Richards RK: Past history and future trends in CME. QRB 4:8, March 1978
20. Sanazaro PJ: Medical audit, continuing medical education and quality assurance. West J Med 125:248, 1976
21. Clute KF: The General Practitioner: A Study of Medical Education and Practice in Ontario and Nova Scotia. Toronto, University of Toronto Press, 1963
22. Peterson OL, Andrews LP, Spain RS, et al.: An analytical study of North Carolina general practice 1953–1954. J Med Educ 31:1, part 2, 1956
23. Williamson JW, Alexander M, Miller GE: Continuing education and patient care research: Physician response to screening test results. JAMA 201:938, 1967
24. Meskauskas JA, Webster GD: The American Board of Internal Medicine recertification examination: Process and results. Ann Int Med 82:577, 1975
25. Youmans JB: Experience with a postgraduate course for practitioners: Evaluation of results. J Assoc Amer Med Coll 10:154, 1975
26. Kotre JN, Mann FC, Morris WC, et al.: The Michigan physician's use and evaluation of his medical journal. Mich Med 70:11, 1971

27. Miller HL: Teaching and Learning in Adult Education. New York, MacMillan, 1964, p 33

28. Gullion DS, Adamson E, Watts MSM: The effect of an individualized practice-based CME program on physician performance and patient outcomes. West J Med 138:582, 1983

29. Stein LS: Your Personal Learning Plan, A Handbook for Physicians. Chicago, Illinois Council on Continuing Medical Education, 1973

30. Sivertson SE, Meyer TC, Hansen R, Schoenenberger A: Individual physician profile: Continuing education related to medical practice. J Med Educ 48:1006, 1973

31. Schneeweiss R: Diagnosis clusters: A new approach for reporting the diagnostic content of family practice residents' ambulatory experiences. J Fam Pract 20:487, 1985

32. Rakel RE: Indexing in office practice: A system for monitoring high-risk patients and filing medical literature. Cont Educ 9:30, 1978

33. Metcalfe DHH, Mancini JC: Critical event outcome studies used as a teaching tool. J Med Educ 47:869, 1972

34. Geyman JP, Brown TC, Lee PV: Perceptions of formal in-training evaluation by family practice residents. J Fam Pract 5:869, 1977

35. Rosenblatt RA, Gaponoff M. The microcomputer as a vehicle for continuing medical education. J Fam Pract 18:629, 1984

36. Stinson ER, Mueller DA: Survey of health professionals' information habits and needs. JAMA 243:140, 1980

37. Croeger RJ: Medical literature filing systems in family practice residency programs. J Fam Pract 16:621, 1983

38. Geyman JP: A new look at continuing medical education in family practice. J Fam Pract 2:119, 1975

9 Clinical Content of Family Practice

The mainspring of family practice is people—well people, sick people, babies, children, adults, and the elderly. The needs of these patients fill the day of the family physician. Most of the people seen by family physicians each day are well known to them, and many of them have become friends. Others present as new patients with acute or chronic complaints, often without previous medical care relative to these complaints. Family physicians are in a unique position to assess their patients as individuals and as members of family units. This knowledge forms a basis for interpretation of the patient's symptoms and clinical findings as well as for management of the patient's particular illness.

Family practice is thus a field more committed to the continuing needs of individuals and their families for primary health care than to any specific content area per se. At the same time, some basic patterns and variables can be identified to describe the clinical content of family practice and the daily work of family physicians.

Until recent years little was known about the content of the practices of primary care physicians. This was partly due to a relative lack of interest in research in primary care in the United States and partly due to a lack of adequate research methods to describe and analyze the content of primary care. Coding systems, for example, initially related to the clinical problems of hospitalized patients, not the clinical problems encountered by physicians in ambulatory care. The major classification system used in this country until recently was the ICDA (International Classification of Disease Adapted for Use in the United States), which did not afford classification of at least 25 percent of the clinical problems encountered by family physicians in everyday practice. The most recent ninth revision (ICD-9-CM) and ICHPPC-2 (International Classification of Health Problems in Primary Care), a widely used adaptation of that classification, alleviate many of the earlier coding problems for primary care.

The purpose of this chapter is threefold: (1) to outline some of the variables which influence the clinical content of family practice; (2) to characterize the content of ambulatory and hospital practice of family physicians based on available studies to date in this country, including studies of referral patterns; and (3) to compare the clinical content of family practice with the other primary care specialties. This chapter is focused on the clinical problems of individual patients. The next chapter will examine the clinical problems of families; these two chapters must be considered together in viewing the clinical content of family practice.

SOME VARIABLES AFFECTING PRACTICE CONTENT

Although there are many similarities in the clinical content of family practice from one part of the country to another, a number of variables may influence the actual practice content of individual family physicians as well as the characteristics of family practice in different regions of the country. Brief consideration of some of these variables illustrates the potential magnitude of these variations.

Some fundamental features of family practice are shown in Table 9-1.[1] Even cursory reflection on these features suggests that the content of family practice in any one setting depends on such factors as the characteristics of the patient population, environmental factors, physician variables, regional differences in health care delivery, and related factors.

Many features of the practice population directly affect the spectrum of clinical problems seen by the family physician. These include age and other demographic characteristics of the population, socioeconomic factors, mobility of the population, and cultural factors, particularly as they influence health-seeking behavior of the population. Thus an older, stable population will involve the family physician in the care of an increased proportion of chronic illness and lesser involvement with obstetric and pediatric care as compared with a younger, more mobile population.

Environmental factors likewise may influence the content of family practice in different parts of the country, including geographic, climatic, industrial, occupational and related factors. Parasitic infestations, for an obvious example, are encountered less often by family physicians in Minnesota than in Louisiana.

Physician variables may produce significant differences in the practices of individual family physicians. The training and experience of family physicians in obstetrics, for example, affects whether or not a given family physician includes obstetrics in his/her practice, which may further influence the age spectrum and proportion of pediatric care in the practice. Another important physician variable relates to the philosophy of the physician concerning the value and need for preventive care.

Regional differences in patterns of medical care may alter the practice content of family physicians considerably in some respects. The involvement of family physicians in obstetrics in the Northeastern United States, for example, has been relatively limited for some years compared to patterns of family practice elsewhere in the country.

TABLE 9-1. CHARACTERISTICS OF FAMILY PRACTICE

1. The pattern of illness approximates to the pattern of illness in the community, i.e., there is:
   a. A high incidence of transient illness.
   b. A high prevalence of chronic illness.
   c. A high incidence of emotional illness.
2. The illness is undifferentiated, i.e., it has not been previously assessed by any other physician.
3. Illnesses are frequently a complex mixture of physical, emotional, and social elements.
4. Disease is seen early, before the full clinical picture has developed.
5. Relationship with patients is continuous and transcends individual episodes of illness.

(From McWhinney IR: Problem solving and decision-making in primary medical practice. Canad Fam Phys 18:11, 111, 1972, with permission.)

Patients seen by family physicians do not readily lend themselves to precise categorization. As pointed out by Malerich:[2]

> [Family practice] defies categorization or fragmentation because its essence is the care of the whole person in relation to his family and environment. In reality, a patient visit frequently includes more than one aspect of illness or concern.

When patients are seen for multiple problems at a single visit, only some of the problems may be coded for reporting purposes, and some problems (especially behavioral problems) may be underreported for a variety of reasons as will be seen in the next chapter.

Despite these variables, however, it is still worthwhile to review some attempts to describe the clinical content of family practice, for certain patterns of illness emerge as major components in the practice of any physician providing primary health care to entire families.

SOME STUDIES OF CLINICAL CONTENT

As pointed out in an earlier chapter, the content of medical practice in the community is quite different from that encountered in most teaching settings to which medical students and residents have been exposed. In their studies of the ecology of medical care in the United States, White and colleagues demonstrated that 750 of 1000 adults at risk during an average month will experience one or more illnesses or injuries. Of course, 250 will consult a physician; of these, 9 will be hospitalized (8 at a community hospital and 1 at a university medical center) and 5 will be referred for consultation to another physician.[3] A similar study in Canada examined the experience of 1000 people over 1 year. Of these, 800 had some illness and 730 consulted a physician; 590 had some disability during the year, 160 were hospitalized, and only 200 were well throughout the year.[4]

During the last 15 years there have been a number of content studies in family practice, but until recently all have had significant limitations preventing generalizability for the entire field. Some excellent studies of the content of family practice have been done in several states, but even collectively these have incompletely described the work of the family physician because of regional variations. Although the National Ambulatory Medical Care Survey provides a wealth of information on office practice for all specialties, many important aspects of ambulatory practice are not included, and hospital practice is totally excluded.

In 1982 a landmark national study of the structure and content of family practice was reported which for the first time provides a comprehensive and definitive view of the field.[5] Through the support of the Robert Wood Johnson Foundation a research group at the University of Washington performed an indepth analysis of several national data sets. The principal data source was derived from the Medical Activities and Manpower Project at the University of Southern California, which carried out a log-diary study in 1977 of a national sample of over 1000 general and family physicians. This data base was supplemented with other information gathered by the federal government—the Area Resource File and the National Ambulatory Medical Care Survey. The USC survey involved separate surveys of self-identified "general practitioners" and "family physicians." These two groups obviously overlap, however, since many general practitioners have become board-certified in family practice and many self-reported "family physicians" have neither completed family practice residency training nor been certified by the American Board of Family Practice. For the purposes of this study, these two groups were therefore combined, though many of the analyses differentiated residency-trained and board-certified family physicians from nonresidency-trained and non-board-certified general practitioners.

The previously mentioned diagnosis cluster technique was used to characterize both the ambulatory and hospital content of family practice in a representative sample of general/family physicians in the United States. The diagnosis clusters are compatible with ICDA-8, ICD-9-CM, ICHPPC, and ICHPPC-2. They were derived from all office-based specialties, and therefore permit both intraspecialty and interspecialty comparisons. A great advantage of the cluster method is the reduction in the number of diagnostic rubrics to a manageable number resulting in less variation when aggregate data sets are compared.[6]

Office Practice

Twenty-five diagnosis clusters were found to comprise 70 percent of all ambulatory visits, as shown in Table 9–2. It can be noted that age of the physician has a major influence on the diagnostic spectrum of the practice. Older physicians tend to see older patients, encounter more chronic illness, and are less likely to do obstetrics. Board-certification seems to have little effect on the diagnostic content of office practice. Residency-trained family physicians record the diagnoses of anxiety and depression more frequently than nonresidency-trained physicians.

Further variations in the diagnostic content of office practice have been demonstrated on the basis of differences in geographic location. Family physicians in the Northeast, for example, see more chronic illness but much less obstetrics than those elsewhere in the country. Obstetrics represents an especially large part of family practice in the North Central region, while trauma comprises a larger part of office practice in the West than in other parts of the country. Differences in practice arrangement have little effect on the diagnostic content of office practice, but the extent of urbanization does have such an effect; rural family physicians record more than twice the number of obstetric visits than their urban counterparts.

Since the above findings are based primarily on a 3-day log-diary study of participating physicians conducted by the Medical Activities and Manpower Project at the University of Southern California, it is useful to compare the results of this study with those from two other large data sets. The National Ambulatory Medical Care Survey (NAMCS) is an ongoing survey of office-based physicians sponsored by the National Center for Health Statistics, and involves a random sample of physicians in all specialties recording data over 1 week of office practice. The Virginia Study reported on the ambulatory and hospital visits to 36 family physicians and 82 family practice residents in Virginia over a 2-year period from 1973 to 1975.[7]

In their analysis of these data sets, Rosenblatt and his colleagues noted striking similarities between the USC and NAMCS data as validation of the USC study, while commenting on the Virginia comparison as follows:[5]

> In sum, the Virginia Study data present a profile of family medicine in one area of the country. Major differences emerge in the specific frequency of individual diagnoses in the Virginia Study when compared with a national sample. As contrasted with the NAMCS-USC comparison, in which only 2 of the most common 30 rubrics differed from one another by more than 50 percent, 15 of 30

TABLE 9-2. FREQUENCY OF MOST COMMON DIAGNOSIS CLUSTERS FOR OUTPATIENT FAMILY PRACTICE BY PHYSICIAN AGE, BOARD CERTIFICATION, AND RESIDENCY TRAINING (WEIGHTED PERCENT)[a]

Cluster	All Family Physicians	Physician Age (yr)			Board Certified		Residency Completed	
		45	45–54	55+	Yes	No	Yes	No
1. General medical examination	14.5	12.7	16.1	13.7	13.1	15.1	11.9	14.8
2. Acute upper respiratory tract infection	7.9	9.5	8.6	6.7	8.5	7.7	7.1	8.0
3. Hypertension	7.0	5.5	6.2	7.4	5.9	7.4	8.6	6.8
4. Soft tissue injuries	3.9	3.7	3.2	4.7	3.4	4.2	2.8	4.1
5. Acute sprains, strains	3.1	3.1	3.3	2.9	3.2	3.1	2.5	3.2
6. Prenatal and postnatal care	3.0	4.2	3.9	1.6	3.7	2.6	3.1	2.9
7. Depression/anxiety	2.9	2.6	2.3	3.7	3.0	2.9	4.6	2.8
8. Ischemic heart disease	2.6	1.7	2.3	3.3	2.4	2.7	1.9	2.7
9. Diabetes	2.4	2.4	1.9	3.0	2.4	2.4	2.2	2.4
10. Dermatitis/eczema	2.1	1.6	2.1	2.3	1.4	2.4	1.6	2.2
11. Degenerative joint disease	2.0	1.6	1.1	3.1	1.2	2.1	2.2	2.0
12. Urinary tract infection	2.0	1.5	2.1	2.2	1.6	2.2	1.7	2.1
13. Obesity	1.7	1.0	1.8	1.9	1.2	1.9	2.1	1.7
14. Acute lower respiratory tract infection	1.7	2.3	1.2	2.0	2.0	1.6	1.6	1.7
15. Nonfungal skin infection	1.6	1.9	1.3	1.8	1.6	1.6	1.2	1.7
16. Infectious diarrhea/gastroenteritis	1.5	1.4	1.3	1.7	1.5	1.5	1.3	1.6
17. Vaginitis, vulvitis, cervicitis	1.3	1.2	1.2	1.4	1.5	1.2	2.4	1.2
18. Fractures/dislocations	1.2	1.3	1.5	1.0	1.5	1.2	1.2	1.3
19. Otitis media	1.2	1.8	1.3	0.9	1.2	1.2	1.4	1.2
20. Emphysema, chronic bronchitis, chronic obstructive pulmonary disease	1.2	1.7	1.3	0.8	1.6	1.0	1.5	1.1
21. Medical/surgical aftercare	1.1	1.4	1.1	2.0	1.5	1.0	1.5	1.1
22. Peptic ulcer diseases	1.0	1.2	0.8	1.1	1.2	1.0	0.5	1.1
23. Headache	0.9	0.9	0.6	1.1	0.8	0.8	0.7	0.9
24. Bursitis, synovitis, tenosynovitis	0.8	0.8	0.8	0.8	0.8	0.8	0.9	0.8
25. Low back pain	0.8	0.7	0.8	0.9	0.8	0.8	0.8	0.8

[a]Based on 38,511 patient encounters recorded in USC data by office-based physicians.
(From Rosenblatt RA, Cherkin DC, Schneeweiss R, et al.: The structure and content of family practice: Current status and future trends. J Fam Pract 15:681, 1982, with permission.)

TABLE 9-3. FIFTY MOST COMMON HOSPITAL DIAGNOSES BY OFFICE-BASED GENERAL AND FAMILY PHYSICIANS (n = 7830)

Diagnosis (Ranked by Frequency in USC Data)	ICDA-8 Code	Weighted Percent	Cumulative Percent
1. Acute myocardial infarction without hypertensive disease	410.9	3.5	3.5
2. Acute, ill-defined cerebrovascular disease without hypertension	436.9	2.7	6.2
3. Pneumonia, unspecified	486.0	2.7	8.9
4. Congestive heart failure	427.0	2.7	11.6
5. Diabetes mellitus without acidosis or coma	250.9	2.6	14.2
6. Chronic ischemic heart disease without hypertensive disease	412.9	2.5	16.7
7. Emphysema	492.0	2.4	19.1
8. Medical/surgical aftercare—other	Y10.5	1.9	21.0
9. Back sprain, strain—unspecified	847.9	1.7	22.7
10. Postpartum observation	Y7.0	1.6	24.3
11. Single born without immaturity	Y20.0	1.5	25.8
12. Diaphragmatic hernia without obstruction	551.3	1.4	27.2
13. Back sprain, strain—other	847.8	1.3	28.5
14. Cholecystitis, cholangitis without calculus	575.0	1.2	29.7
15. Gastroenteritis, colitis	9.2	1.2	30.9
16. Other diseases of intestines, peritoneum—other	569.9	1.2	32.1
17. Acute appendicitis with peritonitis	540.0	1.1	33.2
18. Essential benign hypertension	401.0	1.1	34.3
19. Inguinal hernia without obstruction	550.0	1.0	35.3
20. Delivery without complication	650.0	1.0	36.3
21. Diverticula of colon	562.1	0.9	37.2
22. Fracture of neck or femur—other and unspecified—closed	820.4	0.8	38.0
23. Uterine fibroma	218.0	0.8	38.8
24. Prenatal care without associated nonobstetric condition	Y6.0	0.8	39.6
25. Uterine prolapse	623.4	0.8	40.4
26. Appendicitis, unqualified	541.0	0.8	41.2
27. Fracture of vertebral column without spinal cord lesion—unspecified	805.6	0.8	42.0
28. Calculus of kidney and ureter	592.0	0.7	42.7
29. Malignant neoplasm of large intestine—unspecified	153.8	0.7	43.4
30. Ulcer of duodenum—other and unspecified	532.9	0.7	44.1
31. Abdominal pain	785.5	0.7	44.8
32. Other disease of respiratory system—other	519.9	0.7	45.5
33. Gastritis and duodenitis	535.0	0.7	46.2
34. Gangrene NEC[a]	445.9	0.7	46.9

TABLE 9-3. (continued)

Diagnosis (Ranked by Frequency in USC Data)	ICDA-8 Code	Weighted Percent	Cumulative Percent
35. Intestinal obstruction without hernia—other and unspecified	560.9	0.7	47.6
36. Pain referable to urinary system	786.0	0.7	48.3
37. Asthma	493.0	0.6	48.9
38. Displacement of intervertebral disc— unspecified	725.9	0.6	49.5
39. Fracture of ankle—closed	824.0	0.6	50.1
40. Metabolic diseases—other and unspecified	279.0	0.6	50.7
41. Malignant neoplasm—other	199.1	0.6	51.3
42. Vaginal bleeding	629.5	0.6	51.9
43. Diseases of jaw—inflammatory conditions	526.4	0.6	52.5
44. Cholelithiasis—other and unspecified	574.9	0.6	53.1
45. Anemia, unspecified	285.9	0.6	53.7
46. Pelvic inflammatory disease	616.0	0.6	54.3
47. Malignant neoplasm of bronchus and lung	162.1	0.5	54.8
48. Malignant neoplasm of breast	174.0	0.5	55.3
49. Malignant neoplasm of kidney excluding pelvis	189.0	0.5	55.8
50. Diabetes mellitus with acidosis or coma	250.0	0.5	56.3

[a]NEC—not elsewhere classified.
(From Rosenblatt RA, Cherkin DC, Schneeweiss R, et al.: The structure and content of family practice: Current status and future trends. J Fam Pract 15:681, 1982, with permission.)

rubrics differed by that amount in the NAMCS-Virginia comparison. There is considerable variation in diagnosis frequency, by region, patient age, and physician age and training. It is this variation that limits the generalizability of any regional or residency-based data on the content of family practice.

Hospital Practice

Analysis of the USC study has yielded the most informative picture of the hospital practice of family physicians throughout the country yet available. Over 96 percent of the study sample (99.5 percent of residency graduates) were found to have an active hospital practice, and the average physician had 23 percent of all patient encounters in the hospital.

Table 9–3 lists the 50 most common diagnoses for hospitalized patients by frequency. Two of the top ten ambulatory diagnoses appear in the top ten of hospital diagnoses—diabetes mellitus and chronic ischemic heart disease.

The use of diagnosis clusters affords an even more graphic perspective of the hospital practice of U.S. family physicians. One-half of all hospital encounters are included in just 14 diagnosis clusters. By means of the cluster method, for example, two major clusters sort out as second and third most common, respectively—pregnancy and malignant neoplasms—neither of which appeared among the nine most common individual diagnosis. Table 9–4 presents these findings, together with

TABLE 9-4. TOP 30 CLUSTERS OF HOSPITAL DIAGNOSES BY OFFICE-BASED GENERAL AND FAMILY PHYSICIANS (n = 7830)

Cluster[a]	Weighted Percent	Cumulative Percent	Weighted Percent		Rank	
			Residency Graduates (n = 1240)	Nongraduates (n = 6590)	Residency Graduates	Nongraduates
1. Ischemic heart disease (including myocardial infarction)	7.9	7.9	5.6	8.0	3	1
2. Pregnancy—normal and complicated	6.2	14.1	12.8	5.8	1	3
3. Malignant neoplasm	6.2	20.3	6.5	6.2	2	2
4. Back pain, radiculopathy	4.3	24.6	2.2	4.5	10	4
5. Cerebrovascular disease	4.0	28.6	5.0	3.9	4	5
6. Pneumonia	3.1	31.7	3.7	3.1	6	6
7. Diabetes mellitus	3.1	34.8	3.8	3.0	5	7
8. Congestive heart failure	2.7	37.5	2.3	2.8	8	8
9. Chronic obstructive pulmonary disease	2.7	40.2	1.6	2.8	13	9
10. Appendicitis/appendectomy	2.3	42.5	0.8	2.4	26	10
11. Fractures and dislocations (except femur)	2.3	44.8	0.8	2.4	27	11
12. Surgical aftercare	2.0	46.8	2.5	2.0	7	12
13. Cholecystitis	1.9	48.7	0.7	1.9	30	13
14. Peptic ulcer disease	1.8	50.5	1.9	1.8	11	14
15. Benign diseases of uterus	1.7	52.2	0.5	1.7	34	15

16.	Fracture of femur	1.6	53.8	0.3	1.7	39	16
17.	Diarrheal disease	1.6	55.4	1.7	1.6	12	17
18.	Hernias of abdominal wall without obstruction	1.4	56.8	0.9	1.5	24	19
19.	Kidney stone	1.4	58.2	0.2	1.5	40	18
20.	Diseases of urinary tract	1.4	59.6	1.0	1.4	22	20
21.	Diseases of intestine and peritoneum (NEC)[b]	1.3	60.9	1.0	1.4	21	21
22.	Upper respiratory tract infection and influenza	1.2	62.1	1.2	1.2	18	22
23.	Essential benign hypertension	1.1	63.2	0.2	1.2	43	23
24.	Abnormal menstrual bleeding	1.0	64.2	0.1	1.0	46	24
25.	Pyogenic infections of skin and subcutaneous tissue	0.9	65.1	1.3	0.9	17	25
26.	Diverticulitis of colon	0.9	66.0	0.4	0.9	35	26
27.	Pelvic inflammatory disease	0.8	66.8	0.1	0.9	45	27
28.	Gastrointestinal obstruction	0.8	67.6	0.7	0.8	31	28
29.	Arthritis	0.8	68.4	0.6	0.8	32	29
30.	Anemia	0.7	69.1	1.3	0.7	15	31

[a]Ranked by frequency of clusters in USC diagnosis data
[b]NEC—not elsewhere classified

(From Rosenblatt RA, Cherkin DC, Schneeweiss R, et al.: The structure and content of family practice: Current status and future trends. J Fam Pract 15:681, 1982, with permission.)

comparative rankings of diagnosis clusters for residency graduates and nongraduates. Residency-trained family physicians tend to be more involved with obstetrics, more complex medical problems, and behavioral/psychiatric problems than are non-graduates, but are less involved with the hospital care of surgical and orthopedic problems.

REFERRAL AND CONSULTATION

A rather complete picture of referral rates in family practice can be pieced together from various studies carried out in different parts of the country over the past 10 years. The average referral rate involves approximately 2 percent of visits for studies in North Carolina,[8] New York,[9] Vermont,[10] California,[11] and Washington.[12] The surgical specialties and medical subspecialties consistently draw most of the referrals, and only occasional consultations are requested from general pediatricians and general internists.

All of the above studies are in single-specialty family practice, fee-for-service settings. One may wonder to what extent referral patterns may vary in multispecialty group practice and in HMO settings. A recent study provides an initial answer to this question. Mayer examined 1-year's experience in a large multispecialty group in Minneapolis, Minnesota which provides both fee-for-service and prepaid medical care to similar populations. He found a 3.2 percent referral rate among 5833 fee-for-service visits and a 4.4 percent referral rate among 6395 HMO visits.[13] Table 9–5 presents the comparative frequency of referrals by specialty, and further compares these findings with single-specialty family practice settings in California and New York. Again, most referrals involve the surgical specialties and medical subspecialties. Economic factors were considered the most likely influence on the slightly higher referral rate observed in this particular HMO, which pays for all services of member physicians thereby involving no economic disincentive to referral.

Presently available evidence therefore shows that family physicians provide definitive care for at least 97 percent of patient visits in their everyday practice. At the same time, consultation and referral represent an essential mechanism for providing the highest quality of patient care and constitute an important method of continuing medical education for family physicians.

COMPARATIVE CONTENT BY SPECIALTY

Rosenblatt and colleagues recently extended their diagnosis cluster method to the analysis of ambulatory care for all office-based specialties in the United States. Their study classified 96,332 ambulatory diagnoses recorded by 3222 physicians responding to the National Ambulatory Medical Care Survey (NAMCS) during 1977 and 1978. Their findings provide the most accurate portrait of the distribution of ambulatory care by specialty yet available.[14]

Table 9–6 displays the distribution of ambulatory visits by patient age and physician specialty. It can be seen that general/family physicians account for three-eighths of all visits, representing more than three times the ambulatory volume of internal medicine, and even exceeding the combined ambulatory volume of general internal medicine, pediatrics, and obstetrics–gynecology. Interestingly, general/fami-

TABLE 9-5. COMPARATIVE FREQUENCY OF REFERRALS IN DIFFERENT PRACTICE SETTINGS

	Fee-for-Service Plymouth			HMO Plymouth			Geyman et al Fee-for-Service			Metcalf and Sischy Fee-for-Service		
	No.	%	Order	No.	%	Order	No.	%	Order	No.	%	Order
General surgery	29	17.3	1	42	14.8	1	26	20.6	1	26	25.5	1
Otolaryngology	22	13.1	2	38	13.4	2	3	2.4	9	10	9.8	3.5
Orthopedics	21	12.5	3	23	8.1	5.5	20	15.9	2	10	9.8	3.5
Obstetrics/gynecology	18	10.7	4	27	9.5	4	15	11.9	3	11	10.8	2
Dermatology	15	8.9	5	30	10.6	3	0	0	—	7	6.9	7
Opthalmology	9	5.4	6	7	2.5	12.5	14	11.1	4	6	5.9	8
Cardiology	8	4.8	7.5	17	6.0	8	4	3.2	8	1	1.0	12
Neurology	8	4.8	7.5	15	5.3	9.5	8	6.3	6	8	7.8	5.5
Mental health	7	4.2	9.5	20	7.1	7	7	5.6	7	3	2.9	9
Allergy	7	4.2	9.5	15	5.3	9.5	0	0	—	2	2.0	10
Pediatrics	5	3.0	11.5	9	3.2	11	0	0	—	1	1.0	12
Gastroenterology	5	3.0	11.5	6	2.1	14	2	1.6	10	0	0	—
Urology	3	1.8	14	23	8.1	5.5	10	7.9	5	8	7.8	5.5
Rheumatology	3	1.8	14	7	2.5	12.5	0	0	—	0	0	—
Nephrology	3	1.8	14	1	0.4	16	0	0	—	0	0	—
Endocrinology	2	1.2	16	2	0.7	15	1	0.8	11	1	1.0	12
Others	3	1.8	—	1	0.4	—	16	12.7	—	8	7.8	—
Total	168			283			126			102		

(From Mayer TR: Family practice referral patterns in a health maintenance organization. J Fam Pract 14:315, 1982, with permission.)

TABLE 9-6. DISTRIBUTION OF AMBULATORY VISITS TO OFFICE-BASED U.S. PHYSICIANS, BY PATIENT AGE AND PHYSICIAN SPECIALTY (PERCENT)

Physician Specialty	Patient Age				
	< 17	17–44	45–64	> 65	All Ages
General and family practice	32.6	38.0	39.1	40.0	37.4
General internal medicine	1.5	8.6	17.9	22.1	11.6
Pediatrics	44.5	0.7	0.1	0.0	9.6
Obstetrics and gynecology	1.0	18.8	4.4	1.3	8.7
General surgery	2.8	6.0	7.9	7.7	6.1
Psychiatry	0.6	4.6	2.6	0.6	2.6
Other specialties	17.3	23.3	28.0	28.3	24.0
Total	100.0	100.0	100.0	100.0	100.0

(From Rosenblatt RA, Cherkin DC, Schneeweiss R, et al.: The content of ambulatory medical care in the United States: An interspecialty comparison. N Engl J. Med 309:892, 1983, with permission.)

ly physicians account for almost twice the number of ambulatory visits for the geriatric population than provided by general internists.

Fifteen diagnosis clusters were found to comprise 50 percent of all ambulatory care visits. Only a few specialties handle the majority of all ambulatory visits. General/family physicians, general internists, and general pediatricians together account for well over one-half of all patient visits for the 15 most common medical problems combined. The three primary care specialties together account for 58.6 percent of all office visits to physicians and 65.9 percent of all visits for the 15 most common diagnosis clusters. General/family physicians alone account for more than one-quarter of the visits in 12 of the 15 most common diagnosis clusters. Figure 4–5 in an earlier chapter displays the comparative contributions of the various specialties to the ambulatory care of patients presenting with problems included in the 15 most common diagnosis clusters. Of special interest are the findings that general/family physicians account for more than one-half of all office visits for six of the most common diagnosis clusters, including hypertension, diabetes mellitus, acute upper and lower respiratory infections, soft tissue injury, and acute sprains and strains.

Another striking finding of this study is the extent to which the various specialties differ in terms of the spectrum of their workload. Figure 9–1 illustrates the proportional ambulatory workload by diagnostic cluster and by specialty for one-half of office visits to these specialties. It is readily apparent that psychiatry, pediatrics, obstetrics–gynecology, and dermatology are the least varied for one-half of their workload, with no more than two diagnosis clusters (one in psychiatry) making up that amount of their office practice. General/family practice, general internal medicine, and general surgery on the other hand, are the most varied, each with 11 diagnosis clusters making up one–half of their respective office practices.

Much less information is available concerning interspecialty comparisons for hospital practice. One study, however, provides some information on this subject. Garg and colleagues studied the problems of hospital care of over 4500 patients in 9 Ohio hospitals in 1975. They found that general/family physicians played an ac-

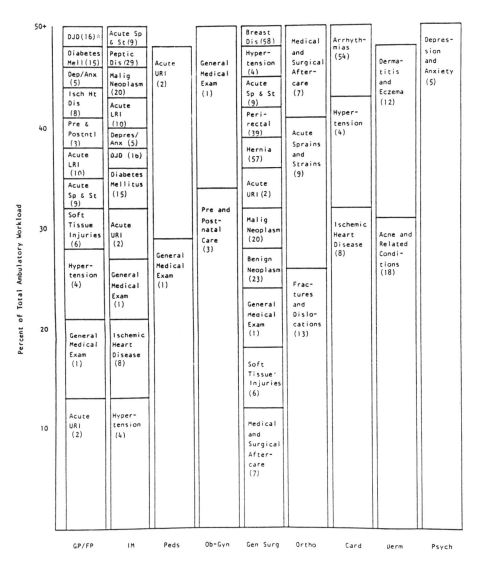

* Numbers in parentheses represent the rank order of the accompanying diagnosis for all visits to all specialties.

Figure 9-1. Diagnostic clusters accounting for majority of ambulatory visits to selected physician specialties, United States, 1977–78.
(From Rosenblatt RA, Cherkin DC, Schneeweiss R, et al.: The content of ambulatory medical care in the United States: An interspecialty comparison. N Engl J Med 309:892, 1983, with permission.)

tive role in inpatient care, and had the most varied inpatient experience. They noted less variety for the other primary care specialties—42 percent of pediatricians' patients were hospitalized for respiratory illness and 33 percent of internists' patients were hospitalized for diseases of the circulatory system.[15] Table 9–7 shows the distribution of patient discharges by physician specialty, length of stay, and number of patient visits each day in the hospital.

TABLE 9-7. DISTRIBUTION OF PATIENT DISCHARGES BY PHYSICIAN SPECIALTY, MEAN NUMBER OF DAYS HOSPITALIZED, AND MEAN NUMBER OF PATIENTS SEEN PER DAY

Specialty	Physicians Number (Percent)	Percent of Physician Discharges per Year	Mean Number of Discharges per Year per Physician	Mean Number of Days Hospitalized	Mean Number of Patients Seen per Day per Physician
All	532 (100%)	100	150	8.7	3.6
Primary care	282 (53%)	45	133	9.6	3.5
Internal medicine	70 (13%)	13	145	12.1	4.8
General and family practice	185 (35%)	28	129	8.9	3.1
Pediatrics	27 (5%)	4	133	6.6	2.4
Other specialties	237 (45%)	52	168	7.9	3.6
Unspecified and unknown	13 (2%)	3	202	8.9	4.9

(From Garg ML, Skipper JK, McNamera MJ, Mulligan JL: Primary care physicians and profiles of their hospitalized patients. AJPH 66:4, 390–392, 1976, with permission.)

COMMENT

The most current information available on the clinical content of medical practice in the ambulatory setting clearly demonstrates that general/family practice serves by far the largest segment of the population's needs of any specialty, and indeed represents the foundation of the present health care system. In addition, an active inpatient role is also played by general/family physicians in the United States. These findings dispel several misperceptions held by some—e.g., that family practice is predominantly involved with minor illness, is largely an ambulatory field, acts as a triage field to the nonprimary care specialties, and plays a comparatively limited role in the health care system.

The clinical content of family practice, in summary, is featured by breadth, flexibility and variations by individual family physicians and by needs of the communities in which they practice. The daily work of the family physician is characterized by variety—variety of clinical problems encountered, variety of stages of care (from health maintenance to terminal care), variety by stages in the life cycle of families and the endless variety of the needs and responses of people in various stages of health and illness.

REFERENCES

1. McWhinney IR: Problem solving and decision-making in primary medical practice. Canad Fam Phys 18:11, 109, 1972
2. Malerich JA: What constitutes family practice in West St. Paul. GP 40:163, 1969
3. White KL, Williams F, Greenberg B: Ecology of medical care. N Engl J Med 265:885, 1961
4. Kohn R: The Health of the Canadian People. Ottawa, Queen's Printer, 1965, p 113
5. Rosenblatt RA, Cherkin DC, Schneeweiss R, et al.: The structure and content of family practice: Current status and future trends. J Fam Pract 15:681, 1982
6. Schneeweiss, R, Rosenblatt RA, Cherkin DC, et al.: Diagnosis clusters: A new tool for analyzing the content of ambulatory medical care. Med Care 21:105, 1983
7. Marsland DW, Wood M, Mayo F: A data bank for patient care, curriculum, and research in family practice: 526,196 patient problems. J Fam Pract 3:25, 1976
8. Hansen JP, Brown SE, Sullivan RJ, et al.: Factors related to effective referral and consultation process. J Fam Pract 15:651, 1982
9. Metcalfe DHH, Sischy D: Patterns of referral from family practice. J Fam Pract 1:34, 1974
10. Ruane TJ: Consultation and referral in a Vermont family practice: A study of utilization, specialty distribution, and outcome. J Fam Pract 8:1037, 1979
11. Geyman JP, Brown TC, Rivers K: Referrals in family practice: A comparative study by geographic region and practice setting. J Fam Pract 3:163, 1976
12. Moscovice I, Schwartz CW, Shortell SA: Referral patterns of family physicians in an underserved rural area. J Fam Pract 9:677, 1979
13. Mayer TR: Family practice referral patterns in a health maintenance organization. J Fam Pract 14:315, 1982
14. Rosenblatt RA, Cherkin DC, Schneeweiss R, et al.: The content of ambulatory medical care in the United States: An interspecialty comparison. N Engl J Med 309:892, 1983
15. Garg ML, Skipper JK, McNamera MU, Mulligan JL: Primary care physicians and profiles of their hospitalized patients. AJPH 66(4):390, 1976

10 | The Family in Family Practice

It is axiomatic that family practice as a specialty is involved with the comprehensive, ongoing care of individual patients and their families over the full course of the family life cycle. It is also axiomatic that the family is the basic unit of care in family practice, but this deceptively simple concept bears further examination. By this do we mean that the family physician cares for all members of the family as individuals, with due consideration of the family environment as a factor which may modify his/her care of the individual family member? Or does the family physician also care for the family itself as the patient, involving diagnostic and therapeutic efforts oriented to family problems, not just individual problems? Most family physicians accept the first question as a matter of course; but there is less agreement and understanding of the dimensions of the second question.

Although many in family medicine accept the family as a patient as an article of faith, there is a considerable gap today between this conceptual goal and actual practice. As Carmichael says: "to care for the patient in the context of the family is one thing; to turn the family into the object of care is another."[1]

A common clinical example encountered in everyday practice illustrates this gap. Many family physicians are skilled in recognizing depression as a primary problem or as a problem associated with concurrent organic illness. But how many family physicians take the next step toward diagnosis and management of related, or even causative, problems within the family itself, such as a marital problem, a parent-adolescent relationship problem, or other major dysfunction of the family? In order to accomplish this task, a conceptual shift is needed to perceive the family itself as the patient, and to develop and apply a set of clinical strategies that apply to family problems.

Since family physicians have the unique responsibility and opportunity to care for the entire family, they are obliged to know as much as possible about the family as a functional unit and about the patterns of illness in families. The purpose of this chapter is fourfold: (1) to describe briefly the changing roles of the American family; (2) to outline family development in terms of the family life cycle; (3) to discuss the nature of illness within families; and (4) to present diagnostic and management approaches to family problems which are applicable in family practice, together with some perspective as to the extent to which it is reasonable to care for the family unit per se as the unit of care.

CHANGING ROLES OF THE AMERICAN FAMILY

Behavioral scientists consider that our rapidly moving technologic society has produced changes in the role of the family which engender many family conflicts. What is usually recognized as the traditional model for the modern American family evolved in a predominantly agricultural economy with a majority of the population living in rural or semi-rural communities. William Ogburn, a sociologist, has enumerated six basic functions of the traditional family which have been essentially lost in recent decades:[2]

1. The Economic Function: Until about 50 years ago all members of the family shared in producing most of what the family consumed. Today, the husband invariably works outside the home and his role in daily family life is much less dominant. Children usually have little understanding of his working role, and often see him in his nonworking hours in the home as someone too tired to take an active interest in their activities. In order to contribute to the family's income, today's wife, who works outside the home, often feels conflict between her desire to share in the family's economic life and the inevitable decrease in her involvement with the growth and development of her children.
2. The Protective Function: Families no longer directly have to protect their own members from bodily harm, but instead rely on police, sheriffs, and others. In times of illness, disability, and unemployment the personal responsibility of the family has been replaced by public mechanisms such as unemployment compensation, social security, health insurance, and other programs. Care of chronic illness, especially in the aged, has often shifted from the home to the convalescent hospital and nursing home.
3. The Religious Function: Compared with the central role of religious teaching and custom in the earlier traditional family, formal religion plays a much diminished role in the home of today's family. Religious training is more the responsibility of the church which itself has perhaps a weaker influence on many of the younger generation than in the past.
4. The Recreational Function: The home is no longer the place for recreation for the entire family. Outside facilities and commercial entertainment are now more likely to attract one or two members of the family than the entire family. Television provides a common entertainment in the home, but is usually enjoyed more on an individual than a family basis, and competes for time available for intrafamily communication.
5. The Educational Function: Children's education has almost entirely shifted from the family to the schools, even including sex education. Family conflicts frequently arise when the standards of behavior and speech learned at school are at variance with those of the family.
6. The Status-Conferring Function: In the past, the family to a large extent determined the individual's socioeconomic status. In small communities, families were well known and had a definite place in the social structure. Now the husband's job more often defines the family's status.

While other institutions (e.g., the church, schools, political and social systems) have at least partly taken over many of the functions of the traditional family, one function has remained as central and vital—that of providing emotional support for family members. As Spanier observes:[3]

Humans have a great need for intimacy. As society becomes more urban, industrial, and mobile, it also becomes more impersonal. In short, a growing need for personalization is found in a society that is becoming more impersonal, and one looks to the family to meet this need. Love is sought from parents, children, and other intimate companions because it is unlikely that this need will be met elsewhere. Perhaps paradoxically, then, the family may become stronger and more valuable as other social institutions such as the church and state erode its traditional responsibilities.

Livsey has observed that the changes causing increasingly specialized functions of the family parallel the evolutionary changes of society in general at a given time and at a given place.[4] That these changes have resulted in new conflicts, confusion of roles, and personal and family problems cannot be denied.

Though our American society and family structures are admittedly undergoing many changes, all evidence leads us to believe that the family is here to stay, albeit in more varied forms than the traditional nuclear family. About one-half of the population lives in the nuclear unit including two parents and their children. There is also an increasing number of single-parent families; during the 1970s households maintained by a woman alone, and by a man alone, with children increased by twofold and by over 60 percent, respectively.[5] At the same time, the number of unmarried couples living together more than doubled during the 1970s.[6]

Although the divorce rate has doubled over the last 20 years, there are proportionately more married people in the United States now than at any time in the history of reliable census data. When divorce occurs, there is a strong tendency toward remarriage; one-quarter of divorced people remarry within 1 year and one-half do so within 3 years.[7] Moreover, as reflected by such statistics as suicide rates, it has been amply demonstrated that family life is more directly correlated with satisfactory living adjustments than is the unmarried state. Most behavioral scientists feel the giving and receiving of affection within the family are functions which no other institution can adequately perform. Curry takes this one step further in viewing the family as the basic unit of humanity. He sees each person as:

> . . . [a] human being because of all the relationships he has about him, all the feelings that exist between others and himself, especially with members of the nuclear family, the simple family, the extended family, and even the community. It is, in the last analysis, our relationships with others which make our lives happy and meaningful, which give us our humanity.[8]

FAMILY LIFE CYCLE

The concept of the family life cycle is based on several basic assumptions: (1) that families within our culture tend to have a beginning and an end; (2) that a number of distinct sequential phases can be recognized; and (3) that various phase-specific tasks can be delineated within each stage.[9]

The family life cycle has been described in a number of ways and has usually been viewed as including 5 to 12 recognizable stages. Regardless of the particular classification of the family life cycle which one finds most useful, they all have in common five basic developmental phases for every elementary family:

1. Birth of family: Elementary family originates with marriage of couple.
2. Phase of expansion: Begins with birth of first child and continues until the

youngest child reaches adulthood. This phase includes the period of fertility, the period of physical and social maturation of children.

3. Phase of dispersion: Begins when the first child achieves adult status and continues until all children have grown and left home.

4. Phase of independence: Begins when all children have reached adulthood and left home so that the parents again live alone.

5. Phase of replacement: Begins when the parents retire from their major life roles and ends with their death. Usually includes a dependency stage of variable length.

Within each stage of the family life cycle, a number of predictable stage-specific tasks occur. As observed by Worby, "these tasks arouse considerable stress within the family system and require of all family members a continuous mutual and reciprocal set of readjustments."[10] Table 10-1 outlines some of the important stage-specific tasks for each stage of the family life cycle as described by Duvall.[10]

Within the family life cycle, some interesting observations have been made of both marital and individual development. Rollins and Feldman, for example, studied levels of marital satisfaction over the family life cycle, and demonstrated similar highs and lows for both wives and husbands with troughs of lesser satisfaction during the midportion of the cycle.[11]

The family life cycle represents the composite of the individual developmental changes of family members, the evolution of the marital relationship, and the cyclic development of the evolving family as a unit. The life cycle of the family is one of constant change as its individuals grow and develop and as their roles and interrelationships within the family change.

STRESS AND TRANSITIONAL CRISES

The course of the family life cycle involves multiple stress points, particularly associated with major change in the family unit and transition from one stage to the next. Critical events such as divorce or death of a spouse precipitate crisis within the family with resultant disequilibrium and need for reorganization. Previous roles and rules of intrafamily relationships frequently fail to maintain satisfactory family organization, and new relationships among family members are often established.

As a result of his work with a social readjustment rating scale, Holmes has concluded that generalizations can be made about the relative stress on family life caused by various life crises. For example, "normative" crises, such as marriage, pregnancy, and retirement, are especially stressful, while divorce, separation, and death are the most stressful among "nonnormative" crises. Table 10-2 shows the relative stress ratings which have been derived from continued research over the years by Holmes and colleagues for various life events.[12]

The process of family reorganization is often unpredictable and potentially disruptive. While the reorganized family may function as well as or better than before the crisis, the result of reorganization frequently may be increased family dysfunction. Figure 10-1 graphically displays the response of a family to crisis resulting in a new level of family function.[13]

Depending on the outcome of the response of individual family members and the family as a whole, a given "normal" crisis may or may not cause a clinical problem perceived by the individual, the family, or the physician as requiring care. Table

TABLE 10-1. STAGE-CRITICAL FAMILY DEVELOPMENT TASKS THROUGH THE FAMILY LIFE CYCLE

Stage of the Family Life Cycle	Positions in the Family	Stage-Critical Family Developmental Tasks
1. Married couple	Wife Husband	Establishing a mutually satisfying marriage Adjusting to pregnancy and the promise of parenthood Fitting into the kin network
2. Childbearing	Wife–mother Husband–father Infant daughter or son or both	Having, adjusting to, and encouraging the development of infants Establishing a satisfying home for both parents and infant(s)
3. Preschool-age	Wife–mother Husband–father Daughter–sister Son–brother	Adapting to the critical needs and interests of preschool children in stimulating, growth-promoting ways Coping with energy depletion and lack of privacy as parents
4. School-age	Wife–mother Husband–father Daughter–sister Son–brother	Fitting into the community of school-age families in constructive ways Encouraging children's educational achievement
5. Teenage	Wife–mother Husband–father Daughter–sister Son–brother	Balancing freedom with responsibility as teenagers mature and emancipate themselves Establishing postparental interests and careers as growing parents
6. Launching center	Wife–mother–grandmother Husband–father–grandfather Daughter–sister–aunt Son–brother–uncle	Releasing young adults into work, military service, college, marriage, etc., with appropriate rituals and assistance Maintaining a supportive home base
7. Middle-aged parents	Wife–mother–grandmother Husband–father–grandfather	Rebuilding the marriage relationship Maintaining kin ties with older and younger generations
8. Aging family members	Widow/widower Wife–mother–grandmother Husband–father–grandfather	Coping with bereavement and living alone Closing the family home or adapting it to aging Adjusting to retirement

(From Duvall EM: Family Development (4th ed). Philadelphia, J.B. Lippincott, 1977, p 151, with permission.)

TABLE 10-2. THE SOCIAL READJUSTMENT RATING SCALE

	Life Event	Mean Value
1.	Death of spouse	100
2.	Divorce	73
3.	Marital separation	65
4.	Jail term	63
5.	Death of close family member	63
6.	Personal injury or illness	53
7.	Marriage	50
8.	Fired at work	47
9.	Marital reconciliation	45
10.	Retirement	45
11.	Change in health of family member	44
12.	Pregnancy	40
13.	Sex difficulties	39
14.	Gain of new family member	39
15.	Business readjustment	39
16.	Change in financial state	38
17.	Death of close friend	37
18.	Change to different line of work	36
19.	Change in number of arguments with spouse	35
20.	Mortgage over $10,000	31
21.	Foreclosure of mortgage or loan	30
22.	Change in responsibilities at work	29
23.	Son or daughter leaving home	29
24.	Trouble with in-laws	29
25.	Outstanding personal achievement	28
26.	Wife begin or stop work	26
27.	Begin or end school	26
28.	Change in living conditions	25
29.	Revision of personal habits	24
30.	Trouble with boss	23
31.	Change in work hours or conditions	20
32.	Change in residence	20
33.	Change in schools	20
34.	Change in recreation	19
35.	Change in church activities	19
36.	Change in social activities	18
37.	Mortgage or loan less than $10,000	17
38.	Change in sleeping habits	16
39.	Change in number of family get-togethers	15
40.	Change in eating habits	15
41.	Vacation	13
42.	Christmas	12
43.	Minor violations of the law	11

(From Holmes TH, Rahe RH: The social readjustment rating scale. J Psychosom Res 11:213, 1967, with permission.)

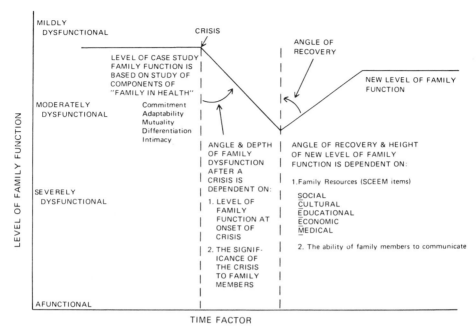

Figure 10-1. Schema for evaluation of family in crisis. *(From Smilkstein G: The family in trouble—How to tell. J Fam Pract 2:19, 1975, with permission.)*

10–3 illustrates various kinds of clinical problems which can occur in response to critical events which commonly occur in the course of a family's life cycle.

This kind of conceptual framework can be useful to family physicians in everyday practice by increasing their awareness of potential future crises in the individual patient and his/her family. It is well known that individuals with certain stress problems have a greater likelihood of developing other problems as a result of future

TABLE 10-3. EXAMPLES OF MAJOR CRISES

Stage	"Normal" Crises	Clinical Problems
Birth of family	Early sexual adjustment	Sexual problems
Expansion of family		
Early (Preschool)	Birth of child	Postpartum depression
Middle (School)	Separation anxiety	Hyperactive child
Late (Adolescence)	"Empty nest" syndrome	Last fling
	Teenage identity crisis	Juvenile delinquency
Dispersion	Career stagnation	Depression
Independence	Menopause	Depression
	Marital readjustment	Alcoholism
	Death of parents	
Replacement	Physical disability	Organic brain syndrome
	Retirement	Depression
	Death of mate	Suicide
	Loneliness	

crises. Thus, the physician caring for an obstetric patient with postpartum depression would observe her more closely 5 years later for signs of separation anxiety. This framework also illustrates that two or more individual "crises" may be concurrent at any given time in a family's development; for example, depression and an "empty nest syndrome" in a 45-year-old wife and mother may coexist with a teenage identity crisis in her 18-year-old son and with postretirement depression in her 66-year-old father.

NATURE OF ILLNESS WITHIN THE FAMILY

General Considerations

Any discussion of the nature of illness within the family is necessarily an extremely complex subject, so that all that will be attempted here is a brief overview of some of the important principles involved in the care of families in health and illness. As already noted, the family is a continuously evolving unit with a life cycle of its own. The occurrence and response of the family to illness are influenced by such diverse factors as the socioeconomic, cultural, environmental, genetic, and educational background of the family; the presence of chronic disease within the family; the level of function of the family as a unit; and previous patterns of health and illness in the family. The family milieu is further complicated by a wide range of complex interactions between the sick family member and the family.

The broad concerns of family physicians bring additional complexity to the subject. They are involved with the full spectrum of health care including health maintenance, preventive and anticipatory care, recognition and management of acute disease, care of chronic illness, rehabilitation, and, ultimately, care of the terminally ill. Family physicians are also involved with illness in the family as a unit as well as illness in a family member as an individual. Family physicians therefore must apply their knowledge of the family, understanding of family dynamics, and clinical knowledge and skills in order to recognize and manage the varied problems encountered in everyday practice.

Incidence

The incidence of illness within the family is determined by a number of interrelated factors which may alter considerably the incidence of illness which is encountered in the individual patient. Some of the more important factors modifying the incidence of illness in the individual include genetic and familial factors, the transmission of infectious disease, and the effect of psychosocial factors.

The occurrence of infectious disease in families has been correlated with several features of family structure and function. Meyer and Haggerty, for example, studied the incidence of streptococcal infections in 16 families over a 1-year period. They found that mothers developed streptococcal illness more often than fathers, and that the incidence of streptococcal infections was highest between ages 2 to 5 years, in family members sleeping in the same room, and in families with acute or chronic stress. They even demonstrated that the likelihood of developing antistreptolysin-0 titer rise depended on the level of stress within the family.[14]

The frequent association of organic and functional problems has been well recognized for years, and often clouds the distinction between organic and functional illness. Somatization (i.e., the presentation by the patient of a physical complaint such as backache, fatigue, or dizziness on the basis of emotional problems and psychosocial stress) provides a classic example of this difficulty. Somatization is encountered in a range of clinical situations including depression, anxiety reactions, malingering, chronic pain disorders, and psychophysiological reactions. It may be precipitated and reinforced by family problems.[15]

There is abundant evidence that psychosocial factors play a major role in the occurrence of illness within families. Medalie and his colleagues, for example, studied the incidence of angina pectoris among 10,000 men, and demonstrated markedly increased incidence of this condition in men with relatively low levels of wives' love and support and in men with families with the most family problems.[16,17]

Although various kinds of family problems, such as marital problems and other family relationship problems, are common in the experience of all family physicians, they tend to be underreported,[18] and their true incidence is not well understood. It has been documented, however, that the sudden increased use of health care services within families is often a signal to the physician that a family problem exists.[19]

Presentation of Illness

The presentation of illness in families is also marked by recognizable features and patterns. Figure 10–2 illustrates the variations which often occur within families as a result of a primary nondifferentiated respiratory infection in one family member. Striking variations in symptomatology, timing and duration of illness are demonstrated among family members.[20]

Peachey has studied the incidence of illness in 25 families of a rural family practice. She has demonstrated four basic patterns of illness—constant illness, regular periodicity, clustering, and simultaneity, and suggests that such patterns may hold predictive value.[21]

The social interactions of a person who is sick or who thinks he/she is sick can be described as "illness behavior." Such behavior may be appropriate or inappropriate according to the circumstances. Examples of inappropriate illness behavior could take the form of an individual with severe and apparent organic disease refusing to assume the sick role, as well as the other side of the issue whereby an individual without organic disease may acquire a sick role.

All practicing physicians, particularly those involved in primary care, can recall many patients who presented with a chief complaint which was not the real reason for seeking care but a kind of "ticket" which was felt by the patient to be "legitimate" in medical terms. It takes a perceptive physician to uncover the real

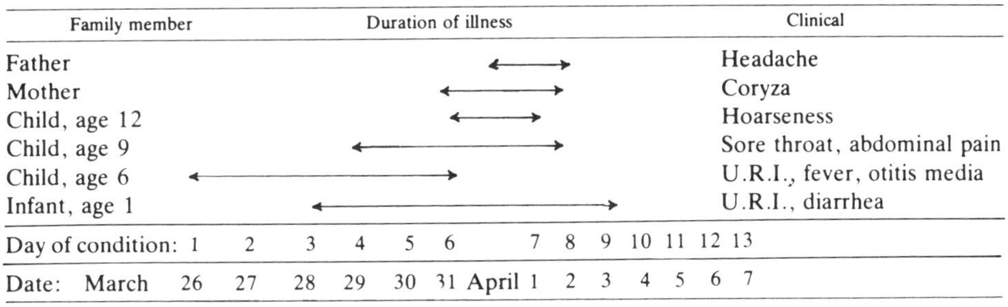

Family member	Duration of illness	Clinical
Father	←——→	Headache
Mother	←————→	Coryza
Child, age 12	←———→	Hoarseness
Child, age 9	←—————→	Sore throat, abdominal pain
Child, age 6	←————————→	U.R.I., fever, otitis media
Infant, age 1	←—————————→	U.R.I., diarrhea
Day of condition: 1 2 3 4 5 6 7 8 9 10 11 12 13		
Date: March 26 27 28 29 30 31 April 1 2 3 4 5 6 7		

Figure 10-2. Nondifferentiated respiratory infection: Primary, secondary, and tertiary cases. *(From Medalie JH: Family medicine—Principles and Applications. Baltimore, Williams & Wilkins, 1978, p 86, with permission.)*

problem in these situations, and in many instances it is related to causative or associated family conflicts. In addition, even when the patient's complaints are valid and undisguised, there may be forces within the family which favor the patient's continued sick role and failure to respond to medical management.

Impact of Individual's Illness on Family

As already noted, a major illness in an individual family member usually precipitates crisis within the family with resultant disequilibrium and need for reorganization. Previous patterns of intrafamily relationships are challenged and often break down when a family member is in the hospital, in danger of dying, disabled, or making new demands on the family.

A family's reaction to crisis has been divided by Hill into three basic phases: (1) initial period of denial; (2) period of confusion, anxiety, and frequently resentment toward the sick family member; and (3) period of recovery and reorganization.[23] While the reorganized family may function as well as or better than before the crisis, the result can often be serious emotional pain or functional disability in one or more family members other than the one who is ill. New relationships between family members will have evolved which the physican should understand. In addition to the possible need for treatment of other members of the family, the physician may find that the recovery or rehabilitation of his/her patient may be unfavorably affected by family reorganization. This underscores the importance of considering the entire family when treating an individual patient with a serious disease or disability.

Olsen has observed that "serious illness is a family affair—the family, not just the patient, has the illness."[23] The family is thrown into disequilibrium, acute illness or exacerbations of chronic illness may be precipitated in other family members, and the family will attempt to shift toward a new homeostasis which will be more tolerable. Serious emotional problems or impairment of functional ability may occur in other family members which will call for further intervention beyond the care of the individual patient with the initial illness.

Examples of these concepts are commonly observed. Klein, Dean, and Bogdanoff have demonstrated an increase in somatic complaints in the spouse of the sick individual.[24] Downes has shown that some chronic diseases, such as hypertensive vascular disease and arthritis, have appeared in both husband and wife at a rate significantly higher than expected.[25] Family members have even been found to go through stages associated with cancer similar to those the sick family member experiences, including shock and anger at the diagnosis, guilt for missed past appointments, and a period of anticipatory grief and hope.[26]

Impact of Family on Individual's Illness

Just as illness in the individual can have profound impact on the family, so can the family as a unit have significant influence on the course of illness in the individual family member. This influence can operate in both positive and negative directions in terms of the individual's illness.[27]

On the positive side, the support of other family members (especially the spouse) can greatly improve the outcome of illness in the individual family member. Both patient compliance and control of hypertension have been shown to be enhanced when the spouse participates in the treatment program of patients with hypertension.[28] A strong association has been demonstrated between family reinforcement and the response of patients to rehabilitation programs.[29] A protective effect of marriage has been documented vis-a-vis the average annual death rates from such diseases as tuberculosis and arteriosclerotic heart disease.[30]

On the negative side, there are likewise abundant examples of unfavorable impact of the family upon individual illness. One study in North Carolina showed marked increases in morbidity and mortality from cerebrovascular disease in blacks correlated with increased disorganization of the family.[31] Another study has documented increased complication rates during pregnancy in women with the combination of high stress and low family support.[32] A further negative example is graphically illustrated by the following observations of Rosen and colleagues in commenting upon the situation of a depressed patient with somatizing complaints:[15]

> When the somatic symptoms of an untreated depression continue over a long period of time, a radical change may occur in family structure and function. A depressed man may be unable to work due to musculoskeletal problems, which may result in his receiving increased nurturance from the family and his wife returning to work. Possible consequences of this scenario are that the "illness" may provide an unconscious solution to chronic anxiety and tension associated with work and unmet intrapsychic needs and may provide the spouse with increased self-esteem and power. Therefore, the family may unconsciously undermine treatment that would return it to its former state of social functioning. Hence even with a "cure" of the disease, the illness may continue.

The potential influences of a given family on the illness of a family member depend in large part on the existing level of function of the family as a unit, whether healthy or dysfunctional. Olsen has noted four features of healthy families which are adapting well to stress and change.

1. There is a clear separation of the generations so that the parents are satisfying each other's emotional needs or, in case of conflict, are able to fight straight.
2. There is a flexibility within and between roles so that shifting can be tolerated with relative comfort.
3. There is a tolerance for individualization. The family can accept and enjoy differences and can tolerate the anxiety of disequilibrium in the system as the members grow and change.
4. Communications among the family members are direct and consistent and tend to confirm the self-esteem of each.

THE FAMILY AS THE UNIT OF CARE

General Considerations

There is presently considerable debate within family medicine as to the extent to which the family per se can or should become the patient in family practice as contrasted with the traditional emphasis on the individual as the patient.[33-36] There is general consensus that the individual patient should remain as the principal focus in the physician–patient relationship in family practice, and that a family orientation and knowledge about the family assists the family physician in caring for individual family members. A variety of specific issues have been raised, however, when the focus shifts to the family unit itself as the patient. These issues include philosophic, technical, educational, and ethical considerations. Some of the objections to the family as patient in its own right include the following:

- Most existing family practices, for a variety of reasons, fall far short of including all family members in the practice.[37,38]
- Patients usually place a higher priority on the care of their individual problems rather than their family problems.[39–41]
- Existing methods for diagnosis and management of family problems per se are still rudimentary.
- There are many potential and actual situations in which the individual family member's interests are in conflict with those of the family and where the family physician may be caught in the middle of this conflict.[42,43]

Despite these difficulties, since there is broad agreement that the family physician needs to know as much as possible about the family regardless of the nature of his/her intervention, it is useful to briefly highlight some of the promising approaches to diagnosis and management which are currently being developed.

Diagnostic Approaches

Several recently developed approaches to gather and record various kinds of information concerning the family are of interest and seem to have practical relevance to family practice.

1. Family Health Tree. Prince–Embury has developed a useful technique designed to assist in the identification of physical symptom patterns within the family. The Family Health Tree consolidates in one form four types of information—simultaneity of symptoms, similarity of symptoms across family members, any dominant physical symptom within the family, and extent of focus versus distribution of symptoms among family members. Figure 10–3 illustrates this method.[44]
2. Genogram. Various methods of recording genograms have been described for application in family practice for recording both genetic and informa-

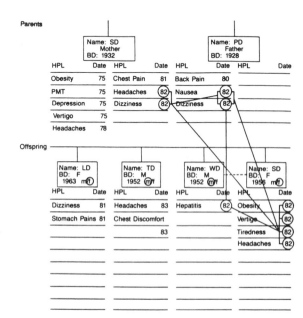

Figure 10-3. Excerpt from family health tree demonstrating simultaneity of symptoms clustering among four family members after marriage of son. *(From Prince-Embury S: The Family Health Tree: A form for identifying physical symptom patterns within the family. J Fam Pract 18:75, 1984, with permission.)*

tion about interpersonal relationships among family members. Figure 10–4 presents an example of such a genogram, together with a listing of genogram symptoms intended to simplify the convenient recording and interpretation of this information.[45]

3. Family APGAR. Smilkstein has developed the Family APGAR as a brief screening questionnaire designed to elicit a data base which assesses the level of family function in terms of five important components—adaptation, partnership, growth, affection, and resolve. A small number of carefully selected open-ended questions can yield basic family function information for each component. An APGAR scoring system is then applied which ranges from a highly functional family (APGAR 7 to 10) to a severely dysfunctional family (APGAR 0 to 3).[46] This technique has seen extensive use since its introduction in 1978, and its reliability and validity have been demonstrated in a number of studies in different population groups.[47]

   Smilkstein suggests that the workup of the dysfunctional family should include, in addition to the Family APGAR, two additional diagnostic approaches: (1) identification and evaluation of the family's crises, present and past; and (2) assessment of the family's resources.[46]

4. Family Assessment Schema. Arbogast and colleagues have recently described another method to assess family function which is presently being used by the Family Medicine Program at the University of Maryland.[48] They have developed a short family interview questionnaire which gathers information on the family life cycle, family process, and the family's social milieu (Table 10–4).

5. Family Circle Method. This method is a simple process in which individual family members are asked to make a family circle drawing representing his/her personal view of family relationships. These drawings provide a graphic view of patterns of closeness and distance, of power and decision making, and of family alliances and boundaries. They can be quite helpful in readily acquiring added perspective on family dynamics.[49]

6. Family Problem-Oriented Medical Record. In order to facilitate and organize pertinent information concerning the family, a practical method for maintaining a family-oriented medical record is also required. Two similar methods have been found useful in community-based family practice, including a family problem list and family tree data.[50,51]

Management Approaches

Although management approaches to problems of dysfunctional families are not as yet well developed, some broad principles can be briefly outlined which allow for a varied set of treatment options adapted to the particular needs of each family. Crucial to the effectiveness of any approach, however, is the family physician's understanding of the family's problem(s) and the family dynamics in process, together with his/her own skills as a "therapeutic instrument."

The family physician's effectiveness in dealing with family problems is enhanced by the following attributes:

1. Capacity to listen as an active process
2. Ability to observe and interpret interactions among family members
3. Knowledge of family dynamics in health and illness
4. Ability to communicate clearly, to facilitate communication between family members, and to present an empathetic, open self to the family

194

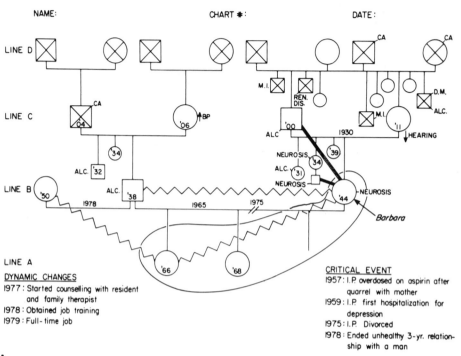

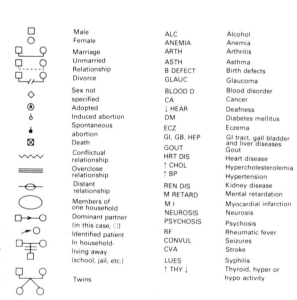

Figure 10-4. A. Completed genogram for Barbara. **B.** Genogram symbols. *(From Jolly N, Froom J, Rosen MG: The genogram, J Fam Pract 10:251, 1980, with permission.)*

TABLE 10-4. FAMILY INTERVIEW QUESTIONNAIRE

Family Life Cycle
- (I)[a] 1. How many are there in the family?
- (I)   2. Who lives at home?
- (A)   3. In what phase of the family life cycle is this family?
- (I)   4. What problems does this raise for them presently?
- (I)   5. What major problems has this family had in the past (inquire about death, separation, major physical or mental illness, financial crisis, etc.)?
- (I)   6. Does this family feel these problems were dealt with satisfactorily?

Family Process or Psychosocial Interior
- (I)   1. Who are the major decision makers in the family?
- (I)   2. Who can each person talk to most easily?
- (I)   3. What are the family members expectations of each other? Are these expectations being achieved? (Are they realistic?)
- (I)   4. How does each member of this family get attention?
- (A)   5. How much tolerance for individual difference and self-expression is there in the family?

Social Milieu
- (I)   1. How much contact do you have with relatives? Are they helpful? Do they create problems?
- (I)   2. Do the family members have many friends in their neighborhood? To what groups or clubs do family members belong?
- (I)   3. What sort of community resources has the family used? Would they use them again?
- (I)   4. What is the educational level and the financial status of the parents of the family?

[a]I = Inquire; A = Assess. *(From Arbogast RC, Scratton JM, Krick JP: The family as patient: An assessment schema. J Fam Pract 7:1151, 1978, with permission.)*

5. Ability to be nonjudgmental and to avoid entangling alliances with individual family members
6. Appreciation of sociocultural and environmental influences on family life styles
7. Recognition of the family life cycle as the evolving milieu for health and illness in the family
8. Capacity to integrate behavioral science principles and care of family problems into the traditional medical care of clinical problems of individual patients
9. Understanding and awareness of oneself as a therapeutic agent
10. Ability to individualize the care of individual patients and their families based upon the unique circumstances and needs of each family.

Once the family physician has identified a specific family problem, he/she is then faced with the need to select a particular kind and style of intervention. Consideration must be given to frequency and duration of future visits, inclusion of other family members in addition to the identified individual patient(s), and possible participation of other health professionals.

The family physician's interventions will most commonly involve short-term counseling, including selected family members as appropriate. Ornstein recommends that the family physician develop his/her own personal skills and methods as a "therapeutic instrument" rather than attempt to apply traditional "psychiatric" styles of intervention.[52] Cathell echoes this advice, noting that the family physician is more directive, authoritative, problem-oriented, and pragmatic than the psychiatrist, and suggesting that the family physician's methods should be based on these differences and the particular nature of his practice.[53]

Much can be accomplished by the family physician in the course of office visits linked to other forms of treatment. In the case of a depressed patient being treated for duodenal ulcer, for example, it takes little time to palpate for epigastric tenderness and evaluate response to drug and dietary management. An excellent opportunity is available to uncover sources of stress and related problems in the patient's life and family.

Brief crisis intervention counseling is a technique especially well suited to the management of many common problems encountered in family practice. Schwenk and Bittle have suggested a number of situations amenable to this approach as listed in Table 10-5.[54]

Involvement of other family members may vary from a series of formal counseling sessions for a couple with a marital problem to intermittent visits involving

TABLE 10-5. CRISIS AMENABLE TO CRISIS INTERVENTION

Precipitating Event	Classification[a] Biologic	Environmental/	Adventitious	Type of Loss[b] Sexual/Self-Esteem	Role	Mastery/Nurturing
Small child starting school	X					X
Adolescent maturation (pubertal)	X				X	X
Death of a close relative	X					X
Menopause	X			X	X	
Retirement	X			X	X	
Child outside of marriage		X		X	X	X
Promotion to new job		X				X
Adopted child		X		X		
Divorce		X		X		X
Birth of premature child			X	X	X	
Diagnosis of chronic illness			X	X		
Rape			X	X	X	
Alcoholism in parent			X			X
Impotence			X	X	X	
Myocardial infarction			X		X	
Attempted suicide in relative			X	X		X

[a]Cumming J, Cumming E: Ego and Mileau. Chicago, Aldine, 1962.
[b]Stickler and LaSor: Ment Hyg 54:2, 1970.
(From: Schwenk TL, Bittle SP: Applicability of crisis intervention in family practice. J Fam Prac 8:1151, 1979, with permission.)

two or more family members, and occasionally a conference of the entire family may be useful. Schmidt has recently proposed a set of indications for convening the family,[57] which is based upon a reasonable probability of associated family problems (Table 10–6).[58–94] Counseling visits need not be lengthy—much can be ac-

TABLE 10-6. INDICATIONS FOR CONVENING THE FAMILY

Medical Condition	Associated Family Situation Problem(s)	Supporting Data
Pregnancy	High stress, low support, complications; fathers have symptoms	Nuckolls;[58] Lipkin, Lamb[59]
Failure to thrive	General, unspecified	Mitchell et al.[60]
Recurrent childhood poisoning	Stressful life event in context of emotional instability	Rogers[61]
Preschool behavior problems	Strained marital relationships	Richman[62]
School behavior problems	Marital disharmony	Whitehead[63]
Adolescent maladjustment	Effective parental coalition and clear intergenerational boundaries required for growth	Kleinman[64]
Major depression	Somatization, spouse and children become ill	Calling;[65] Widmer et al.;[66] Crook, Raskin;[67] Aneshensil et al.[68]
Chronic illness	Hidden patients within the family	Downes,[69] Klein et al.[70]
Diabetes	Marital stress, nondiabetic child suffers, parents unnecessarily restrict activity and career aspirations	Downes;[71] Crain et al.[72] Katz;[73] Crain et al.;[74] Kronenfeld, Ory[75]
Arteriosclerotic heart disease, coronary bypass surgery	Family support improves medical and psychological outcomes	Medalie et al.;[76] Zyzanski, Schmidt;[77] Segev, Schlesinger[78]
Poor adherence to medical regimen	Family's attitudes greatly influence patient adherence	Steiell;[79] Cooper, Lynch;[80] Heinzelmann, Bagley;[81] Oakes;[82] Litman;[83] Schulz[84]
High "inappropriate" use of health services	Family stress, health behavior is learned from the family, low support associated with high utilization	Mechanic;[85] Mechanic;[86] Blake et al.[87]
Terminal illness	Spouse develops physical problems	Guillo;[88] Bertman[89]
Bereavement	Increased morbidity and mortality, little support from family when a neonate dies	Kraus, Lilienfield;[90] Rees, Lutking;[91] Parkes, Brown;[92] Parkes et al.;[93] Helmrath, Steinitz[94]

(From Schmidt DD: When is it helpful to convene the family? J Fam Pract 16:967, 1983, with permission.)

TABLE 10-7. CONTRAST BETWEEN WORKING WITH FAMILIES IN FAMILY MEDICINE AND FAMILY THERAPY

Family Medicine	Family Therapy
Focus on prevention and on normal developmental tasks of family rather than dysfunction	Focus on treatment of family dysfunction
If change occurs, initiative comes from within the system. No contract for change	Change dependent on intervention from outside system
Longer contact (in years) with family over time	Therapy for 3 to 12 months is usual
Briefer (half-hour) and fewer (1 to 3 average) sessions with whole family perhaps several weeks apart	Longer (1 hour) and more (weekly) sessions with whole family (7 to 10 minimum)
Individual contacts can add to overall picture of family in less threatening manner (focus may be on physical symptom)	Whole family or subsystems usually seen. Resistance may be high; many families refuse family therapy
Broader focus available through familiarity with the extended family over time, and with the community	Only immediate family members known to the therapist and focus is on limited problem areas
Clinician has often joined with members separately prior to whole family interview	"Joining" may take several months
Relationship facilitated by dependence on clinician's medical expertise	Credibility as someone with expertise on family may be higher
Lack of expertise in managing difficult family problems and exceeding limits of training may result in problems if family refuses to see family therapist	Much greater expertise and experience with difficult families makes crisis into occasions for change

(From Christie-Seely J Jr: Teaching the family system concept in family medicine. J Fam Pract 13:391, 1981, with permission.)

complished in a series of visits, each as short as 20 or 30 minutes. Christie-Seely has compared the process and content of family counseling as practiced by family physicians with that of family therapy as summarized in Table 10–7.[95]

Some reports have documented the value of family sessions. Liebman, Silbergleit and Farber, for example, have found a family conference of value in the care of the patient with cancer,[96] while Hoebel has found brief family-interactional therapy effective in the management of cardiac-related high-risk behaviors.[97]

Future family practice groups are likely to develop a variety of organizational approaches to deal with family problems. Some may involve other health professionals on either a part-time or full-time basis in the care of these problems within the group setting. Many family practice residency programs are already involving others, such as clinical psychologists and medical social workers, in the management of family problems. Whatever approach family physicians take to these kinds of problems, the overriding requisite is that they be sensitive to ways in which their added knowledge of the family can help in providing better care for individual family members, and in some instances, to the family as a unit.

REFERENCES

1. Carmichael LP: The family in medicine, process or entity? J Fam Pract 3:562, 1976
2. Ogburn WF: Quoted in understanding the changing role of the family today. Patient Care Management Concepts, Vol. 3, Oct. 31, 1969 p 22
3. Spanier GB: The changing profile of the American family. J Fam Pract 13:61, 1981
4. Livsey CG: Family therapy: Role of the practicing physician. Modern Treatment 6:808, 1969
5. Household and family characteristics. In: Bureau of the Census (Suitland, Md.): Current Population Reports, series P-20 No. 352, Government Printing Office, 1980
6. Marital status and living arrangements. In: Bureau of the Census (Suitland, Md.): Current Population Reports, series P-20, No. 349. Government Printing Office, 1980
7. Number, timing, and duration of marriages and divorces in the United States. In: Bureau of the Census (Suitland, Md.): Current Population Reports, series P-20, No. 297. Government Printing Office, 1976
8. Curry HB: The family as our patient. J Fam Pract 1:70, 1974
9. Worby CM: The family life cycle: An orienting concept for the family practice specialist. J Med Educ 46(3):198, 1971
10. Duvall EM: Family Development (4th ed). Philadelphia, J. B. Lippincott, 1971, p 151
11. Rollins BC, Feldman H: Marital satisfaction over the family life cycle. J Marriage and Family 32:25, February 1970
12. Holmes TH, Rahe RH: The social readjustment rating scale. J Psychosom Res 11:213, 1967
13. Smilkstein G: The family in trouble—how to tell. J Fam Pract 2:19, 1975
14. Meyer RJ, Haggerty RJ: Streptococcal infections in families: Factors altering individual susceptibility. Pediatrics 29:539, 1962
15. Rosen G, Kleinman A, Katon W: Somatization in family practice: A biopsychosocial approach. J Fam Pract 14:493, 1982
16. Medalie JH, Goldbourt U: Angina pectoris among 10,000 men. II. Psychosocial and other risk factors as evidence by a multivariate analysis of a 5-year incidence study. Am J Med 60:910, 1976
17. Medalie JH, Snyder M, Groen JJ, et al.: Angina pectoris among 10,000 men. Am J Med 55:583, 1973
18. Stewart WL: Clinical evidence of the Virginia study. J Fam Pract 3:30, 1976
19. Mechanic D: The influence of mothers on their children's health attitudes and behavior. Pediatrics 33:444, 1964
20. Medalie JH: Family Medicine—Principles and Applications. Baltimore, Williams and Wilkins, 1978, p 86
21. Peachey R: Family patterns of illness. GP 27:82, 1963
22. Hill R: Social stresses on the family. Social Case Work 39:139, 1958
23. Olsen EH: The impact of serious illness on the family system. Postgrad Med 172, February 1970
24. Klein R, Dean A, Bogdanoff M: The impact of illness upon the spouse. J Chron Dis 20:241, 1968
25. Downes J: Chronic disease among spouses. Milbank Mem Fund Quarterly 25:334, 1947
26. Bruhn JG: Effects of chronic illness on the family. J Fam Pract 4(6):1057, 1977
27. Richardson HB: Patients have families. New York, Commonwealth Fund, 1945
28. Schmidt DD: The family as the unit of care. J Fam Pract 7:303, 1978
29. Litman TJ: The family and physical rehabilitation. J Chron Dis 19:211, 1966

30. Kraus A, Lilienfeld A: Some epidemiologic aspects of the high mortality rate in the young widowed group. J Chron Dis 10:207, 1959

31. Smith H: North Carolina Mental Health Planning Staff: A comprehensive mental health plan for North Carolina. Vol. 1, Attach. 3, Raleigh, N.C., N.C. Dept. of Mental Health, 1965, p 35

32. Nuckolls K: Life crises and psychosocial assets: Some clinical implications. In Kaplan BH, Cassel JC (eds): Family and Health. Chapel Hill, N. C., Institute for Research in Social Science University of North Carolina, 1975

33. Schwenk TL, Hughes CC: The family as patient in family medicine: Rhetoric or reality? Soc Sci Med 17:1, 1983

34. Merkel WT: The family and family medicine: Should this marriage be saved? J Fam Pract 17:857, 1983

35. Carmichael LP: Forty families—A search for the family in family medicine. Fam Systems Med 1:12, 1983

36. Ransom DC: On why it is useful to say that "The family is a unit of care" in family medicine: Comment on Carmichael's essay. Fam Systems Med 1:17, 1983

37. Fujikawa LS, Bass RA, Schneiderman LJ: Family care in a family practice group. J Fam Pract 8:1189, 1979

38. Wall EM, Shear CL: Characteristics of patients seeking family-oriented care. J Fam Pract 17:665, 1983

39. Kiraly DA, Coulton CJ, Graham A: How family practice patients view their utilization of mental health services. J Fam Pract 15:317, 1982

40. Schwenk TL, Clark CH, Jones GR, et al.: Defining a behavioral science curriculum for family physicians: What do patients think? J Fam Pract 15:339, 1982

41. Hyatt JD: Perceptions of the family physician by patients and family physicians. J Fam Pract 10:295, 1980

42. Williamson P. McCormick T, Taylor T: Who is the patient? A family case study of a recurrent dilemma in family practice. J Fam Pract 17:1039, 1983

43. Brody H: Ethics in family medicine: Patient autonomy and the family unit. J Fam Pract 17:973, 1983

44. Prince-Embury S: The Family Health Tree: A form for identifying physical symptom patterns within the family. J Fam Pract 18:75, 1984

45. Jolly N, Froom J, Rosen MG: The genogram. J Fam Pract 10:251, 1980

46. Smilkstein G: The family APGAR: A proposal for a family function test and its use by physicians. J Fam Pract 6:1231, 1978

47. Smilkstein G, Ashworth C, Montano D: Validity and reliability of the family APGAR as a test of family function. J Fam Pract 15:303, 1983

48. Arbogast RC, Scratton JM, Krick JP: The family as patient: An assessment schema. J Fam Pract 7:1151, 1978

49. Thrower SM, Bruce WE, Walton RF: The Family Circle method for integrating family systems concepts in family medicine. J Fam Pract 15:451, 1982

50. Grace NT, Neal EM, Wellock CE, Pile DD: The family-oriented problem-oriented medical record. J Fam Pract 4:91, 1977

51. Ruth DH, Rigden S, Brunworth D: An integrated family-oriented medical record. J Fam Pract 8:1179, 1979

52. Ornstein PH: The family physican as a "therapeutic instrument." J Fam Pract 4:659, 1977

53. Cathell JL: Somehow, "GP-style" psychotherapy works. Consultant 8:12, 1968

54. Schwenk TL, Bittle SP: Applicability of crisis intervention in family practice. J Fam Pract 8:1151, 1979

55. Cumming J, Cumming E: Ego and Mileau. Chicago, Aldine Publishing, 1962

56. Strickler M, LaSor B: The concept of loss in crisis intervention. Ment Hyg 54:2, 1970
57. Schmidt DD: When is it helpful to convene the family? J Fam Pract 16:967, 1983
58. Nuckolls K: Life crisis and psychosocial assets: Some clinical implications. In Kaplan BH, Cassel JC (eds): Family and Health. Chapel Hill, N.C., Institute for Research in Social Science, University of North Carolina, 1975
59. Lipkin M, Lamb GS: The couvade syndrome: An epidemiologic study. Ann Intern Med 96:509, 1982
60. Mitchell WG, Gurrell MA, Greenberg RA: Failure-to-thrive: A study in a primary care setting, epidemiology and follow up. Pediatrics 65:971, 1980
61. Rogers J: Recurrent childhood poisoning as a family problem. J Fam Pract 13:337, 1981
62. Richman N: Behaviour problems in pre-school children: Family and social factors. Br J Psychiatry 131:523, 1977
63. Whitehead L: Sex differences in children's responses to family stress: A re-evaluation. J Child Psychol Psychiatry 20:247, 1979
64. Kleinman JI: Parental coalition and optimal psychosocial function of male adolescents. The relationship of family structure to psychosocial health in "healthy" and "normal" adolescent males, dissertation. Garden City, N.Y., Adelphi University, 1976
65. Calling A: The sick family. JR Coll Gen Pract 14:181, 1964
66. Widmer RB, Cadoret RJ, North CS: Depression in family practice: Some effects on spouses and children. J Fam Pract 10:45, 1980
67. Crook T, Raskin A: Parent–child relationships and adult depression. Child Dev 52:950, 1981
68. Aneshensil CS, Fredericks RR, Clark VA: Family roles and sex differences in depression. J Health Soc Behav 22:379, 1981
69. Downes J: Illness in the chronic disease family. Am J Public Health 32:589, 1942
70. Klein R, Dean A, Bogdonoff MD: The impact of illness upon the spouse. J Chronic Dis 20:241, 1978
71. Downes J: Chronic disease among spouses. Milbank Mem Fund Qu 25:334, 1947
72. Crain JA, Sussman MB, Weil WB: Effects of a diabetic child on marital integration and related measures of family functioning. J Health Hum Behav 7:122, 1966
73. Katz AM: Wives of diabetic men. Bull Memminger Clin 33:279, 1969
74. Crain JA, Sussman MB, Weil WB: Family interaction, diabetes, and sibling relationships. Int J Soc Psychiatry 12:35, 1966
75. Kronenfeld JJ, Ory MG: Familial perception of juvenile diabetes. Postgrad Med 70:83, 1981
76. Medalie JH, Synder M, Groen JJ, et al.: Angina pectoris among 10,000 men—Five year incidence and univariate analysis. Am J Med 55:583, 1973
77. Zyzanski SJ, Schmidt DD: Family support following coronary bypass surgery: Psychologic and medical correlates. Presented to the North American Primary Care Research Group, Columbus, Ohio, May 19, 1982
78. Segev U, Schlesinger Z: Rehabilitation of patients after acute myocardial infarction: An interdisciplinary, family-oriented program. Heart Lung 10:841, 1981
79. Steiell JH: Medical condition, adherence to treatment regimens, and family functioning. Arch Gen Psychiatry 37:1025, 1980
80. Cooper NA, Lynch MA: Lost to follow up: A study of non-attendance at a general paediatric outpatient clinic. Arch Dis Child 55:765, 1979
81. Heinzelmann F, Bagley R: Response to physical activity programs and their effects on health behavior. Public Health Rep 85:905, 1970
82. Oakes TW: Family expectations and arthritis patient compliance to a hand-resting splint regimen. J Chronic Dis 22:757, 1970
83. Litman TJ: The family and physical rehabilitation. J Chronic Dis 19:211, 1966

84. Schulz SK: Compliance with therapeutic regimens in pediatrics: A review of implications for social work practice. Soc Work Health Care 5:267, 1980
85. Mechanic D: The influence of mothers on their children's health attitudes and behavior. Pediatrics 33:444, 1964
86. Mechanic D: The experience and report of common physical complaints. J Health Soc Behav 21:146, 1980
87. Blake RL, Roberts C, Mackey T, Hosokawa M: Social support and utilization of medical care. J Fam Pract 11:810, 1980
88. Guillo SV: A study of selected psychological, psychosomatic, and somatic reactions in women anticipating the death of a husband, dissertation. New York, Columbia University, 1981.
89. Bertman SL: Lingering terminal illness and the family: Insights from literature. Fam Process 19:341. 1980
90. Kraus AS, Lilienfield AM: Some epidemiologic aspects of the high mortality rate in the young widowed group. J Chronic Dis 10:207, 1959
91. Rees WD, Lutking SG: Mortality of bereavement. Br Med J 1:13, 1967
92. Parkes CM, Brown RJ: Health after bereavement—A controlled study of young Boston widows and widowers. Psychosom Med 34:449, 1972
93. Parkes CM, Benjamin B, Fitzgerald RG: Broken heart: A statistical study of increased mortality among widowers. Br Med J 1:740, 1969
94. Helmrath TA, Steinitz EM: Death of an infant: parental grieving and the failure of social support. J Fam Pract 6:785, 1978
95. Christie-Seely J Jr: Teaching the family system concept in family medicine. J Fam Pract 13:391, 1981
96. Liebman A, Silbergleit, I, Farber S: Family conference in the care of the cancer patient. J Fam Pract 2:343, 1975
97. Hoebel FC: Brief family-interactional therapy in the management of cardiac-related high-risk behaviors. J Fam Pract 3:613, 1976

11 Practice Patterns of Family Physicians

The last two chapters have examined the clinical content of family practice from two vantage points—the individual patient and the family as patient. The focus so far has therefore been on What is seen in family practice, not how this kind of care is actually provided in the community. Against this background, it is now of interest to look at the process of care in family practice.

The purpose of this chapter is twofold: (1) to describe some basic patterns of family practice in the United States from several perspectives; and (2) to compare family practice with other specialties in terms of practice patterns, including workload, practice style, and practice satisfaction.

SOME PATTERNS OF PRACTICE

Organizational Structures
One of the striking features of changing medical practice in most fields of medicine in this country in recent years is the steady growth of group practice. The American Medical Association defines group practice as:

> the application of medical services by three or more physicians formally organized to provide medical care, consultation, diagnosis and/or treatment through joint use of equipment and personnel, and with the income from medical practice distributed in accordance with methods previously determined by members of the group.

The number of groups in the United States doubled between 1965 and 1975, while the proportion of organizational forms represented by partnerships decreased from 77.8 percent in 1965 to 27.7 percent in 1975. During the same 10-year period, the average size of all types of group practice increased—by 1975 family practice groups* averaged 3.5 physicians per group and multispecialty groups averaged 13 physicians per group.[1] By 1983, among office-based physicians in all specialties, about 60 percent were in solo practice, 10 percent in partnerships, and the rest in various forms of group practice (with 13 percent in large groups with more than 15 physicians each).[2]

With the growth of group practice among family physicians, partnership and

---

*A Family Practice Group is defined by the American Medical Association as one composed predominantly of general/family physicians.[1]

solo practice have steadily decreased. That this trend will continue unabated is reflected by the choices being made by today's family practice residency graduates—only about 16 to 18 percent of graduates have opted for solo practice during the last 10 years. Dramatic differences were found by physician age in choices of group, partnership, and solo practice among respondents to the previously described USC study, with solo practice declining from over 92 percent of general/family physicians over 65 years of age to about 45 percent of those less than 35 years old.[3] By comparison, among all active members of the American Academy of Family Physicians (AAFP) in 1983, 43 percent were in solo practice and 11.5 percent were in partnerships.[4]

The USC study examined comparative workloads and hours worked by general/family physicians in solo, single-specialty, and multispecialty group practice. Table 11–1 shows rather similar figures for these three types of practice, and

TABLE 11-1. PATIENT ENCOUNTERS, PROFESSIONAL HOURS WORKED, AND PATIENTS SEEN PER PROFESSIONAL HOUR BY PHYSICIAN, PRACTICE, AND ENVIRONMENTAL CHARACTERISTICS

	Total Patient Encounters Weekly (Weighted Mean) (n = 577)	Total Professional Hours Worked Weekly (Weighted Mean) (n = 546)	Patients Seen Per Professional Hour (n = 514)
Physician characteristics			
Residency graduate			
Yes	141.0	52.5	2.70 ⎤
No	169.8	49.2	3.44 ⎦
Board certified			
Yes	164.6	50.8	3.16
No	168.5	49.0	3.46
Age			
Under 45 yr	156.8	49.3	3.32
45–54 yr	187.7	50.7	3.62
Over 54 yr	154.9	48.6	3.20
Practice characteristics			
Arrangement			
Solo	166.8	49.5	3.34
Single-specialty group	171.0	49.0	3.57
Multispeciality group	164.9	50.7	3.29
Urbanization level			
SMSA	155.6 ⎤	48.5	3.22
Adjacent to SMSA	202.2 ⎦	51.5	3.81 ⎤
Not adjacent to SMSA	181.8	51.3	3.58 ⎦
Region			
Northeast	156.3	49.7	3.18
North Central	160.7	49.7	3.22
South	191.8 ⎤	50.5	3.81
West	130.9 ⎦	45.9	2.85

Note: Brackets denote statistically significant differences at 0.05 level using two-tailed unpaired t test with 10 degrees of freedom using standard errors corrected for design defects.
(From Rosenblatt RA, Cherkin DC, Schneeweiss R, et al.: The structure and content of family practice: Current status and future trends. J Fam Pract 15:681, 1982, with permission.)

further compares them with comparable figures accounting for differences in regional location, age, residency training, and board certification.[3]

There are many advantages to group practice. The group can allow frequent consultation among its members, emergency coverage of nights and weekends on a rotating basis, and many fringe benefits. Vacation and continuing education time can be readily scheduled within the group. Overhead expenses can be shared, and more staff and facilities can be afforded than by the individual practitioner. Retirement and pension plans are available, as well as life insurance at a lower cost, and one can enter practice without an initial capital outlay. But there are some disadvantages to group practice, which for some individuals in some communities would make other methods of practice preferable. There may be professional, business, or personality causes of disagreement among physician–members for many reasons. Occasionally older members of larger groups tend to take advantage of their seniority, which becomes a progressive cause of friction and discontent. Income distribution may not correlate well with the productivity of individual members. Group physicians may not set their own pace as easily as if they were in solo or partnership practice. In some multispecialty groups, the family physician may not have the opportunity to practice the full range of his skills and interests.

Partnership with another family physician often affords an excellent method of practice, especially if the two partners have had comparable levels of training and share a similar philosophy of practice. Another common approach is that of expense-sharing agreements, which in a sense are hybrid partnerships/groups. Such arrangements may allow solo practitioners in adjoining offices to share many overhead expenses, as well as provide emergency coverage of each other's practice on nights and weekends. The individual physician can thereby achieve some of the advantages of group practice while alleviating some of the disadvantages of solo practice.

Solo practice allows maximal independence and a full sense of individuality to one's practice. But the increasing need for more complex facilities and staff in family practice, together with the essential need for adequate coverage during time away from the practice, will probably result in a continuing trend away from solo practice for most family physicians.

Although the trend is toward more group practice by family physicians, the variations among individual family physicians and community settings will likely foster the continuation of partnership practice and, to a lesser extent, solo practice.

Practice Settings

As already noted in earlier chapters, family practice is a flexible form of medical practice which directly meets the needs of the community in all types of practice settings, whether urban, suburban, or rural. Family physicians may organize their practices along any of the lines which have just been described, and may practice in either the private sector or in a variety of environments within the public sector.

One of the recently developing important trends is the increasing variability in practice arrangements among family physicians, including the growing trend toward one form or another of salaried practice. In 1980, 84 percent of AAFP active members were in private, fee-for-service practice. By 1983, this group had decreased to 73 percent, whereas 15.5 percent of those in nongovernmental practice were on straight salary, with another 9.5 percent working for salary plus percentage. At that time, 10 percent were in HMOs, 7.5 percent in IPAs, 3.8 percent in PPOs, and 2.2 percent in free-standing episodic care centers.[4] In 1981, among all general/family physicians in the United States, 14 percent were working under contracts with hospitals,[5] usually based in hospital or satellite clinics. As a growing number of hospitals become more active in expanding their primary care networks, this figure is certain to increase.

Group practice for some years has been growing by about 8 percent per year, but many expect more rapid growth in the 1980s the "decade of group practice." Some of the current trends in group practice include an emphasis on marketing; increasing size of groups, both for single-specialty and multispecialty groups; increasing emphasis on networking, including satellite clinics; increasing preference of young physicians to join groups; and increasingly common use of incentive plans as opposed to equal-distribution plans.[2]

The public sector continues to attract a sizable number of physicians in various settings, including the National Health Service Corps (NHSC), Indian Health Service, and a variety of other governmental ambulatory and hospital settings.

A number of studies have demonstrated some interesting patterns of choice of specific practice settings by physicians. As one example, Cooper and colleagues studied the factors influencing the location decision of 1161 physicians in the primary care specialties. They found that a wide range of personal and professional considerations are involved in this decision, to the extent that no one factor was ranked as the most important factor by over 50 percent of respondents. Table 11–2 lists the frequency of factors listed first, second, or third in importance in decision making. It can be noted that the opportunity to join a desirable partnership or group practice was the most influential single factor by this group.[6]

Age Spectrum of Practice

The USC study has provided an interesting overview of the age spectrum of the patient population in family practice.[3] These findings are almost identical to those of the National Ambulatory Medical Care Survey. Several differences were demonstrated by age of physician, extent of residency training, and region of the country:

- Younger physicians see a higher proportion of children and women in the child-bearing years, while the overall age of the practice population tends to age as the physician ages.
- Though older family physicians have an older practice, virtually all general/family physicians have an active patient population in both pediatric and geriatric age groups (i.e., "age specialization" rarely occurs).
- Residency-trained family physicians (i.e., younger physicians) see proportionately more women of child-bearing age and fewer pediatric and geriatric patients than nonresidency-trained physicians.
- Rural physicians showed the opposite pattern, seeing more pediatric and geriatric patients and fewer women in their child-bearing years than do urban physicians.
- Western physicians see more women of child-bearing age and fewer pediatric and geriatric patients, while northeastern physicians have the opposite pattern.
- Demographic features are the most important factors influencing the practice population of U.S. family physicians, demonstrating that family practice does in fact adapt to the needs of the population it serves.[3]

TABLE 11-2. FREQUENCY OF FACTORS RANKED FIRST, SECOND, OR THIRD, BY ALL PRIMARY CARE PHYSICIANS[a]

Factor	No.	%
Opportunity to join a desirable partnership or group practice	499	43.0
Climate or geographic features of area	402	34.6
Availability of clinical support facilities and personnel	251	21.6
Preference for urban or rural living	250	21.5
Income potential	192	16.5
Opportunity for regular contact with a medical school or medical center	184	15.9
Influence of wife or husband (her/his desires, career, etc.)	181	15.6
Having been brought up in such a community	163	14.0
Having gone through medical school, internship, residency, or military service near area	143	12.3
Recreational and sports facilities	139	12.0
High medical need in area	136	11.7
Quality of educational system for children	119	10.3
Opportunity for regular contact with other physicians	113	9.7
Influence of family or friends	107	9.2
Access to continuing education	103	8.9
Cultural advantages	91	7.8
Opportunity to work with specific institution	68	5.9
Opportunities for social life	40	3.5
Prosperity of community	30	2.6
Organized efforts of community to recruit physicians	22	1.9
Advice of older physician	21	1.8
Prospect of being more influential in community affairs	20	1.7
Influences of preceptorship program	12	1.0
Payment of forgiveness loan	11	1.0
Availability of good social service, welfare, or home care services	11	1.0
Availability of loans for beginning practice	9	0.8

[a] N = 1,161.
(From Cooper JK, Heald KS, Coleman S: Rural or urban practice: Factors influencing the location decisions of primary care physicians. Inquiry 12:18, 1975, with permission.)

Team Practice

Another dimension of changing health care in many fields is the growing emphasis upon "team practice." For all office-based physicians in the United States the average number of nonphysician personnel per physician increased from 1.7 to 2.1 between 1975 and 1981.[5] Family practice groups include a larger staff of allied health personnel per physician (2.57) compared with other specialties.[1] This is not surprising in view of the broad range of services and relatively high patient volume characteristic of family practice.

"Team practice" is not as new a concept as some would have us believe. Certainly it can be argued that physicians working together in a group represent one form of team practice. It is also evident that various kinds of allied health personnel have worked closely with physicians for many years on a teamwork basis. There is, however, a trend toward increased diversity of disciplines contributing to today's patient care, together with greater amounts of responsibility being delegated by physicians to allied health professionals for certain aspects of patient care.

The previously described physician extender represents an important new addition to family practice in many settings. Although functionally comparable in terms of training and roles, physician extenders in primary care represent two basic groups: physician's assistant (including Medex) and nurse practitioner. As a group, Medex graduates have been most directly involved with family practice and with rural locations. Other physicians' assistants and nurse practitioners have gravitated more toward urban and institutional settings, although about one-fifth of them have located in rural areas in association with family physicians.[7] Over 40 percent of all physicians' assistants in practice are working under the supervision of family physicians.[8]

Over one-half of Medex are employed in solo or partnership practices, whereas nurse practitioners and other physicians' assistants are most frequently associated with groups or other more organized practice settings.[9] Overall comparisons between the percentage employed and workload of these three groups are shown in Table 11–3.[7]

As physician extenders have become integrated in everyday medical practice, the development of protocols for the care of specific clinical problems has facilitated their active role in patient care. The use of protocols by well-trained physician extenders can save physician time and facilitate the evaluation of medical care without compromising the quality of care (which may be improved in the process).

It is likely that other disciplines will in the future contribute more actively, especially on a part-time and consultative basis, to comprehensive care in family practice settings. Blanchard and Kurtz have described the involvement of a medical social worker in family practice, with a particular focus on preventive and early

TABLE 11-3. SELF-REPORTED ACTIVITIES OF PHYSICIAN EXTENDER GRADUATES[a]

	Physician's Assistants	Medex	Nurse Practitioner (Certificate)	Nurse Practitioner (Master's)
Percentage employed	89	96	90	98
Median number of patients seen daily	24	> 25	12	11
Median patient care hours worked per week as NHP	48	48	31	39

Note: response rates vary for each item

[a]Adapted from Nurse Practitioner and Physician Assistant Training–Deployment Study. Bethesda, Md., System Sciences, Inc., Sept. 30, 1976. Final Report on Contract No. (HRA) 230-75-0198.

(From Kane RL, Wilson WM: The new health practitioner—The past as prologue. West J Med 127:258, 1977, with permission.)

interventional services.[10] Clinical psychologists may participate with family physicians in individual group therapy.[11] Clinical pharmacists may provide drug information, consultation, and related services in family practice groups.[12,13]

Utilization of Community Resources

Recent years have been a growing proliferation of health-related community resources at local, state, regional, and national levels. These resources and agencies often have much to contribute to the health care of patients with chronic illness, psychosocial problems, and many other problems. The family physician plays a vital role in linking individuals and families in their practices to appropriate community resources when needed, and in coordinating the total health care of their patients. This requires the family physician to be knowledgeable of available resources within the community and to be skilled in the utilization thereof.

Farley and Treat recommend that family physicians develop and maintain an up-to-date index of community resources on the basis of need. They suggest that the following categories be used as the nucleus for an index system.[14]

1. Adoption
2. Aging
3. Alcoholism
4. Birth control
5. Blindness
6. Cancer
7. Chronic illness
8. Communicable disease control
9. Counseling services
10. Drug addiction
11. Handicapped children or adults
12. Mental illness
13. Nursing care
14. Poison control
15. Psychological testing

Referral of patients to community agencies should involve personal contact by the family physician whenever possible. Werblun and Twersky suggest the following approaches for family physicians making referrals to community agencies:[15]

1. Identify the specific physical and/or psychosocial problem
2. Identify the patient's (and/or family's) perception of the problem
   a. What does the patient or family want to do about it?
   b. What has already been done?
   c. What resources have been used in the past?
3. Identify the patient's available resources
   a. Personal, family, and social support systems?
   b. Financial resources available?
4. Determine community resources available
   a. Patient's eligibility (e.g., financial, age, geographic location, disability)?
   b. Accessibility to the patient?
   c. Patient's ability to meet a "fee-for-service" requirement?
   d. Waiting period?
   e. Will the services meet the patient's needs?

5. Function as a facilitator in the referral process
6. Act as the patient's advocate as needed
7. Evaluate success of referral
   a. Utilize a consent for mutual exchange of information
   b. Obtain feedback from patient, family, and agency

Hospital Privileges

The subject of hospital privileges for family physicians has attracted considerable interest and, on occasion, some controversy as the supply of physicians and competition among physicians have increased. Some of the concerns which have been raised relate to the potential influence on hospital privileges of such factors as regional differences, urban versus rural location, residency training, and cost of malpractice liability insurance. Several national studies have been reported within the last 4 years which provide a rather complete picture of present trends in hospital privileges for family physicians.

A large national study in 1980 involving more than 5200 active AAFP members and an 84 percent response rate showed that 95.6 percent of the responding family physicians had hospital admission privileges in one or more hospitals. Table 11–4 displays the extent of hospital privileges in obstetrics and surgery by region and geographic location (SMSA versus non-SMSA).[16] Overall, 37 percent of U.S. family physicians were found to include obstetrics in their practices, while more than one-half (55.5 percent) first assisted in surgery. A majority (58.5 percent) had no privileges in major surgery because they did not request them. Considerable regional and geographic differences were demonstrated, with a higher level of surgical and obstetric privileges in the western states and nonmetropolitan areas than in the eastern states and metropolitan areas.

At the same time the AAFP completed a national study of the hospital privileges of more than 3000 graduates of family practice residency programs. Table 11–5 shows their hospital privileges in comparable areas, again by region and geographic location. Almost two-thirds (64.3 percent) of the residency graduates practice obstetrics and 62.2 percent first assist in surgery. Differences in hospital privileges by region and geographic location were similar to those observed for nonresidency graduates.[17]

Further information on hospital privileges in the areas of intensive and coronary care is provided by a large study comparing hospital privileges in New England states and eight Rocky Mountain states. Table 11–6 summarizes the extent of hospital privileges in these two areas and documents greater access to intensive and coronary care units in New England than might have been expected.[18]

Of all types of hospitals, university hospitals as tertiary care centers present the most difficulty to any of the primary care specialties in obtaining hospital privileges. A recent study by Weiss, however, has revealed that 78 percent of university-based family practice programs hospitalize all or some of their patients at the university hospital, where family physicians have hospital privileges with the following overall frequencies: general medical (94 percent), adult ICU (50 percent), coronary care (65 percent), general pediatrics (81 percent), pediatric ICU (29 percent), normal newborn nursery (79 percent), intensive care nursery (12 percent), routine obstetrics (77 percent), and high-risk obstetrics (31 percent).[19]

Some interesting comparisons can be made between the patterns of hospital privileges for AAFP members in 1969 and in 1980. A national survey of almost 20,000 AAFP members in 1969 (then the American Academy of General Practice) showed,

TABLE 11-4. PERCENTAGE OF AAFP ACTIVE MEMBERS IN DIRECT PATIENT CARE, OFFICE BASED WHO CARE FOR PATIENTS IN VARIOUS CATEGORIES BY STANDARD METROPOLITAN STATISTICAL AREA (SMSA) VS NON-SMSA WITHIN REGION, DECEMBER 1980

	Perform Obstetric Routine Care	Perform Obstetric Complicated Delivery	Perform Obstetric High Risk	Perform Cesarean Sections	Perform Surgery Assisting	Perform Surgery Intermediate	Perform Surgery Major
New England[b]							
SMSA (312)	12.8	2.9	2.2	1.3	33.0	16.0	2.6
Non-SMSA (169)	32.5[a]	11.8[a]	9.5[a]	1.8	49.1[a]	19.5	4.1
Middle Atlantic							
SMSA (416)	9.3	1.7	1.8	0.2	15.5	5.5	1.2
Non-SMSA (64)	16.9	7.8[a]	7.8[a]	0.0	35.6[a]	9.4	1.6
East North Central							
SMSA (302)	35.9	12.6	10.7	3.8	48.4	25.2	6.5
Non-SMSA (148)	64.1[a]	43.6[a]	32.5[a]	24.0[a]	83.9[a]	46.3[a]	20.6[a]
West North Central							
SMSA (192)	67.3	25.3	17.5	10.2	68.3	45.5	9.9
Non-SMSA (302)	81.2[a]	59.4[a]	43.1[a]	37.1[a]	84.7[a]	58.4[a]	28.5[a]
South Atlantic							
SMSA (278)	9.3	2.9	2.3	1.8	14.1	6.0	3.7
Non-SMSA (195)	31.8[a]	20.0[a]	17.9[a]	10.8[a]	33.9[a]	20.6[a]	10.8[a]
East South Central							
SMSA (223)	14.8	9.4	5.4	3.6	31.4	17.9	6.3
Non-SMSA (270)	43.8[a]	32.0[a]	22.7[a]	21.4[a]	60.8[a]	38.4[a]	21.2[a]
West South Central							
SMSA (289)	24.2	16.2	12.7	14.1	62.5	44.1	27.2
Non-SMSA (173)	62.0[a]	48.3[a]	35.7[a]	43.7[a]	81.7[a]	63.7[a]	38.0[a]
Mountain							
SMSA (244)	28.9	8.0	2.9	4.5	76.2	32.8	10.6
Non-SMSA (218)	72.0[a]	52.7[a]	41.4[a]	40.7[a]	82.4	63.9[a]	42.5[a]
Pacific							
SMSA (408)	27.5	10.1	5.2	8.6	81.0	39.7	14.0
Non-SMSA (103)	66.5[a]	49.0[a]	29.0[a]	43.3[a]	88.2	64.2[a]	30.5[a]
Total							
SMSA (2664)	25.5	9.6	6.8	5.4	48.1	25.6	9.2
Non-SMSA (1642)	57.7[a]	40.8[a]	30.1[a]	27.6[a]	70.3[a]	46.0[a]	23.6[a]

[a] Proportions are statistically significant at $P < .05$.
[b] Extreme care should be used in comparing SMSA vs non-SMSA in New England, since SMSAs are defined using the town as the primary unit rather than the county.
(From Clinton C, Schmittling G, Stern TL, et al.: Hospital privileges for family physicians: A national study of office-based members of the American Academy of Family Physicians. J Fam Pract 13:361, 1981, with permission.)

TABLE 11-5. PERCENTAGE OF FAMILY PRACTICE RESIDENCY GRADUATES IN SMSAs/NON-SMSAs BY REGION HAVING VARIOUS HOSPITAL PRACTICE PRIVILEGES, 1979

	Routine Obstetric Care	Complicated Obstetric Care	Cesarean Sections	Surgery First Assist	Minor Surgery	Major Surgery
New England[b]						
SMSA	38.9	9.3	3.7	37.0	3.7	0.0
Non-SMSA	61.0[a]	28.0[a]	6.1	54.9[a]	14.6[a]	0.0
Middle Atlantic						
SMSA	29.5	5.7	0.4	15.5	6.4	0.0
Non-SMSA	49.3[a]	20.3[a]	5.8[a]	49.3[a]	11.6	4.3[a]
East North Central						
SMSA	75.2	28.7	2.4	61.2	35.8	0.9
Non-SMSA	86.1[a]	67.1[a]	12.1[a]	91.9[a]	49.5[a]	5.2[a]
West North Central						
SMSA	88.9	51.9	6.8	81.5	63.0	4.3
Non-SMSA	96.8[a]	84.9[a]	36.5[a]	94.1[a]	74.0[a]	21.9[a]
South Atlantic						
SMSA	26.4	10.2	2.2	23.2	13.4	1.0
Non-SMSA	45.9[a]	24.3[a]	3.3	32.6[a]	17.7	1.1
East South Central						
SMSA	55.7	18.0	3.3	42.6	21.3	1.6
Non-SMSA	65.0	50.0	20.0[a]	68.3[a]	43.3[a]	8.3
West South Central						
SMSA	61.8	38.2	19.1	65.6	48.1	12.2
Non-SMSA	88.0[a]	70.7[a]	57.3[a]	93.3[a]	76.0[a]	28.0[a]
Mountain						
SMSA	66.7	33.3	9.6	78.1	42.1	4.4
Non-SMSA	91.4[a]	70.3[a]	39.1[a]	89.8[a]	74.2[a]	22.7[a]
Pacific						
SMSA	66.8	34.8	16.2	77.3	50.7	8.8
Non-SMSA	83.8[a]	64.1[a]	41.5[a]	93.0[a]	70.4[a]	23.2[a]
Total						
SMSA	56.3	25.4	7.0	53.0	32.9	3.7
Non-SMSA	77.0[a]	57.3[a]	24.8[a]	76.3[a]	51.2[a]	13.3[a]

[a]Differences are statistically significant at $P < .05$.
[b]Care should be used in comparing SMSA vs non-SMSA in the New England region, since SMSAs are defined using the town as the primary unit rather than the county.
(From: Stern TL, Schmittling G, Clinton C, et al.: Hospital privileges for graduates of family practice residency programs. J Fam Pract 13:1013, 1981, with permission.)

for example, that the proportions of respondents with hospital privileges in obstetrics, surgical assisting, and major surgery were 67, 64, and 40 percent, respectively. In 1980, the AAFP overall study of active members showed declines in all three areas, with obstetrics decreasing to 37 percent, surgical assisting to 55 percent, and major surgery to 14 percent.[16,20,21] At the same time, however, graduates of family practice residencies in 1980 reported hospital privileges in obstetrics, surgical assisting, and major surgery to be 64, 62, and 7 percent, respectively. In comparison with their 1969 AAGP counterparts, they had comparable involvement in obstetrics and

TABLE 11-6. EXTENT OF PRIVILEGES GRANTED TO FAMILY PHYSICIANS IN INTENSIVE AND CORONARY CARE[a]

		Region I			Region VIII			
		Full	*Some*	*None*	*Full*	*Some*	*None*	*P Value[b]*
Intensive care unit	Urban	19	60	21	30	61	9	NS
	Rural	35	60	5	54	45	1	<.03
Coronary care unit	Urban	18	59	23	27	59	14	NS
	Rural	35	60	5	54	44	2	<.04

[a]All figures in percentages.
[b]Difference between Regions I and VIII. ***P value <0.05 is statistically significant.
NS = Not significant.
(Adapted from Sundwall DN, Hansen DV: Hospital privileges for family physicians: A comparative study between the New England states and the Intermountain states. J Fam Pract 9:885, 1979, with permission.)

surgical assisting, a sharply decreased role in major surgery, and an increased role in intensive/coronary care (90 versus 50 percent).[20,21]

Of further interest are the reasons for lack of hospital privileges in specific areas based on the two recent national AAFP studies. The overwhelming majority of family physicians without privileges in certain categories did not request them. Denial of privileges is uncommon. In 1980 only 3.6 percent of active AAFP members felt their privileges were unduly restricted, [16] whereas denial of privileges affected 1 percent or fewer of residency-trained family physicians in medicine, pediatrics, and obstetrics, and only 1.8 percent and 3.6 percent of residency graduates requesting privileges in ICU/CCU and complicated obstetrics, respectively.[20] Likewise, prohibitive liability insurance costs are not a major factor. Even in the Pacific region, where these rates are highest, this was a reason for not having privileges in obstetrics and major surgery for only 9 to 14 percent of active AAFP members[16] and less than 4 percent of residency-trained family physicians in 1980.[20]

A major development facilitating appropriate inpatient roles of family physicians has been the organization of clinical departments of family practice in approximately one-third of short-term stay hospitals in the United States. The generalist role within the medical staffs of hospitals has traditionally lacked an organizational or scientific base. The customary organizational structure in the past has been the administrative department of general practice. These departments have usually been weak and loosely organized, lacking both a recognized clinical service and formal mechanisms for assessment of quality of care by their members. Since the advent of the American Board of Family Practice in 1969 and the subsequent widespread growth of 3-year family practice residency programs, however, this situation has been abruptly altered. Departments of family practice have been established as clinical departments in both community hospitals and academic medical centers. With respect to hospital privileges, AAFP guidelines recommend the following process.[22]

> Privileges should be assigned to members of the family practice department by the executive committee of the family practice department after interview and thorough evaluation of the applicant. If the applicant requests privileges in another clinical department, privileges will be assigned in the same manner with the approval of the appropriate clinical department.

Changes made by the Joint Commission on Accreditation of Hospitals in 1977 specifically charged the department chairman with the responsibility of recommending to the medical staff the criteria for the granting of privileges in the department.[23] Although the ultimate responsibility for delineation of hospital privileges for physicians in any specialty rests with the Executive and/or Credentials Committees of the medical staff and the governing board of the hospital, the review of applicants' qualifications and recommendations for privileges within departments is central to this process.

Present guidelines of the Joint Commission on Accreditation of Hospitals (JCAH) state that . . . "Privileges granted shall be commensurate with the training, experience, competence, judgment, character, and current capability of the candidate."[24] Mechanisms are now in place in most hospitals involving an active role of departments of family practice in recommending and monitoring the hospital privileges of their members. In the event of denial of privileges, a candidate has the right of due process including established appeal procedures as described in an excellent recent review by Pugno.[25]

Consultation and Referral

All physicians have their own individual limitations which must be acknowledged and not exceeded. Early in practice, family physicians should become acquainted with physicians in all other specialty fields from whom they can seek advise and help. They will thereby develop patterns of consultation which will depend on their own training and experience, the availability of medical resources within the community, and their proximity to consulting specialties.

There are many methods of consultation used by family physicians. The simplest, and perhaps the most common, is the informal consultation in the hall or doctor's room of the hospital with colleagues in family practice or other fields. Another common form of consultation is by telephone, where the family physician may be advised of further steps in patient care which may or may not involve referral of the patient to the consultant. Still another form is mandatory consultation as required in some hospitals for certain clinical problems.

Referral of patients can take several forms, and it is important that both the family physician and consultant know what each expects of the other. A referral may be (1) for confirmation of diagnosis, with return of the patient to the family physician for treatment; (2) for a "second opinion" in any aspect of diagnosis or therapy; and (3) for diagnosis and/or treatment by the consulting physician with return of the patient to the family physician upon conclusion of care for the given clinical problem. Most referrals in family practice are for assistance with treatment rather than for diagnostic opinion. When a patient has been referred to a consultant for a specific problem, the family physician most commonly will continue to play an active role in the care of the patient. Examples of such continued involvement include ongoing management of concurrent medical problems, assisting at surgery, and postoperative care.

The process of consultation and referral is a potentially complicated one which requires of the family physician the same level of concern and effort as would be involved in other kinds of prescriptions for the patient. Rudy and Williams have examined the effects of this process on therapeutic outcome, and have identified the following pitfalls to be addressed by referring physicians:[26]

1. Resistance to consultation/referral by the referring physician
2. Resistance to consultation/referral by the patient

3. Failure to follow through
4. Failure to adequately interpret the patient/family complex to the consultant
5. Failure to define for the consultant desired objectives of the consultation
6. Reticence toward critical evaluation of the consultation by the referring physician

Froom and his colleagues in a recent paper called attention to various risks of referral, especially those resulting from miscommunication between the referring physician and consultant, incomplete information and lack of involvement by the principal parties in clinical decision making. In their words:[27]

> The family physician should provide the consultant with pertinent information and take part in both diagnostic and therapeutic decisions. (In addition), the patient must be made an active participant in the decision process. Uncertainties about diagnosis and therapeutic outcome should be shared with the patient. What is ultimately involved is making decisions under conditions of uncertainty in which both the probabilities of outcomes and the values of the patient must be taken into account. The family physician can play an important, possibly unique role in such principled gambling because of his knowledge of the patient and his family, the shared trust that has developed over time, and his defined role as an advocate for the patient. Although referral risks may not be entirely eliminated, a trio of patient, consultant, and referring physician can reduce these risks and contribute to increased satisfaction for all parties.

The family physician's skillful use of consultation not only results in the best possible patient care, but also affords an important avenue of continuing medial education. Good rapport and working relationships based on mutual respect with consultants in all fields enhances the family physician's own enjoyment of the practice of family medicine, and is in the best interest of his/her patients.

COMPARATIVE PATTERNS AMONG SPECIALTIES

Workload and Related Factors
The new Socioeconomic Monitoring System (SMS), initiated by the American Medical Association in late 1981, provides an excellent updated view of comparative characteristics of the various specialties in the United States as derived from quarterly telephone surveys of physicians. Table 11-7 provides a composite comparison of ten characteristics of the major specialties in 1982.[5]

Several overall observations stand out from these findings. The work week in terms of hours devoted to all professional activities and patient care activities are quite similar among the major specialties. General/family physicians and pediatricians spend the most time in the office, with correspondingly less time involved in hospital rounds. General/family practice accounts for the largest number of total patient visits and office visits, with pediatrics second and obstetrics–gynecology third on both counts. Internal medicine and surgery account for the largest number of hospital visits, with general/family practice third. Internal medicine and general/family practice in that order, record the longest length of stay per hospitalized patient. Fees and income are highest in the surgical specialties and lowest in the primary care specialties.

TABLE 11-7. COMPARATIVE WORK LOAD AND RELATED FACTORS BY SPECIALTY FOR 1982

	All Physicians[a]	General and Family Practice	Internal Medicine	Surgery	Pediatrics	Obstetrics
All Professional Activities[b] (mean number of hours per week)	56.8	57.4	58.9	57.0	57.2	58.4
Patient Care Activities[c] (mean number of hours per week)	51.0	53.4	52.7	51.4	51.3	53.5
Office Hours (mean number of hours per week)	26.4	33.1	26.2	22.1	32.1	26.9
Hospital Rounds (mean number of hours per week)	9.4	8.4	15.2	9.6	8.5	6.4
Total Patient Visits[d] (mean number per week)	131.8	160.6	118.9	118.8	134.9	128.2
Office Visits (mean number per week)	81.8	115.0	61.6	69.2	100.8	93.7
Hospital Visits (mean number per week)	34.1	30.7	45.0	42.8	23.6	27.9
Length of Stay (mean number of days per patient)	6.6	5.9	7.3	4.9	4.1	3.8
Fee for Office Visit (Established Patient) (mean fee in dollars)	21.60	17.48	25.30	23.57	21.10	25.76
Net Income from Medical Practice (mean net income in thousands of dollars)	99.5	71.9	86.8	130.5	70.3	115.8

[a]Includes physicians in specialties not listed separately.
[b]Includes all patient care activities, administrative activities connected with medical practice and other professional activities that do not involve patient care such as medical staff functions, teaching, and research.
[c]Includes direct patient care and activities related to patient care, such as interpreting laboratory tests and x-rays and consulting with other physicians.
[d]Includes visits in the office, on hospital rounds, in hospital emergency rooms and outpatient clinics, and in all other settings.
(*From Reynolds RA, Abram JB: Socioeconomic characteristics of medical practice 1983. Chicago, American Medical Association 1983, pp 48, 50, 56, 60, 66, 70, 74, 94, 96, 116, with permission. Copyright 1983, American Medical Association.*)

Practice Style

Several descriptors of comparative practice styles by specialty are of some interest, including differential rates of adopting new procedures, changing patterns of ambulatory surgery, and approaches to clinical problem solving. The American Medical Association's SMS survey for 1982 asked physicians whether they performed during the past year any new diagnostic or therapeutic procedures that reflected recent changes in medical knowledge or technology (excluding the use of new prescription drugs). In view of some of the changing trends in the health care system described in an earlier chapter, it comes as no surprise that more physicians are performing ambulatory surgery than in the past, particularly in general/family practice and surgery[5] (Table 11-8).

McWhinney observed in 1972 that the problem-solving strategy used in a clinical specialty depends on four factors: (1) tacit assumptions about the problems likely to be encountered; (2) the general objectives of the specialty; (3) the utility of individual procedures; and (4) tradition.[28] There is some evidence that the problem-solving strategies of family physicians are quite different from those used by other clinical specialties.

Smith and McWhinney studied two groups of physicians—nine family physicians and nine consulting internists—in terms of their diagnostic approach to three programmed patients simulating three clinical problems: (1) a 32-year-old housewife with fatigue, depression, and mild iron deficiency anemia; (2) a 19-year-old male presenting with sore throat due to infectious mononucleosis; and (3) a 28-year-old male presenting with periodic headaches over many years. They found that family physicians asked fewer history questions, requested fewer items of information from the physical examination, and ordered fewer laboratory tests. The family physicians also asked a higher proportion of questions about mental status and life situation in two of the three cases. There were no significant differences in the final diagnoses obtained by the family physicians and internists.[29] More recently, Noren and colleagues reported the results of a large national study of general/family physicians and internists. They found similar differences in the practice styles of these two specialties. General/family physicians spent an average of 13 minutes per office visit, using laboratory tests and x-rays in 34 and 19 percent of visits, respectively; internists spent an average of 18.4 minutes per office visit, using laboratory tests and x-rays in 73 and 53 percent of visits.[30]

TABLE 11-8. PERCENT OF PHYSICIANS WHO PERFORM SURGERY BY CURRENT AMOUNT OF AMBULATORY SURGERY COMPARED TO 2 YEARS AGO[a]

Specialty	More Than 2 Years Ago	Same As 2 Years Ago	Less Than 2 Years Ago
All physicians	34	57	9
General and family practice	38	53	9
Medical specialties	25	65	9
Surgical specialties	37	55	8
Emergency medicine	12	75	13

[a]Compares 1982 with 1980.
(From Reynolds RA, Abram JB: Socioeconomic characteristics of medical practice 1983. Chicago, American Medical Association 1983, p 11, with permission. Copyright 1983, American Medical Association.)

It is both logical and efficient for the family physician to use time as a diagnostic factor. In contrast to the consultant, who must necessarily emphasize thoroughness and a more extensive diagnostic workup at what may be the only encounter with the patient, the family physician through his/her continuing relationship with the patient can proceed in steps with additional workup for persistent and/or new symptoms or for lack of response or treatment.[31]

Practice Satisfaction

Although satisfaction with medical practice involves innumerable factors and individual variations by specialty and by physician, some patterns emerge from available studies. The Medical Economics Continuing Survey of 1976 showed that greater ease of practice and more free time were rated by physicians as their chief practice goal regardless of specialty, as had also been the case in 1965. There were more similarities than differences in these findings. Yet some differences could be noted—pediatricians were least satisfied with their income and general surgeons were most likely to desire more specialization. Within the general/family practice field, three times as many general practitioners wanted smaller practices compared to family physicians in 1976, when national data for family practice showed a weekly average of 190 patient visits in contrast to 163 patient visits per week for general practice.[32]

Malpractice Liability

Since recent trends in the malpractice liability area represent an increasingly difficult problem for medicine as in other professions and fields, it is useful to briefly consider some of these trends and their effects on the various specialties. Among the major trends, the following stand out:[33]

- During the late 1960s and early 1970s, claims frequency grew at an average annual rate of 12 percent while paid claim severity increased by 10 percent per year.
- The national malpractice problem was widely perceived to peak in 1975 as a crisis, prompting many states to pass various forms of legislation to address the problem.
- The claim frequency after 1975 dropped back to 1971 levels, but the average amounts paid on malpractice claims against physicians more than doubled from 1971 to 1978.
- The number of annual claims per 100 physicians was 3.3 before 1978, and between 1978 and 1983 jumped to 8 per 100 physicians.[34]
- More than one-quarter of all malpractice claims against physicians arise from surgery-related incidents, while the highest awards for damages involve birth-related problems.[35]
- Legislation involving medical malpractice in the various states since 1975 has included provision for voluntary binding arbitration (13 states), modification or abandonment of the collateral source rule (16 states), limits on contingency fees (17 states), clarification of informed consent (23 states), authorization of screening panels (30 states), and limits on statutes of limitation (38 states); of these, caps on awards and mandatory offset of collateral compensation have had the greatest impact on reducing claims severity.
- The most common responses of physicians to malpractice risks, according to the American Medical Association's SMS program, have been to keep

more detailed patient records (45 percent), and to order more diagnostic tests (41 percent).[34]

- The proportion of physician-owned insurance companies has steadily increased in recent years; of the 20 largest medical liability insurance carriers in 1983, 10 were physician-owned.[36]

The impact of these trends has varied considerably by specialty. Table 11–9, for example, summarizes the incidence of physician liability claims by specialty, region, type of practice, and sex. It is readily apparent that psychiatry is most insulated[5] from malpractice liability problems, followed by the primary care specialties (especially pediatrics); the surgical specialties and obstetrics–gynecology have been heavily impacted by recent trends in the malpractice liability area.

COMMENT

Several aspects of the preceding discussion warrant additional comment. The first is the nature of organizational forms of family practice. In view of the diversity of community needs and environments reflected in different practice settings, from

TABLE 11-9. AVERAGE INCIDENCE OF PHYSICIAN LIABILITY CLAIMS BY SPECIALTY, REGION, TYPE OF PRACTICE AND SEX

	Annual Claims per 100 Physicians	
	1976–1981	*Prior to 1976*
All physicians	6.2	2.9
Speciality		
General/family practice	5.1	2.3
Internal medicine	5.2	2.1
Surgical specialty	9.2	4.5
Pediatrics	3.6	1.5
Obstetrics/gynecology	14.0	5.3
Radiology	5.9	3.1
Psychiatry	1.9	1.0
Anesthesiology	5.2	2.6
Other	3.7	2.1
Region		
Northeast	7.6	3.1
North Central	6.2	2.5
South	5.2	2.3
West	6.4	4.2
Type of practice		
Solo	5.8	3.0
Partnership	7.5	3.4
Group	6.9	3.1
Other	4.9	1.9
Sex		
Male	6.5	3.0
Female	3.2	2.3

(From Reynolds RA, Abram JB: Socioeconomic characteristics of medical practice 1983. Chicago, American Medical Association 1983, p 11, with permission. Copyright 1983, American Medical Association.)

large urban centers on the one hand to isolated rural areas on the other, family practice will necessarily develop varied organizational patterns ranging from large multispecialty groups to solo practice. In my view, however, the relatively small family practice group including three- to six-family physicians will emerge as the single most common organizational structure for family practice, particularly in medium and smaller-sized communities. Such a group can adapt well to the needs of a majority of practice settings in the community, and affords the full advantages of group practice to physicians, staff, and patients alike without the added complexities of larger organizational structures. In many instances, these groups will likely have contractual arrangements in one form or another in certain specialties such as surgery and obstetrics–gynecology.

Another area requiring further comment is the projected viability of various types of team practice which are currently being developed and tested. As pointed out in an earlier chapter, there is considerable confusion and controversy today surrounding the role of physician extenders in primary care, particularly with regard to their autonomy in patient care and the nature of physician supervision of their activities. These issues are perhaps best illustrated by the emphasis by some in nursing upon "joint practice" as opposed to "team practice" whereby the nurse practitioner is envisioned as an independent clinician with many of the same roles and skills as the physician. At the conceptual level the concept of "joint practice" has blurred the distinctions between medical practice and nursing practice.[37,38] At the practical level, application of this concept has led some physician extenders to develop "a practice within a practice" in various primary care settings where they function more as physicians and less as team members contributing their special skills to the entire practice.

Although some early results of the deployment of physician extenders are encouraging, it is still too early to extrapolate their widespread utilization in primary care. Support for the expanded roles of physician extenders seems to be steadily waning in the medical community in recent years, especially as the physician supply continues to increase. One study, for example, involving a 60 percent response of all pediatricians in Arizona showed that the role of the pediatric nurse practitioner is perceived as competitive rather than collaborative.[39] Another study by Breslau of patient perceptions and evaluations of the role of the pediatric nurse practitioner showed that patients do not perceive the nurse practitioner to have expertise in an exclusive domain of health problems and tended not to consider her addition to the office to have improved the physician's services.[40]

A final comment is in order concerning the vital importance of maintaining the highest possible quality of the physician–patient relationship in family practice regardless of the organizational form or setting of the practice. The physician–patient relationship today is being affected by such issues as an increasing emphasis on cost–benefit in health care, complexities of third-party billing procedures, questions about confidentiality of records, changing roles of the physician in various forms of team practice, and the threat of malpractice suits for a broader range of results than actual malpractice. Our population is more mobile than in the past, expects more from medicine, and finds health care increasingly fragmented, more costly, and often less accessible and less personal. The primacy of the person as the reason for health care needs to be defended and reinforced. The threat of depersonalization of health care poses a critical challenge to the entire medical profession, but is a fundamental concern in family practice as that specialty taking responsibility for the ongoing care of individuals and their families.

REFERENCES

1. Goodman LJ, Bennett EH, Odem RJ: Group Medical Practice in the U.S., 1975. Center for Health Services Research and Development. Chicago, American Medical Association, 1976.
2. Group practice. Med Economics, Oct. 3, 1983, p 214
3. Rosenblatt RA, Cherkin DC, Schneeweiss R, et al.: The structure and content of family practice: Current status and future trends. J Fam Pract 15:681, 1982
4. Practice patterns. AAFP Reporter 11(1):12, January 1984
5. Reynolds RA, Abram JB: Socioeconomic characteristics of medical practice 1983. Chicago, American Medical Association 1983, p 11
6. Cooper JK, Heald K, Samuels M, Coleman S: Rural or urban practice: Factors influencing the location decision of primary care physicians. Inquiry 12:18, 1975
7. Kane RL, Wilson WM: The new health practitioner—The past as prologue. West J Med 127:254, 1977
8. Light JA, Crain MJ, Fisher DW: Physician assistant: A profile of the profession, 1976. PA Journal 7(3):109, 1977
9. Morris SB, Smith DB: The distribution of physician extenders. Med Care 15(12): 1054, 1977
10. Blanchard LB, Kurtz B: The social worker in a family practice setting. Primary Care 5(1):173, 1978
11. Friedman WH, Jelly E, Jelly P: Group therapy in family medicine. J Fam Pract 6(5): 1015, 1978
12. Maudlin RK: The clinical pharmacist and the family physician. J Fam Pract 3(6):667, 1976
13. Davis RE, Crigler WH, Martin H: Pharmacy and family practice: Concept, roles and fees. Drug Intell Clin Pharm 11:616, 1977
14. Farley ES, Treat DF: Utilization of community resources. In Conn HF, Rakel RE, Johnson TW (eds): Family Practice. Philadelphia, W.B. Saunders, 1973, p 118
15. Werblun MN, Twersky RK: Use of community resources. In Rosen G, Geyman JP, Layton RH (eds): Behavioral Science in Family Practice. New York, Appleton-Century-Crofts, 1980
16. Clinton C, Schmittling G, Stern TL, et al.: Hospital privileges for family physicians: A national study of office-based members of the American Academy of Family Physicians. J Fam Pract 13:361, 1981
17. Stern TL, Schmittling G, Clinton C, et al.: Hospital privileges for graduates of family practice residency programs. J Fam Pract 13:1013, 1981
18. Sundwall DN, Hansen DV: Hospital privileges for family physicians: A comparative study between the New England states and the Intermountain states. J Fam Pract 9:885, 1979
19. Weiss BD: Hospital privileges for family physicians at university hospitals. J Fam Pract 18:747, 1984
20. Black RR, Schmittling G, Stern TL: Characteristics and practice patterns of family practice residency graduates in the United States. J Fam Pract 11:767, 1980
21. GP and the hospital (editorial). Hosp Pract 5:112, 1970
22. Family Practice in Hospitals. Kansas City, Mo., American Academy of Family Physicians, 1977
23. Accreditation Manual for Hospitals. Chicago, Joint Commission on Accreditation of Hospitals, 1977
24. Porterfield JD: Accreditation problems. Hospitals, Feb. 16, 1977

25. Pugno PA: Hospital privileges for family physicians: Rights, rationale, and resources. J Fam Pract 17:77, 1983
26. Rudy DR, Williams T: The consultation process and its effects on therapeutic outcome. J Fam Pract 4(2):361, 1977
27. Froom J, Feinbloom RI, Rosen MG: Risks of referral. J Fam Pract, in press, 1984
28. McWhinney IR: Problem solving and decision making in primary medical practice. Albert Wander Lecture. Proc R Soc Med 65:934, 1972
29. Smith DH, McWhinney IR: Comparison of the diagnostic methods of family physicians and internists. J Med Educ 50(3):264, 1975
30. Noren J, Frazier T, Altman I, et al.: Ambulatory medical care: A comparison of internists and family-general practitioners. N Engl J Med 302:11, 1980
31. Curry HB: Phoenix in flight: All systems go! JAMA 222(7):821, 1972
32. Owens A: What doctors want most from their practices now. Med Econ, March 7, 1977, p 88
33. Danzon PM: The frequency and severity of malpractice claims. Institute for Civil Justice. Santa Monica, Calif., Rand Corporation, 1982
34. American medical association special task force on professional liability and insurance. Report I—Chicago American Medical Association, 1984, p 65
35. Where malpractice suits are most likely to occur. Med Econ, Sept. 19, 1983, p 244
36. Doctor carriers now dominate the malpractice market. Med Econ, Jan. 10, 1983, p 13
37. Geyman JP: Is there a difference between nursing practice and medical practice? J Fam Pract 5(6):935, 1977
38. Levinson D: Roles, tasks and practitioners. N Engl J Med 296(22):1291, 1977
39. Bergeson PS, Winchell D: A survey of Arizona physicians' attitudes regarding pediatric nurse practitioners: Rejection of the concept. Clin Ped 16(8):679, 1977
40. Breslau N: The role of the nurse practitioner in a pediatric team: Patient definitions. Med Care 15(12):1014, 1977

12 Family Practice as a Career Option

What is the most painful and devastating question that can be asked about modern medical practice? It is not whether most doctors are up to date in their knowledge or in their techniques but whether too many of them know more about disease than about the person in whom the disease exists. The physician celebrates computerized tomography. The patient celebrates the outstretched hand.

Norman Cousins[1]

With the disappearance of the free-standing internship and the continued emergence of more kinds of career options in medicine during recent years, today's medical students are confronted with difficult career decisions at an early stage in their medical education. Because of the lead time requirements of the National Intern and Residency Matching Program (NIRMP) and the need to arrange interview visits to potential residency programs during the preceding 3 to 6 months, medical students now find it necessary to make choices among specialties by the end of their third year or start of their fourth year in medical school. For many, this pressure for early career choice may be premature since it is not possible to experience all, or even most, of the various medical career options by that time.

Over the years I have been impressed with the frequency of certain misconceptions, concerns, and questions expressed by medical students with respect to family practice as a career option. The purpose of this chapter is therefore fourfold: (1) to clarify some of the common misconceptions; (2) to discuss some of the personal satisfactions in family practice; (3) to outline some of the requisites for prospective family physicians; and (4) to suggest an approach to selection of graduate training in the field.

SOME MISCONCEPTIONS ABOUT FAMILY PRACTICE

Most misconceptions seem to relate to just a few aspects of family practice. Seven of these will be addressed here.

Patients Usually Prefer a Subspecialist When They Are Sick

It is a common observation among physicians practicing in most types of communities that patients evaluate their physicians more by their availability and personality than by any certificates on the walls of their consultation room. Patients in the general population usually want care for their illnesses by the most direct route, and rate highly a physician who is readily accessible and can provide initial and follow-up everyday care of their health problems.

Patients frequently want a doctor for the entire family and often become resentful of the expense and inconvenience involved in episodic care of multiple illnesses in family members by many other specialists. As they get to know their family physicians, they tend to consult them initially for most health problems within the family. In fact, it is not uncommon for patients to resist referral to a consultant or to call their family physician from a medical center in a distant city for his/her opinion of recommendations made by a specialist whom they do not know. Table 12–1 lists the priorities as ranked by patients in choosing their family physician on the basis of one statewide study.[2]

That the public's demand for the services of the family physician remains at a high level is reflected by Table 12–2, which shows the experience of the American Medical Association's Physician's Placement for the first 2 months of 1985.[3] It can be seen that the greatest number of practice opportunities was general/family practice.

Family Practice Is So Involved With Minor Illness That It Lacks Intellectual Challenge

The clinical content and patterns of family practice were described in some detail in Chapters 9 and 11, which provide ample evidence of the breadth and depth of the family physician's everyday practice. It has been shown that family physicians definitely manage about 97 percent of all of their patient visits, including a wide variety of acute and chronic diseases ranging from minor to terminal illness. Family physicians frequently encounter medical, surgical, and psychiatric emergencies, and are constantly challenged by the problems of early diagnosis, the management of multiple-system disease, and the care of patients with various combinations of organic and functional illness.

TABLE 12-1. FACTORS IN CHOOSING A FAMILY DOCTOR

	Very Important (%)	Important (%)	Not Very Important (%)	Not Important (%)
Willingness to talk about your illness	59	41	0	0
Length of time to get an appointment	35	53	11	1
Access to a hospital you want	34	55	9	2
Personality and appearance	29	55	14	2
Fees	27	48	22	3
Years of experience	24	49	24	3
Office location	18	48	29	5
Weekend and evening office hours	14	52	30	4
Doctor's involvement in civic organizations	5	32	46	17
Listing in Yellow Pages and other directories	6	24	51	19

(From Medical Association of the State of Alabama. Patients will choose doctors who talk to them. Med Econ, Nov. 8, 1982, p 174, with permission.)

TABLE 12-2. AMA PHYSICIANS' PLACEMENT SERVICE STATISTICAL REPORT FOR JANUARY/FEBRUARY 1985. PHYSICIAN PLACEMENT REGISTER/OPPORTUNITY PLACEMENT REGISTER

	Physicians		Opportunities	
Specialties	**No.**	**%**	**No.**	**%**
Allergy	3	0.2	2	0.2
Anesthesiology	102	6.5	9	1.1
Dermatology	17	1.1	7	0.8
General/family practice	170	10.9	269	32.2
Internal medicine	274	17.6	102	12.2
Neurology	23	1.5	16	1.9
Neurosurgery	7	0.4	8	1.0
Obstetrics & gynecology	77	5.0	79	9.4
Ophthalmology	44	2.8	21	2.5
Orthopedic surgery	49	3.1	59	7.1
Otolaryngology	20	1.3	29	3.5
Pathology	36	2.3	1	0.1
Pediatrics	106	6.8	47	5.6
Psychiatry	38	2.4	21	2.5
Radiology	23	1.5	5	0.6
Surgery, general	166	10.6	43	5.1
Urology	55	3.5	14	1.7
Miscellaneous	349	22.7	103	12.1
Total	1559	100.2	835	99.6

(From Physicians' Placement Service. Chicago, Ill., American Medical Association, 1985, with permission.)

Family physicians do not equate severe or rare illness with being more "interesting." Instead, their main satisfaction comes from the understanding of patients and their families as people, and their ability to manage the great majority of illnesses acquired by these families.

Family Physicians Will Not Receive Appropriate Hospital Privileges

The large majority of hospitals in this country continue to be "open-staff" hospitals. Hospital privileges on the various services are extended on the basis of training and demonstrated ability, which is as it should be. The extent of hospital privileges for family physicians does vary somewhat from one geographic area to another and by size of the community, and reflects the pattern of practice for the involved locale. Only a few hospitals are "closed-staff," limiting privileges on more arbitrary grounds to certain categories of physicians. Earlier chapters have documented very high levels of satisfaction with hospital privileges among active AAFP members and family practice residency graduates.[4,5] Table 12-3 presents ratings of practice and career satisfaction recently reported by a national sample 876 residency-trained family physicians.[6] Hospital privileges are clearly not at issue for the vast majority of residency-trained family physicians.

TABLE 12-3. FAMILY PHYSICIANS' RATINGS OF SATISFACTION WITH VARIOUS
ASPECTS OF THEIR CAREERS AND PRACTICE

	Mean ± SD	Very Satisfied (6–7)[a] No. (%)	Moderately Satisfied or Neutral (4–5)[a] No. (%)	Dissatisfied (1–3)[a] No. (%)
The hospital privileges I have	6.1 ± 1.2	679 (78)	150 (17)	41 (5)
The respect I receive from my patients	5.9 ± 1.0	653 (75)	192 (22)	27 (3)
The adequacy of the residency training I received	5.8 ± 1.2	631 (72)	191 (22)	50 (6)
The consultant relationships I have with specialists	5.6 ± 1.2	548 (63)	275 (31)	49 (6)
My work in general	5.5 ± 1.0	525 (60)	307 (35)	40 (5)
The adequacy of my office and support staff	5.5 ± 1.3	521 (60)	277 (32)	71 (8)
The hospital facilities in my community	5.5 ± 1.4	536 (61)	243 (28)	92 (11)
The physical resources and facilities in my office	5.4 ± 1.3	479 (55)	296 (34)	97 (11)
The extent to which I have presently achieved my overall professional goals	5.2 ± 1.2	416 (48)	378 (43)	77 (9)
The opportunity I have for professional contact with physicians in other specialties	5.2 ± 1.5	460 (53)	287 (33)	124 (14)
The opportunity I have for professional contact with other family physicians	5.1 ± 1.4	407 (47)	328 (38)	135 (15)
The organization and management of my practice	5.0 ± 1.4	374 (43)	363 (42)	134 (15)
The amount of time my practice requires	4.8 ± 1.5	315 (36)	352 (41)	203 (23)
The time I have for continuing medical education	4.7 ± 1.5	295 (34)	358 (41)	219 (25)
The time I have for leisure and relaxation	4.2 ± 1.6	220 (25)	338 (39)	314 (36)
The time I have for my family	4.2 ± 1.6	231 (27)	316 (36)	320 (37)
The financial costs involved in operating my practice	3.8 ± 1.6	136 (16)	340 (39)	390 (45)

[a]Responses on a scale from 1 (very dissatisfied) to 7 (very satisfied) were grouped into three main categories of satisfaction.
(From McCranie EW, Hornsby IL, Calvert JC: Practice and career satisfaction among residency trained family physicians: A national survey. J Fam Pract 14:1107, 1982, with permission.)

Inappropriate restriction of hospital privileges should not constitute a major problem for future family physicians, who will be well trained in many aspects of hospital care. Clinical departments of family practice are playing an active role, in liaison with the other specialty departments, in the designation of hospital privileges for family physicians and in the monitoring of quality of care and physician performance.

Family Practice Is More Needed in Rural Than Metropolitan Areas

In metropolitan areas and larger communities, the substantial use of hospitals' emergency rooms bears witness to a failure of available primary care. Such care as is received by this method is episodic, fragmentary, impersonal, and expensive. As the urban and suburban population grows and as more people demand health care for all four of the James' stages of disease, there will be a continuing need for family physicians in any community regardless of size. A physician entering family practice today has many opportunities to associate with other family physicians in urban, suburban, and rural communities anywhere in the country. Whether he/she starts practice alone or in association with one or more other physicians, he can expect to be busy within a matter of months. The latest available data from the American Academy of Family Physicians show that the intended practice locations of 1984 graduates of family practice residency programs represent a broad spectrum of communities (Table 14–2).

I Would Be Too Busy in Family Practice

Many physicians are too busy in practice, but this cannot be well correlated with the clinical discipline. Internists, pediatricians, obstetricians, surgeons, and other physicians can all develop uncontrolled practices, which can compromise unduly their own personal and family life.

When physicians get too busy, it is usually due to such factors as inefficient organization of their practices, lack of education of their patients, insufficient coverage by other physicians, or their own masochistic drive to overwork. The work week in family practice is comparable in hours to that of most other specialties. Many family physicians are able to practice 50 hours a week and share night and weekend calls with other physicians whether they be solo, in an expense-sharing relationship with one or more other physicians, in partnership, or in group practice. A further increase in group and partnership practice can be expected, so that all future family physicians should be able to control their practices.

I Cannot Possibly Learn It All

A common remark expressed by medical students is that family practice is too broad to "learn it all." It is, of course, true that one cannot learn all about each of the component elements of family practice, but this is equally true in any of the clinical disciplines. In the final analysis, one cannot possibly learn all there is to know about any field.

So, in family practice, the goal is not to "learn it all." Rather the goal is to master a specific body of knowledge and acquire a specific range of skills which relate to the prevention, diagnosis, treatment, and rehabilitation of common illnesses of the family. In the course of a 3-year family practice residency program, residents cut across territorial lines between all clinical disciplines, developing proficiency as required by their intended location and type of practice. The practice of family medicine becomes a balance of knowing and doing; one maintains competency in many technical skills through their repetitive application to common clinical problems.

As observed by McWhinney, it is quite evident that the family physician caring for 1500 people cannot match the consultant, who selects his/her patients from a population of 50,000 or more, in detailed mastery of one field. But "the deepest and most vital knowledge—the knowledge that determines how information will be used—does not 'explode' or 'have a half-life of five years' as the catchwords have it. . . . By caring for the whole family, the family physician stands to gain personal knowledge that can be gained in no other way."[7]

Besieged as they are with an overload of information, frequently presented in a context where the relevance to common clinical problems is unclear or lacking, medical students often feel insecure about their capacity to master the knowledge and skills required of a broad specialty. The range, however, of knowledge and skills required by the practicing family physician is not endless, but is finite and allows one to develop and maintain a high level of competence.

Family Practice Is More Suited to Men Than Women

There is ample evidence that women physicians traditionally have been unevenly distributed among the various specialties in medicine. In 1971, for example, when women represented 7.1 percent of all active physicians in the United States, they comprised 21.3 percent of the pediatricians, 18.8 percent of the public health physicians, 14.3 percent of the anesthesiologists, and 13.1 percent of the psychiatrists, but only 7.2 percent of the obstetrician–gynecologists, 4.4 percent of the general/family physicians, 1.1 percent of the general surgeons and 0.5 percent of the orthopedists.[8] There is also evidence of stereotypic thinking among physicians with respect to the believed suitability of medical specialties for women physicians. This has led to attitudes that certain fields are preferable for women which (1) involve more limited time commitments (e.g., anesthesiology, dermatology, rehabilitation medicine, and pathology), and (2) call for qualities and aptitudes commonly attributed to women (e.g., pediatrics and psychiatry).[9]

The last 15 years have seen major changes in the number of women entering medicine and their interest in the various specialties. The proportion of women enrolled in U.S. medical schools increased from about 10 percent of the total enrollment in 1970 to about 30 percent today. By 1982, major shifts had occurred with respect to the relative proportions of women enrolled in the various specialty residencies. In that year, women residents represented 34.4 percent of obstetrics–gynecology residents, 9.7 percent of general surgery residents, and 3.7 percent of residents in orthopedic surgery, whereas the proportion of women residents in psychiatry and anesthesiology increased to 34.4 and 21.8 percent, respectively.[10] The proportion of women selecting family practice residencies has steadily increased to the present level of 21 percent of first-year resident enrollment.

One study in 1977 examined differences in specialty choice selection and personality among male and female medical students in two medical schools. Increased interest was noted among women physicians in nontraditional fields, especially family practice. Family practice was the only specialty in which men and women selecting the same specialty appeared comparable in personality characteristics.[11] There is no reason to believe that women physicians are categorically less (or more) suited to family practice than to other fields.

PERSONAL SATISFACTIONS IN FAMILY PRACTICE

Although the practice satisfaction of family physicians is necessarily subject to considerable individual variation, some of the reasons can be sketched whereby most family physicians find their practices both interesting and rewarding.

Meeting the Needs

All family physicians can be assured that they are meeting important needs of their patients and families in a direct way. This awareness starts early in the careers of family physicians—when they start looking for locations to start practice. They find many attractive practice opportunities regardless of the size of community or part of the country. Not only are other physicians seeking their association, but often hospital administrators and other community leaders are searching for new family physicians for their communities.

Medical graduates entering family practice today can do so knowing that they are meeting directly the most pressing challenge in modern health care—the delivery of primary and continuing comprehensive health care to a growing population. Despite the increasing physician supply, most family physicians find themselves quite busy within a few months after starting practice.

A Complete Physician

Family physicians are enabled by good residency training to be soundly competent to function well in all four of James' stages of disease, from prevention and early diagnosis of subclinical disease to treatment and rehabilitation of symptomatic disease. Though they have limitations in all fields of medicine, they will at the same time possess substantial competence across a wide range of the traditional specialties. As observed by Stephens, family physicians "do not have what Harvey Cox called the 'permission to ignore' whatever lies outside their specialty, nor can they participate in what Michael Balint called the 'collusion of anonymity' in which the patient has many doctors but none of them is in charge."[12]

It is deeply satisfying to family physicians to be able to initiate care in virtually any emergency situation. Their capabilities in emergency care usually include such diverse skills as management of cardiac arrest, diagnosis of the surgical abdomen after trauma, tube thoracostomy for a pneumothorax, management of poisoning in a child, or care of a psychiatric emergency. Family physicians are trained to evaluate all patients who present to their care, seeking consultation when indicated and after appropriate initial care is rendered. It is likewise rewarding for family physicians to have the opportunity to follow patients and their families where the continuity is measured in years, or even generations.

A Part of People's Lives

Family physicians get close to their patients and their families, and know them better the longer they practice. Many of them become their friends. Family physicians thereby have the privilege of participating in all of the major events of their patients' lives—birth, marriage, serious accidents, and death. They have the opportunity to see them grow and develop as individuals. A preschool examination of a child may recall a breech delivery in the middle of a night 6 years previously. A woman successfully managed through menopausal symptoms may be followed into years of improved adjustment to her life situation, while her husband's hypertension is found to be more easily controlled with reduced medication. A middle-aged man who was resuscitated in the coronary care unit after a cardiac arrest may be later followed through a program of counseling and exercise and return to work, while anxiety symptoms in his wife are treated concurrently.

A Part of the Community

Family physicians, as other physicians in our society, are usually accorded a high level of respect within their communities. The physician is recognized as a well-educated person and is often expected to be expert in fields outside of medicine. Unfortunately, this is often not the case, and the wise physician is aware of the limitations of his/her expertise. By virtue of their broad training, experience, and interests, however, family physicians have much to contribute to community affairs if they are so inclined.

Natural areas for community involvement include school health, sports medicine, health education, environmental improvement, disaster planning, emergency care services, voluntary health organizations, and health planning. In becoming involved in the community, however, physicians must be as careful to avoid overextension as they are to avoid uncontrolled practices.

A Varied Life

Variety is certainly the spice of the family physician's life. Each day is unpredictable, and is a mixture of emergency, acute, chronic, and well-patient care. Each day sees the family physician in the office, in the hospital and its emergency room, and at times in the patient's home. Every day is active and filled with decisions, and family physicians find themselves constantly shifting gears as they adapt to different degrees of urgency and patients with different personalities.

The work of the family physician is concrete, and the results of care are usually apparent. Surprises are not uncommon in family practice. Emergencies have a way of occurring when one is least expecting them. Any given day may include an obstetric delivery, a counseling session for a marital problem, closed reduction of a Colles fracture, management of an acute coronary, and diagnosis of unsuspected hypertension by a routine physical examination. At the end of a day, family physicians can usually feel that they have made a difference in the lives of their patients.

The Constant Challenge

The scope and variety of family physicians' practices provide continual challenge. They must be able to integrate the unexpected into each busy day, remain cool under stress, and be as therapeutic as possible in dealing with patients and their families. The overall responsibilities of family physicians are great—for the lives and optimal health of all their patients. Beyond the wide range of services which they can competently provide, they are responsible for referring their patients to consultants or other community health resources so that any additional problems can be managed appropriately. They must learn the art of timely referral which maximizes the results of care by the consultant.

Another challenge to family physicians is the need to remain objective. They must develop the art of sorting out the significant from the inconsequential in the large volume of clinical information which confronts them each day. They must become skilled at looking beyond the patient's complaints to detect possible underlying reasons for the patient's visit. At the same time, they must be sufficiently thorough and comprehensive in the approach to each patient so that serious organic disease is not overlooked.

The process of relating meaningfully to a wide variety of patient types and ages is another area which takes years to refine, and where improvement is always possible. The incessant talker with somatization complaints may be in one examination room, while in the next is a 16-year-old girl who seems reluctant to give any kind of history or clue as to what prompted her visit to the office.

REQUISITES FOR THE FAMILY PHYSICIAN

Family practice requires of its practitioners a special combination of abilities and interests. Other fields, such as radiology, pathology, general surgery, and psychiatry, have their own special requisites for their practitioners, which in many ways are different from family practice. An understanding of the particular requisites of any specialty is essential if the medical graduate is to find satisfaction and be effective in his/her chosen field. A brief review of some of the requisites important to the family physician is therefore of interest here.

Interest in People
Of top priority for family physicians is a real interest in, and even curiosity about, people. They should like people and seek close contact with patients. They should be able to deal with a wide spectrum of personality types. They should be sufficiently warm with people as to seem approachable with any problem, and be non-judgmental of patients with differing beliefs, behaviors, or habits. They should be able to accept people for what they are, be appreciative of their potential, and tolerant of their faults.

Good Judgment
Family physicians must be well endowed with common sense and good clinical judgment. They will be confronted daily with a large number of patients with a larger number of problems. They must be able to sort out effective avenues of management in a level-headed way. They must be adept at recognizing the relative urgency of situations facing them at a given moment, and be comfortable with dealing with several problems at once, each in a different stage of resolution. Their good judgment should extend to their communicative skills with patients, who are often prone to misinterpret a casual remark, making later management more difficult.

Broad Interests
Family physicians should have more broad interests in clinical medicine than other specialists. A keen interest in the science of medicine is vital to the quality of their care of patients and their active participation in continuing medical education.

Family physicians should enjoy becoming competent in portions of many clinical disciplines, and synthesizing information for application to the common illnesses of all members of the family. In order to gain the necessary levels of competence in numerous fields, family physicians need to have high intelligence. They should be as interested in the science of medicine as in people, and should be interested in patients in their family context, and in families in their community and social context.

Decisiveness

This is an important attribute for family physicians. They see a large number of patients each day (usual average 25 to 35), and many problems encountered require immediate decisions regarding therapy or disposition of the patient. All require some tangible decision as to extent and type of work-up and follow-up. This is particularly challenging since many of the patients seen are unselected and "unlabeled."

A tendency to indecisiveness is incompatible with the role of the family physician. To be effective, family physicians must be able to make frequent decisions throughout a day, based on available information which is often incomplete. As Spooner observes, family physicians need to be comfortable with the uncertainty caused by inadequate data to immediately solve a clinical problem, which is the rule in situations where it is too early in the course of the disease to make a diagnosis.[13]

Assume Responsibility

A hallmark of family practice is the capacity of family physicians to accept total responsibility for patients and their families. Family physicians must feel comfortable with, and enjoy, this degree of responsibility for the many families in their practice.

The responsibility of family physicians to their patients does not end with referrals which they may arrange with consulting specialists. Family physicians usually remain involved in the ongoing care of associated medical problems. In addition, family physicians are responsible for the quality of all requested consultations, and for ensuring that further follow-up is continued as needed when the consultants' tasks are completed.

Family physicians must also be ready to accept responsibility for care of both the terminal patient and the chronically ill patient where scientific cure is not possible. Such patients may be difficult to manage, but the family physician is often in the best position to deal with the patient's complaints, if only on a symptomatic and supportive basis. The important thing is that any patient with a debilitating or terminal illness must not be abandoned, and the family physician is best equipped to manage such patients in their family setting.

Of equal importance to the ability to accept responsibility is the ability to share it. Family physicians must disengage themselves from their practices at regular intervals, and should have a call system for coverage of their patients by other physicians during these periods. There are still too many physicians who find it difficult to share responsibility for their patients' care with other physicians. Solo practice without adequate coverage no longer lends itself to good medical care.

Stability

Family physicians are confronted each day with many pressures and with a greater variety of situations than other practitioners. Their busy days are interspersed with difficult decisions and difficult patients. In their close relationship with patients, they will often act as a target for their hostilities. More commonly, they must serve as an "anxiety sponge" for the many patients with acute and chronic anxiety reactions in their practices.

Emotional stability is therefore an essential asset for family physicians. They must continually strive to maintain equanimity, for in this way they will be most effective in treating their patients.

Sensitivity–Objectivity Mix
Family physicians should have another capability with which not everyone is endowed: the ability to be keenly perceptive and receptive to their patients while, at the same time, maintaining sufficient objectivity to manage the problem at hand. Too much empathy without objectivity makes for ineffective and even hazardous patient care. Too little empathy, on the other hand, in the physician–patient relationship carries the risk of overlooking and neglecting underlying functional illness, which often may be the entire basis for the patient's somatic complaints.

The problem of attaining an appropriate balance between sensitivity and objectivity is most marked when the physician is caring for a personal friend. It can become especially difficult for this physician to carry out an emergency procedure, an operative procedure, or family counseling under such circumstances. To a lesser extent, of course, most or all of family physicians' patients may be their friends, so that this is a situation with which they must frequently deal.

Thinker–Doer
Family practice involves an interesting blend of thinking and doing. Family physicians are usually as involved with treatment, often involving manual skills, as with differential diagnosis, history taking, patient education, and counseling. In their intellectual approach to the science of medicine, they should be as interested in common clinical problems and their variants as in rare and esoteric disease. To the family physician, people themselves are "interesting," as is the care of their everyday illnesses.

Flexibility
Flexibility is another important attribute for family physicians. The need for this quality exists on several levels.

Family physicians must remain as open to a new diagnosis as they are to their patients' feelings. This is a particular problem in the primary care role, for they often see an illness at a stage too early for a definitive diagnosis. At a second or third office visit for a new problem, the family physician must be able to reappraise the patient in the light of new history and clinical findings, and must not become too committed to an earlier presumptive diagnosis.

There is an additional problem in the long-term patient with one or more chronic illnesses who has become well known to the family physician for many years. Here again, it is quite easy to overlook new problems unless one remains open to new findings.

A distinct facet to each day in family practice is the need to constantly adjust to diverse personalities and family situations. There is also the need to be quickly adaptable to different severities of illness and different clinical disciplines: thus, at any given time in the family physician's office, in three examination rooms, there may be a prenatal patient, a patient terminally ill with carcinoma, and a middle-aged man with a 2-hour history of chest pain.

Family physicians must also be able to tailor their treatment to the individual patient, which calls for both flexibility and imagination. From their assessment of the patient's level of intelligence and cooperation, as well as the home setting, they must try to devise a prescription for care which can realistically be followed by the patient. It is well known that many drug prescriptions are either never filled or incompletely taken. Prescriptions for changes in exercise, dietary, or behavior patterns are also not followed unless they are both realistic and understandable to the patient.

Ease With Interpersonal Relationships

Family physicians must be adept at getting along well with their colleagues, office and hospital staffs, and other members of the health team. Many family physicians have come to the view that communicative skills are the key foundation for effective family practice. The role of leadership of the health team itself is becoming an increasingly important task as the care of any patient involves the combined efforts of more allied health workers. New working relationships between the family physician, allied health professions in various fields, and other paramedical assistants are evolving, and the ability to communicate easily is essential to good patient care.

Comprehensive Approach

Family physicians must be able to "gather up" their patient's history, physical examination, and laboratory findings in a comprehensive way. This skill requires broad training, experience, and practice. Family physicians can often refine an intuitive sense of what is important and what is not. They must be on guard to be sufficiently circumspect to avoid overlooking the subtle diagnosis and the therapeutic procedure which can be performed better by a consultant. They must also think in terms of what aspects of diagnosis, treatment, and rehabilitation should be done by other consultants or community resources.

Other Personal Traits of the Family Physician

In order to be an effective family physician and to practice a high quality of medicine, other traits are desirable: stamina, an ability to pace oneself, and a basic attitude of optimism, tact, and self-confidence. In addition, family physicians must enjoy learning new clinical knowledge and developing new skills. They should approach their residency years with enthusiasm, and carry this over later into continuing medical education.

Many of the qualities of the idealized family physician have been outlined, toward which most practicing family physicians strive. That this is a big order is acknowledged, but there are many fine physicians in family practice who show that it is possible, and many medical students now in training appear to be well motivated and capable in these directions.

SELECTION OF RESIDENCY TRAINING

Overall Options

Since a substantial part of family practice involves general internal medicine, some medical students wonder whether they should enter a residency in this field. Others wonder whether a primary care residency, involving internal medicine and pediatrics, might provide a good background. Still others consider the possibility of 1 year in several specialty fields or a flexible first graduate (transitional) year followed by continuing medical education in a group practice.

There are significant limitations to all of these approaches. A residency in internal medicine fails to provide exposure and training in many areas integral to family practice, including pediatrics, obstetrics–gynecology, otolaryngology, orthopedics, minor surgery, the behavioral sciences, and family dynamics. The few primary care residencies that have been started concentrate mainly on internal medicine and pediatrics (usually with exclusive emphasis on one or the other), still leaving major areas uncovered. It is generally not feasible to take 1 year of several specialty residencies, and this too still leaves out important areas. A flexible first graduate (now called transitional) year, equivalent to the old rotating internship, followed by what may be promoted as excellent training in a future group practice, likewise leaves large gap areas. Although the young physician can doubtless learn new knowledge and skills in practice from helpful colleagues, he soon becomes engaged in a practice based largely on existing competencies. It is difficult to pursue a systematic contin- uing education in a busy practice which can substitute for major deficiencies of graduate training.

Family practice residencies have been designed to provide the knowledge, skills, and attitudes needed to practice good family medicine. Such an approach is now the only way to become board-eligible in family practice. A shorter period of graduate training or more narrow training through an alternative pathway is not likely to prepare one adequately for the demands of modern family practice.

Personal Considerations

One cannot choose among the 388 U.S. family practice residency programs without first reflecting upon one's personal goals, interests, and learning style. The general types, structures, and content of family practice residencies have already been out- lined in Chapter 7. The available programs represent a wide spectrum from the university-based program in a large academic medical center to a 150-bed com- munity hospital with a family practice residency as the only graduate training pro- gram. The patient care and learning environments in these various programs are quite different. The university-based program typically relates closely to highly struc- tured teaching services in the other major specialties, and much of the family prac- tice resident's learning may be derived from other housestaff. The family practice residency in a smaller community may involve little or no contact with residents in other specialties, less structured teaching services, and more learning from at- tending physicians in the community. Family practice residents may acquire the same range of clinical competencies over a 3-year program in either setting, but they may be more comfortable in one or the other environment.

Some family practice residencies are designed to prepare their graduates for certain types of future practice settings. A family practice residency located in the inner city, for example, may provide the resident with the experience and back- ground required for urban practice better than a program located in a smaller com- munity. Although a number of family practice residencies in urban areas can adequately prepare graduates for rural practice, a program in a smaller community may provide a more typical patient population and learning environment for residents planning to practice in smaller communities.

In addition to considering their future practice goals, prospective residents need to consider their geographic preferences and related environmental needs. Resi- dent applicants may want to stay in the same community or region where they com- pleted medical school, or move to another part of the country for residency training. The desires of one's spouse may be an important factor with respect to occupational or educational needs.

Evaluating Specific Family Practice Residencies

After prospective residents have considered their own personal interests and needs, the next step is to review the current list of approved family practice residencies.*

---

*A current list can be obtained by writing to the Division of Education, American Academy of Family Physicians, 1740 West 92nd Street, Kansas City, Missouri, 64114.

This list can be narrowed down to a manageable number of possible programs by deciding for or against a university- or community hospital-based program and by geographic region. One's list can be further narrowed by talking with a faculty advisor in the Department of Family Practice.

The next essential step is planning for interview visits, usually during the summer and fall of senior year. There is no substitute for actually seeing programs. One has an opportunity to talk with faculty and residents, to see the facilities, to learn the philosophy and ethos of the program, and to see if the community is where one would like to live for 3 years. Such interview visits allow the applicant to ask specific questions about each teaching program and to crystallize feelings about the kind of program that best will meet one's needs. Taking an elective family practice clerkship during the early part of the senior year is another valuable approach to explore a possible program.

A recent study by Di Tomasso and colleagues examined the factors influencing selection of family practice residencies by medical graduates. Table 12–4 presents a list of factors ranked by their importance by 830 graduates entering family practice residencies in 1981.[14]

Although competition for first-year family practice residency positions has been keen, most applicants have obtained positions. Applicants can feel reasonably confident about obtaining a place, particularly if they take the following steps:[15]

1. Plan the senior year carefully to allow interview visits to programs during the summer and fall (most programs terminate interview visits by December 1, some even earlier).
2. Consider a family practice clerkship in a hospital in which one has particular interest.
3. Apply to at least ten programs. It also may be prudent to "cover the bases" by applying to some flexible first graduate year (transitional) positions, but one should realize that opportunities for second-year positions in family practice residencies are limited to a small number of developing programs and whatever attrition may occur within existing programs.
4. Apply well in advance of deadlines.

TEACHING AND RESEARCH

This chapter would not be complete without brief consideration of teaching and research as an important career option in family practice, either on a part-time or full-time basis. There are more than 1100 family practice faculty involved in full-time teaching in U.S. medical schools plus an additional 1200 full-time physicians associated with family practice residency programs in community hospitals. In addition, there are many thousands of family physicians involved on a part-time and voluntary basis in teaching, particularly as attending physicians in family practice residencies or as preceptors for medical students in their practices. More than one-half of graduates of family practice residency programs are currently involved in some part-time teaching, and an additional 5 percent are in full-time teaching positions.[15]

The medical graduate entering family practice today has a wide variety of potential career options within the field. The family physician involved in full-time practice may become involved with part-time teaching in association with a nearby residency program or medical school. He/she may also participate in clinical

TABLE 12-4. MEAN RATINGS,[a] STANDARD DEVIATION, AND RANKS OF QUESTIONNAIRE ITEMS FOR 830 FIRST-YEAR FAMILY PRACTICE RESIDENTS

Questionnaire Item	Mean	Deviation	Rank
Quality of family practice faculty	4.30	.76	1
Geographic location of program	4.28	.86	2
Impression of program's residents	4.22	.87	3
Satisfaction level of residents	4.20	.88	4
Patient care responsibilities assumed	4.04	.90	5
Opportunity to see variety of medical problems	4.02	.94	6
Community in which program is located	3.91	.86	7
Hospital facility	3.89	.79	8
Family practice center facility	3.84	.81	9
Impression of residency director	3.76	.97	10
Reputation of program	3.60	1.03	11
Community hospital setting	3.57	1.22	12
Volume of patients	3.56	.98	13
Social climate of center	3.55	1.09	14
Medical curriculum	3.51	1.07	15
Interviews with program faculty	3.47	1.00	16
On-call frequency	3.28	1.09	17
Proximity of program to family	3.21	1.45	18
Setting similarity	3.00	1.24	19
Presence of other residencies	2.96	1.41	20
Behavioral curriculum	2.93	1.17	21
Program's years of existence	2.90	1.11	22
Academic affiliation with a university	2.88	1.20	23
Program's success in previous match	2.87	1.27	24
Opportunity to teach	2.80	1.13	25
Benefits	2.73	1.13	26
Salaries	2.73	1.12	26
Moonlighting opportunities	2.53	1.22	28
Perceived practice opportunities in geographic area	2.39	1.20	29
Recommendation of medical school adviser	2.03	1.19	30
Opportunity to conduct research	1.64	.94	31

[a]Based upon a Likert rating scale where 1 = not at all important, 2 = a little important, 3 = as important as it was not, 4 = a good deal important, 5 = extremely important.
(From Di Tomasso RA, DeLauro JP, Carter ST Jr: Factors influencing program selection among family practice residents. J Med Educ 58:527, 1983, with permission.)

research, either on an individual or collaborative basis, as will be discussed further in the next chapter. Family physicians engaged in full-time teaching in community hospital-based family practice residencies have an opportunity to combine part-time practice with active teaching, and may also become involved with clinical investigative efforts. University-based family physicians may be involved in a diverse mix of activities, including patient care, teaching, research, administration, and university service.

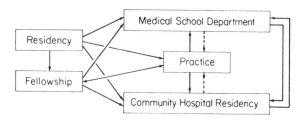

Figure 12-1. Career tracks in family medicine. *(From Geyman JP: Career tracks in academic family medicine: Issues and approaches. J Fam Pract 14:911, 1982, with permission.)*

A recent addition to career options is the development of various kinds of fellowship programs in family medicine. Fellowship programs are available that range in length from several months to 2 years. These provide effective ways for recent residency graduates or family physicians with practice experience to gain background and skills in teaching, curriculum development, and evaluation of teaching programs. Some of these programs, such as the 2-year Family Medicine Fellowship Program sponsored by the Robert Wood Johnson Foundation,* also offer excellent training in such areas as epidemiology, biostatistics, and research design together with practical experience in conducting a research project.

Although a majority of today's family practice faculty entered full-time teaching from practice, an increasing number are now considering academic family medicine as an option following completion of their residency training. Family practice residents with an interest in full-time teaching therefore face a decision as to whether to take fellowship training, enter community practice, or enter full-time teaching directly after residency training. Whether in residency or in community practice, a prospective full-time faculty member needs to weigh the advantages and disadvantages of joining a community hospital program or university-based department. Further, as long-term goals and interests in academic family medicine are considered, possible future shifts in setting and roles may become part of individual career planning. Figure 12-1 illustrates the major pathways within academic family medicine.[16]

There is some debate as to the optimal way for family practice residents to prepare for a career in academic family medicine. Some hold that a preliminary period of 3 to 5 years in active practice in the community is an essential prerequisite to full-time teaching/research. Others feel that adequate clinical experience can be obtained within a teaching or fellowship program as other skills are developed in teaching and/or research. The advantages and disadvantages of these options have been considered elsewhere in a recent paper.[16] There is no single answer to this question, and one's individual approach is entirely a matter of personal choice.

COMMENT

The choice of a specialty in medicine is probably more difficult for a medical student today than ever before, both because of the large number of options available and the pressure toward early, even premature decisions about residency training. Each specialty has its own particular challenges, content, and practice style, and

---

*These programs are now operational at three medical schools: Case Western Reserve University, the University of Missouri, and the University of Washington.

each medical student is confronted by the need to match his/her interests, skills, and goals to a compatible, satisfying field.

Pellegrino has discussed the influence of two ideal types on the influence of internal medicine—the German physician–scientist and the Oslerian scholar-consultant.[17] Today family practice offers medical graduates another kind of model perhaps best described by McWhinney's view of the future family physician:[7]

> They should have a deep commitment to people and obtain their greatest professional fulfillment from their relations with people—to believe, in Lewis Mumford's phrase, in the primacy of the person, to use technology with skill, but to make it always subservient to the interests of the person. . . [Family practice-educators] want physicians who can think analytically when analysis is required but whose usual mode of thought is multidimensional and holistic. They want them to be concerned with etiology in its broadest sense and to be ever mindful of the need to teach patients how to attain and maintain health. They want people who are not afraid of recognizing and talking about feelings: people who know themselves and can throughout their career recognize their defects, learn from experience and continue to grow as people and as physicians.

REFERENCES

1. Cousins N (editorial): The doctor as artist and philosopher. Saturday Review, July 22, 1978, p 56
2. Patients will choose doctors who talk to them. Med Econ, Nov. 8, 1982, p 174
3. Joe Ann Jackson: Personal communication. Chicago, American Medical Association, Dec. 7, 1984
4. Clinton C, Schmittling G, Stern TL, et al.: Hospital privileges for family physicians: A national study of office based members of the American Academy of Family Physicians. J Fam Pract 13:361, 1981
5. Black RR, Schmittling G, Stern TL: Characteristics and practice patterns of family practice residency graduates in the United States. J Fam Pract 11:767, 1980
6. McCranie EW, Hornsby IL, Calvert JC: Practice and career satisfaction among residency trained family physicians: A national survey. J Fam Pract 14:1107, 1982
7. McWhinney IR: Family medicine in perspective. N Engl J Med 293:176, 1975
8. Pennell MY, Renshaw JE: Distribution of women physicians, 1971. J Am Med Wom Assoc 28:181, 1973
9. Ducker DG: Believed suitability of medical specialties for women physicians. J Am Med Wom Assoc 33:25, 1978
10. Crowley AE: Graduate medical education in the United States. JAMA 250:1543, 1983
11. McGrath E, Zimet C: Female and male medical students: Differences in specialty choice selection and personality. J Med Educ 52:293, 1977
12. Stephens GG: Reform in the United States: Its impact on medicine and education for family practice. J Fam Pract 3:510, 1976
13. Spooner MA: Dealing with uncertainty in family medicine. J Fam Pract 2:471, 1975
14. Di Tomasso RA, DeLauro JP, Carter ST Jr: Factors influencing program selection among family practice residents. J Med Educ 58:527, 1983
15. Geyman JP: Evaluating family practice residencies. New Physician 25:35, 1976
16. Geyman JP: Career tracks in academic family medicine: Issues and approaches. J Fam Pract 14:911, 1982
17. Pellegrino ED: The identity crisis of an ideal. In Controversy in Internal Medicine. Ingelfinger FJ, Ebert VE, Finland M, et al. (eds): Philadelphia, W.B. Saunders, 1974, Vol. II, p 41

13 | Research in Family Practice

Any discipline must either grow intellectually or wither. One of the reasons for doing research in family medicine is to add knowledge to a field that lacks answers to many of its questions and which needs an intellectual base that can generate other knowledge as time passes. Another reason for doing research in family medicine is more pragmatic. Family medicine can do its job best if it is accepted as a full partner in the academic world, so that the ideals, goals, and working energies of its practitioners and teachers can influence the course of medical education in positive ways.

Gerald T. Perkoff[1]

Family practice arose on a different basis than most other clinical specialties in medicine. Most fields have developed to encompass new areas of knowledge and/or technology. A majority of the other specialties developed during the period between 1920 and 1950 when the trend toward biomedical research and specialization was particularly active. Family practice, on the other hand, developed in direct response to a broadly perceived lack of adequate primary care, before an active research base was established.

Family practice originated from the background of general practice, lacking both commitment and methods of organized research in the field. The teaching and clinical application of general practice was traditionally derivative in nature—its content was derived from all of the other clinical specialties. The emphasis in general practice has been to distill from the other specialties practical approaches to the diagnosis and treatment of common clinical problems that can be applied in a busy practice. Research has been perceived in a negative light by many general practitioners as lacking relevance to their daily work. Such an attitude has often been reinforced by exposure, during their own medical education, to research activities in other disciplines involving "esoteric" conditions and complex pathophysiologic mechanisms not directly applicable to the everyday practice of the general/family physicians.

Today's circumstances are quite different. With family practice well into its second decade as a specialty, it is an integral part of the formal system of medical education in the United States. Research is becoming recognized as an essential element in the development of the specialty, and the necessary tools for research are being implanted in many teaching and clinical settings throughout the country.

The developing research efforts in family practice raise a number of basic issues with respect to the process of building an ongoing research effort in a broad clinical specialty. There are questions about the content and focus of research in family practice, and how these relate to teaching and patient care. There are questions about applicable methods of carrying out research in the field, and how teaching programs and practicing family physicians can become involved in research. Additional questions relate to how collaborative and consultative linkages can be established within family practice and with related fields, such as epidemiology and biostatistics. This chapter will present an overview of how these kinds of issues are being addressed through the research efforts which are taking place today in family practice.

BACKGROUND

Medical research has traditionally focused heavily on the study of patients admitted to university medical centers and large teaching hospitals. These patients represent only a minute fraction of the population at risk for disease. Although the large majority of all physician–patient contacts takes place in the arena of primary and continuing medical care, this area has received little concerted study.[2] It is therefore clear that research in family practice must develop its own traditions and methods in an essentially uncharted area.

The importance of population-based clinical research in primary care settings is well illustrated by the recent work of Ellenberg and Nelson on the natural history of febrile seizures in children. They conducted an extensive literature review of this common problem with a particular focus on the effects of methods of sample selection on results. They found that clinic-based studies (i.e., especially academic medical centers and referral clinics) reported a range from 2.6 to 76.9 percent for the proportion of children experiencing subsequent nonfebrile seizures after febrile seizures, whereas corresponding figures for population-based studies were consistently low (1.5 to 4.6 percent). Their observations concerning selection bias are probably generalizable to many other health problems:[3]

> Probably most children with febrile seizures are cared for by generalists and community-based pediatricians. Yet, much of the teaching and virtually all of the writing about febrile seizures are done by specialists in academic referral centers. In the recent past, presumably based on their own experience with patients coming to specialized referral centers as well as on the literature stemming from such centers, specialists have often recommended long-term anticonvulsant therapy for all children with febrile seizures. The specialist who sees an occasional child with febrile seizures in whom the outcome is unfavorable has no way of knowing the size of the population from which that child comes and, therefore, does not know the infrequency of the poor outcome.

The word "research" is still a somewhat misunderstood term to many in family practice. Part of this confusion is due to the yet incomplete definition of the form, content, and methods of research being developed in family practice settings. Traditional biomedical definitions of research in other disciplines cannot be transplanted into family practice, for they were designed for different purposes and conditions.

Wood and his colleagues state the situation in this way:[4]

> [The term research] still produces an image of a white-coated, bench-bound physician that induces many negative connotations for the problem-solving, decision-making clinician reveling in the cut and thrust of community practice. The former is only one type of research; observing, recording, and analyzing personal or practice experience over a continuum must be considered another type. It qualifies

by extending the horizons of knowledge for the individual observer, and doubly so if the data are presented in such a way as to allow comparisons with like situations. The hallmark of research is the representation and applicability of the results to other environments, expanding the body of knowledge available.

Webster defines "research" in a fundamental way: "the diligent and systematic inquiry or investigation into a subject in order to discover or revise facts, theories, and applications." Byrne views "research" as "organized curiosity."[5] Whatever definition for the word one accepts, it is clear that research in family practice must be defined broadly.

Family physicians have a wider perspective and experience with health and disease on the community level than any other field in medicine. Because they deal with the everyday problems of patients and families, family physicians have a number of inherent advantages related to research on a patient care level. These include the following:

1. Family physicians see all members of the family, of all ages and both sexes.
2. They have direct experience with primary or first contact care of unselected patients.
3. They have the opportunity to follow most of their patients over a long period of time.
4. They bring a multidisciplinary approach to health care.
5. They see patients in any or all of the James' stages:[6]

    Stage I.   Foundations of disease
    Stage II.   Preclinical disease
    Stage III. Treatment of symptomatic disease
    Stage IV.   Rehabilitation and management of medical conditions for which biologic cure is not possible

McWhinney sees the clinical observation and study of patients in their natural habitat as the center of family practice research:[7]

> Family medicine is, of course, one branch of clinical medicine. Like clinical medicine it has both scientific and technological components. Its scientific subject matter is the phenomena of illness as they present to family physicians; its technological aspect is the development and evaluation of the conceptual, organizational, and material tools used by family physicians. The justification for its independent existence is that the tools are unique to the discipline, not derived from other branches of medicine, and that the phenomena can only be satisfactorily studied from within, rather than outside, the discipline.

SOME BASIC APPROACHES AND METHODS FOR RESEARCH

A Favorable Climate

Perhaps the most important change which has taken place during the last 15 years in family practice with respect to research is the improving climate within the field concerning investigative work. In nonmeteorologic terms, the word "climate" is defined as a particular set of "prevailing attitudes, standards, or environmental conditions of a group, period, or place."[8] There is growing evidence that the necessary attitudes, standards, and environmental conditions within family practice are becoming more facilitative of research activity.

There is an increasing number of family physicians who exemplify the attitudes necessary for investigative work. These include the following kinds of attributes.[9]

1. Curiosity
2. Skepticism
3. Intellectual honesty
4. Awareness of limited knowledge
5. Appreciation of the family physician's role in research
6. Valuing of own observations over time
7. Acceptance of responsibility to help advance the field

The standards of "good practice" in general practice in the past have been largely derived from other clinical specialties in the absence of organized study within the primary care environment. As more is learned from research in family practice settings, and as family physicians increasingly take responsibility for peer review and establishing their own criteria for "good practice," research in family practice will be more directly linked to analysis and improvement of clinical practice.

The environmental conditions in a growing number of family practice settings in the United States further facilitate research activities. These particularly include such basic research tools as the use of the problem-oriented medical record, coding and data retrieval methods, health status indices, and related techniques suited to population-based studies.

Some Basic Research Tools

1. Accepted Classification Systems. Until recently, available classification systems for coding of health problems were based primarily on the diseases of hospitalized patients and were not useful in primary care settings. The last 20 years have seen the development of various classification systems more directly suited to the needs of general/family practice in a number of countries around the world. The International Classification of Health Problems in Primary Care (ICHPPC) has received the most widespread acceptance today, and is endorsed by the World Organization of National Colleges and Academies of General Practice/Family Medicine (WONCA).[10] The ICHPPC-2 is the current version in general use today. It contains 362 diagnostic titles under 18 categories, and permits comparative studies among general/family practice settings around the world.[11] A conversion code has been developed that affords ready conversion from the Royal College of General Practitioners Classification of Diseases (RCGP) to the ICHPPC.[12] ICHPPC-2 is compatible with the two most commonly used classification systems for hospital encounters—ICD-9 and ICD-9-CM.

    A companion classification system to ICHPPC-2 is the NAPCRG Process Classification, developed to facilitate agreement on various services provided by primary care physicians (e.g., procedures, drugs, diagnostic procedures, and type of visit).[13]

2. Glossary of Terms. Another basic need for family practice research is the common acceptance of precise and unambiguous terms for use on encounter forms, and related medical records. An ad hoc committee of the North American Primary Care Research Group (NAPCRG) has addressed this need and formulated a Glossary for Primary Care that has been generally adopted in this country.[14]

3. Problem-Oriented Medical Record. The problem-oriented medical record, originally developed by Weed, has four basic elements:[15,16]
   a. Defined Data Base. This includes any or all of the following: chief complaint, patient profile and related social data, present illness, past history and systems review, physical examination, and reports of laboratory work and special studies. The extent of the data base which is feasible for a given patient in a given practice depends on the limits of time and cost effectiveness.
   b. Complete Problem List. The problem list displays in the front of the patient's chart a complete list of past and present problems, including dates of resolution of inactive problems. A "problem" is defined by Weed as ". . . anything that requires management or diagnostic workup; this includes social and demographic problems."[17]
   c. Initial Plans. Initial plans are listed for each problem, including further diagnostic studies, therapy, and patient education.
   d. Progress Notes. Progress notes are written in a "SOAP" format:
      Subjective: presenting, changing, and resolving symptoms.
      Objective: physical, laboratory, and x-ray findings.
      Assessment: refinement of diagnosis and assessment of progress.
      Plans: additional plans for diagnosis and management. In complicated cases, flow sheets may be used which incorporate frequently monitored observations.

4. Age-Sex Register. An age-sex register in family practice is an important part of a data system that facilitates clinical research as well as improved office management, outreach, and audit.[18] The use of such cards permits profiling of the practice population by age and sex, an essential part of many comparative clinical studies.

5. Diagnostic Index. The diagnostic index is a compilation of patients by diagnosis, and is synonymous to morbidity index, disease index, and problem index. Various types of diagnostic indices have been developed for use in primary care. The E-book is perhaps the most widely used method, first developed by Eimerl in England and introduced into the United States by Wood and Metcalfe.[19]

6. Encounter Form. The encounter form provides essential information for each doctor–patient encounter for both practice management and research purposes. Specific kinds of encounter data which are generally required include the following:
   a. Facility identification
   b. Provider information
   c. Person identification
   d. Source(s) of payment
   e. Date
   f. Patient's reason for visit, symptom, or complaint
   g. Physician evaluation (diagnosis or problem)
   h. Diagnostic, therapeutic or management procedures
   i. Disposition of patient[20]
   A universal encounter form would be highly desirable for administrative, insurance, and research purposes, and there are some efforts in this direction, but common agreement on a minimal basic data set and a logistic design are first required on the part of all concerned parties.[20]

7. Information Management System. An integrated medical information system is required in order to carry out research in primary care settings. Such a system captures patient encounter data by means of an encounter form, and integrates the other record-keeping tools that have just been described into a structured system that can provide ongoing information about the practice as a whole as well as individual patients and single illnesses. An increasing number of family practice offices in both teaching and nonteaching settings have access to microcomputers to facilitate this process.

At this writing about one-half of U.S. family practice residency programs have computers available for research. Table 13–1 shows the extent to which various elements of a medical information management system are operational in these programs.[21]

8. Indices of Health Status. Another important need for research in family practice is for methods that can profile a patient's changing health status over time. Such information is vital to the evaluation of the effects of different modes of therapy on the duration and severity of clinical problems, identification of high-risk patients, and related research purposes. A useful Health Status Index has been developed at Michigan State University.[22] A number of other scales of adult health status have been developed by the Rand Corporation as part of their Health Insurance Study. Some of these were recently applied by the Primary Care Cooperative Information (COOP) Project in New England for measuring functional levels of primary care patients on the basis of selected physical and mental health status scales. Table 13–2 displays validity figures for the various scales used.[23]

9. Library Services. Several recent directions in medical library activities have made literature resources readily accessible to practicing physicians throughout the country. In most states, for example, university medical center libraries have developed excellent interlibrary loan services with libraries in outlying community hospitals.

The National Library of Medicine initiated a new type of monthly bibliography in 1970, the *Abridged Index Medicus*,* especially designed for use by individual physicians and libraries of small hospitals and clinics. This publication is based on articles from 100 English language journals, and allows quick review of the literature on clinical subjects.

The National Library of Medicine has also developed a computer-based system for rapid bibliographic access called MEDLINE (MEDical Literature Analysis and Retrieval System on-LINE). This system draws on a data base containing references to approximately half a million citations from 3000 biomedical journals. MEDLINE is especially designed to locate specific information rapidly. MEDLINE literature searches are available in about 800 institutions and agencies in North America, and searches for less than 30 citations are usually available in 2 working days. When information is needed on an emergency basis, a MEDLINE search will be run immediately during hours when the data base is accessible. Specific details concerning the procedures and nominal costs of MEDLINE searches are available through most medical libraries. A recent innovation in bibliographic retrieval is a computer-based self-service system

---

*The *Abridged Index Medicus* is available on a subscription basis from the United States Government Printing Office, Washington, D.C., 20402; subscription cost in 1985 was $43.00 per year.

TABLE 13-1. PRACTICE DATA SYSTEM ELEMENTS BY PROGRAM TYPE[a]

			% of Programs			
	Community (n = 30)	University Affiliated (n = 155)	University Administered (n = 55)	University (n = 61)	Military (n = 12)	Total (n = 304)
Referral information	47	53	65	68	40	56(170)
Morbidity index	73	63	46	72	27	62(185)
Socioeconomic status	83	61	62	71	34	63(188)
Race	84	68	70	78	50	71(218)
Laboratory data	67	75	78	77	50	74(224)
Visit/productivity data	77	75	72	92	62	77(236)
Procedure data	77	82	84	92	75	83(254)
Age/sex register	97	87	82	92	85	88(269)

[a]Programs with element available or in development.
(From: Culpepper L., Franks P: Family medicine research: Status at the end of the first decade. JAMA 249:63, 1983, with permission. Copyright 1983, American Medical Association.)

TABLE 13-2. RAND SCALES SELECTED TO MEASURE PHYSICAL AND MENTAL FUNCTIONING BY PATIENT SELF-REPORT METHOD

Scale (No. of Items)		Meaning of Scale	Internal Consistency[a]	Test-Retest
		Physical		
Self-care limitations	(1)	Chronic limitations in self-care (e.g., eating, dressing)	Not relevant for single-item scale	0.99[b]
Mobility limitations	(3)	Chronic limitations in mobility (e.g., need help to go out)	0.92	0.99[b]
Physical ability II	(4)	Able to perform moderate-strenuous physical task (e.g., run short distance)	0.89	Not computed
Role activity limitations	(3)	Chronic limitations in role functioning (e.g., can't work)	0.98	0.92[b]
		Mental		
Anxiety	(5)	Feeling anxious, worried, tense during past month	0.88	0.70[c]
Depression	(3)	Feeling depressed, down-hearted, blue during past month	0.84	Not computed
Vitality	(4)	Felt energy, pep, vitality, during past month	0.81	Not computed

[a]Coefficient of reproducibility or Cronbach's alpha.
[b]Correlation between scores on alternate test forms 4 months apart.
[c]Product-moment correlation between alternate forms 1 week apart.
(From: Nelson E, Conger B, Douglass R, et al.: Functional health status levels of primary care patients. JAMA 249:3331, 1983, with permission. Copyright 1983, American Medical Association.)

(Paper Chase) developed at Beth Israel Hospital in Boston in conjunction with the National Library of Medicine.[24] This system is widely used in that hospital, demonstrates the effectiveness of this technique, and may lead to more general use of similar methods elsewhere.

Consultation and Collaboration

Consultation is important with colleagues who have done similar kinds of research and with consultants in such fields as epidemiology, biostatistics, and related fields. Such consultation is more readily available to family physicians than in the past, particularly through linkages established with these disciplines by many family practice teaching programs. It can also be anticipated that collaborative research projects will be carried out with increasing frequency involving departments of family practice in medical schools and practicing family physicians in the community.

Planning a Research Project

Any research project inevitably must begin with a question asked by an individual. The potential range of researchable questions in family practice is extremely wide. What the curious individual does next with respect to ways and means of planning and conducting a research project depends on such variables as the nature of the study, the numbers of subjects required for meaningful results, the availability of time and resources, the need for specialized assistance from other disciplines, and the experience and skills of the prospective researcher.

The planning of any research project is a critical and demanding process which involves progressive refining of the research question before the project itself can be designed and carried out. A useful, stepwise process for planning clinical, social and behavioral research projects has been developed by Gordon.[25] Parkerson and Gehlbach have further identified the specific steps required in the process of refining a research question, as illustrated by the example in Table 13–3.[26]

CONTENT AREAS FOR RESEARCH

The spectrum of needed research in family practice is wide. Although incomplete, Table 13–4 presents a simple taxonomy with four major categories of research, together with sample subject areas in each category.[27]

Spitzer views the directions for potential research in family practice in these terms:[28]

> The family physician has a distinctive perspective and the obligation to study intact human beings in free-living, non-institutionalized populations over long periods of time, observing transitions from health to disease and back to health, with a unique opportunity to observe, on a firsthand basis, many of the concurrent phenomena that affect health and disease, such as family, employment, housing, and exposure to risk factors.
>
> Some subject areas that deserve high priority in family medicine research are calibrational studies focusing on clinical phenomena such as quantification of pain, quantification of the quality of survival, the development of explicit criteria for adequate clinical management of carefully defined conditions, demarcation of presenting complaints and their combinations as distinct from the demarcation of diagnoses, a taxonomy for behavior associated with disease or perceived disease, prognostic stratification of patients, and the calibration of the clinician himself as a reliable observer.

White goes further in proposing the following kinds of important and researchable problems in primary care and family practice:[29]

> What are the situational circumstances associated with the onset of illness?
> What role does separation play in the genesis of illness?
> What events or changes trigger consultation with a physician?
> What role do environmental factors play in the genesis of illness?
> Does the identification and monitoring of high-risk groups reduce morbidity?
> How valid are probabilistic models in primary care?
> What information does each test or X-ray really contribute to the resolution of the patient's presenting complaint?

Still others conceptualize the need and priorities of family practice research from different perspectives. Thus, Cluff stresses the importance of research on the functional status of patients as a neglected measure of patient care outcome;[30] Ramsey calls for a research thrust to describe the relationships between the family system and the body's three major regulatory systems—the nervous, immune, and endocrine systems;[31] and Kleinman calls for the application of medical anthropology to the study of the biopsychosocial model in primary care.[32]

TABLE 13-3. EXAMPLE OF REFINING A RESEARCH QUESTION

(1) General Research Question: Is continuity of care beneficial?

(2) Population to Be Studied	(3) Study Period	Variables to be Measured		(6) Methods of Measurement	(7) Resources Required	(8) Estimate of Feasibility
		(4) Nonspecific	(5) Specific			
Hypertensive patients in a family medicine group practice	2 years	Continuity of care	Return visits to the same physician	Enumerate from medical records	Clerical	Little extra expense— *feasible*
		Beneficial for the patient	Patient satisfaction	Questionnaire	Investigation of other questionnaires. Possible consultants. Printing and mailing.	Expensive but *feasible*
		Control of blood pressure	Blood pressure readings	Medical records	Trained abstractors	Expensive— *not* feasible
		Patient morbidity	List of patient problems	Medical records	Trained abstractors	Expensive— *not* feasible
		Beneficial for the physician	Physician satisfaction	Questionnaire	Same as for first questionnaire (see above)	Expensive— *not* feasible

(9) Refined Research Question: Are hypertensive patients returning to the same physician satisfied with their medical care?

(10) Hypothesis: Hypertensive patients returning to the same physician are satisfied with their medical care.

(From: Parkerson GR, Gehlbach SH: Refining research questions. J Fam Pract 8:859, 1979, with permission.)

TABLE 13-4. A TAXONOMY FOR RESEARCH AREAS IN FAMILY PRACTICE

Epidemiologic and Clinical Research	Health Services Research	Behavioral Research	Educational Research
Single illness studies	Consumers	Doctor-patient relationships	Medical student interest in family practice
Morbidity	Health and illness behavior	Health team and changing roles	Teaching aids for family practice
Natural history	Needs and demands	Impact of societal changes on primary care	Family practice residency programs
Prevention	Consumer participation	Family dynamics	Educational objectives
Early diagnosis	Patient compliance	Normal	Role of problem-oriented record and medical audit
Management	Effects of health education	Abnormal	Program costs
Case reports	Providers	Changing patterns	Model family practice clinic costs and revenue
Practice studies	Numbers and distribution	Developmental aspects of family life cycles	Self-assessment methods
Content	Efficiency (utilization)	Counseling	Family practice residents
Common diseases	Physician performance	Methods	Practicing family physicians
Common problems	Referral patterns	Results	Continuing medical education
Variation with geographic setting	Costs of primary care		Needs of family physicians
Consultation rates	Solo practice		Physician performance
Changing patterns	Family practice group		
Family studies	Multispecialty group		
Morbidity	Allied health manpower studies		
Prevention	Task definition		
Role of genetic counseling	Health team studies		
Crisis intervention	Cost and efficiency studies		
	Drug and laboratory procedure studies		
	Experimental models for delivery of primary care (including comparison of family practice and multi-specialty approaches)		
	Interface		
	Patient outcome studies		
	Costs and incentives		
	Cost-benefit ratios		
	Facilities and utilization		
	Role of health hazard appraisal		

(From: Geyman JP: Research in the family practice residency program. J Fam Pract 5:247, 1977 with permission.)

Regardless of how one conceptualizes the content and focus of needed research in family practice, it is clear that the horizons for such research are necessarily broad. Although a strong clinical base of research in the field is essential, research in health services and educational dimensions of family practice are also required. Ultimately, the priorities for categories and subjects of research will inevitably be based on local and individual interests and capabilities. As a reference point of interest, Figure 13–1 displays the relative proportions of various kinds of research papers published during the first 10 years of *The Journal of Family Practice*, 1974–1983.[33]

CURRENT STATUS, PROBLEMS, AND STRATEGIES FOR RESEARCH

Current Status

Several organizations have made important contributions to the development of research in family practice over the last decade. The North American Primary Care Research Group (NAPCRG) was established in 1972 to provide an open forum for the presentation and discussion of research in primary care.[34] Its meetings have included sufficient critique of each presentation so as to afford useful opportunities for presenters to improve their research skills. Today there are over 700 members of NAPCRG, mostly in family medicine.[21] The Society of Teachers of Family Medicine (STFM) has an active research committee, and has sponsored periodic workshops since 1975 to increase faculty skills in research. The American Academy of Family Physicians (AAFP) has encouraged research activities of its membership, and through the Family Health Foundation has provided grant support to an increasing number of research projects in the field. In addition, the Robert Wood Johnson Foundation has fostered the development of research skills through its 2-year Family Medicine Fellowship Program.

In 1980 a joint study was conducted by STFM and NAPCRG to determine the status of research in U.S. and Canadian family practice teaching programs. Table 13–5 shows the level of interest in research by type of program, and Table 13–6 displays the training and percentage of time spent in research by family medicine

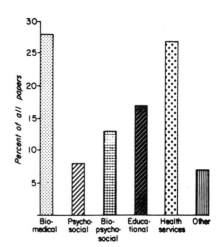

Figure 13-1. Overall percentage of all papers by major content area (1974–1983). *(From Geyman JP, Berg AO: The Journal of Family Practice 1974–1983: Analysis of an evolving literature base. J Fam Pract 18:47, 1984, with permission.)*

TABLE 13-5. ORGANIZATION FOR RESEARCH, BY PROGRAM TYPE

| | % (No.) of Programs | | | | |
| | | | Current Program Emphasis on Research | | |
	Designated Coordinator	Regular Meetings	Little Or None	Emerging	Visible
Community (n = 38)	42	16	26	42·	32
University affiliated (n = 166)	50	16	19	49	33
University administered (n = 63)	52	33	25	46	29
University (n = 72)	64	43	12	31	57
Military (n = 14)	79	29	7	50	43
Total (n = 353)	54(189)	26(88)	19(67)	44(155)	37(131)

(From Culpepper L, Franks P: Family medicine research: Status at the end of the first decade. JAMA 249:63, 1983, with permission. Copyright 1983, American Medical Association.)

faculty. As expected, university programs are the most active in research, and Ph.D., faculty tend to devote more of their time to research than do M.D. faculty. At the same time, 139 of the responding programs identified more than 800 practicing family physicians in the community who were involved in collaborative research in one capacity or another.[21]

A further view of the nature of published research to date is afforded by Figure 13–2, which displays the trends over the last 10 years in types of papers published in *The Journal of Family Practice*. A continuing increase is noted in observational

TABLE 13-6. FACULTY INVOLVED IN RESEARCH (351 PROGRAMS RESPONDING)

| | % of Time Spent in Research | | | | | | |
| | >50 | | 50-10 | | <10 | | Total |
Credentials	No. of Programs	No. of Faculty	No. of Programs	No. of Faculty	No. of programs	No. of Faculty	No. of Faculty
Physicians							
MD/PhD	5	5	11	12	9	10	27
MD/MPH							
or MS	2	4	17	18	12	16	38
MD (other)	3	9	13	18	20	42	69
MD	17	25	51	94	137	292	411
Subtotal	—	43	—	142	—	360	545
Nonphysicians							
PhD	16	25	44	61	40	49	135
Master's							
degree	1	1	6	6	7	7	14
Other	4	6	18	29	17	20	55
Subtotal	—	32	—	96	—	76	204
Total	—	75	—	238	—	436	749

(From Culpepper L, Franks P: Family medicine research: Status at the end of the first decade. JAMA 249:63, 1983, with permission. Copyright 1983, American Medical Association.)

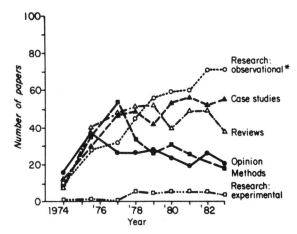

Figure 13-2. Number of papers by type and by year. *(From Geyman JP, Berg AO; The Journal of Family Practice 1974-1983: Analysis of an evolving literature base. J Fam Pract 18:47, 1984, with permission.)*

*Includes case control, cohort, and survey studies

research, a decrease in methods papers, and a consistently low proportion of experimental research papers.[33]

Problems

The joint STFM-NAPCRG study also identified the major problems perceived by family practice programs in carrying out research activities. Table 13-7 presents their experience and perceptions vis-a-vis ten potential impediments to research.[21] It is readily apparent that lack of time and shortage of funding constitute the major limiting factors to research in family practice. This undoubtedly reflects the lack of a "critical mass" of family practice faculty, as pointed out in an earlier chapter, in many programs as needed to carry out research in addition to heavy commitments in patient care, teaching, and administration.

TABLE 13-7. IMPEDIMENTS TO RESEARCH

	% of Programs		
	Not a Problem	*Minor Problem*	*Major Problem*
Lack of faculty time	5	17	78
Lack of funding for faculty time for research	13	26	61
Lack of funding for staff, equipment, supplies	14	38	48
Lack of faculty research skills	10	45	45
Lack of role models	15	42	43
Lack of "rewards"	31	40	29
Lack of faculty interest	23	55	22
Lack of technical support	48	35	17
Lack of practice organization	48	38	12
Lack of practice population	75	20	5

(From Culpepper L, Franks P: Family medicine research: Status at the end of the first decade. JAMA 249:63, 1983, with permission. Copyright 1983, American Medical Association.)

Strategies

In response to these problems and in view of the overriding importance of further developing research in family practice, the Study Group in Family Medicine Research* recently made the following recommendations:[35]

To Individual Practitioners and Teachers of Family Medicine, it is recommended:

1. That full-time practicing family physicians use the problem solving skills they have developed in confronting patient care problems to seek solutions for these problems by conducting research in their own practices
2. That family medicine teachers conduct research themselves and assist full-time practicing family physicians in their practice based research
3. That all persons who practice and/or teach family medicine recognize the importance of research in augmenting the scientific base of their discipline and in improving patient care, support research by others, and apply the results of research as they practice and teach

To Family Medicine Academic Units: Divisions, Departments, and Residency Training Programs, it is recommended:

1. That family medicine curricula provide elective time for research activities by students, residents, and Fellows
2. That family medicine faculty be given protected time for research activities
3. That Family Medicine Research Centers be developed, based upon the demonstrated ability to provide a critical mass of researchers whose principal activity is conducting, teaching, and facilitating research
4. That the Family Medicine Research Centers provide for professionals who practice and/or teach family medicine the following educational and supportive resources:
   A. Training sessions in research methods at introductory, intermediate, and advanced levels
   B. Research fellowships for periods ranging from three months to three years
   C. Teams of health professionals with research expertise, including practicing family physicans, to assist in research activities conducted in practice and teaching sites
   D. Leadership for active collaboration in research activity between professionals in academic centers and full-time practicing family physicians

To Family Medicine Professional Organizations, it is recommended:

1. That family medicine professional organizations perform the following functions:
   A. Raise funds to support the Family Medicine Research Centers and other research endeavors in family medicine, both internally from their own membership and externally from other foundations, corporations, and governmental agencies
   B. Provide opportunities for their members to train for the participation in and the evaluation and rational application of research

---

*An autonomous group organized and supported by the STFM's Task Force on Research Status and Needs; this group was also supported by NAPCRG, the AAFP, the College of Family Physicians of Canada, and the Family Health Foundation of America.

C. Establish mechanisms to provide family medicine researchers ready access to information pertinent to their research, both from the literature and directly from colleagues with like research interests

D. Provide forums for presentation and critique of research as well as peer support and personal interaction between novice and experienced researchers

E. Communicate to other health organizations and constituencies the research activities, resources, and needs of family medicine

2. That the requirements for residency training in family medicine in the United States be modified to require that training programs offer elective opportunities in family medicine research, either directly by each program or through cooperative arrangements with other organizations

3. That the educational objectives for certification in family medicine in Canada be modified to include objectives appropriate for training residents to conduct and/or participate in research studies

OPPORTUNITIES FOR INVOLVEMENT IN RESEARCH

In an excellent paper on this subject, Phillips proposes a spectrum of involvement styles by which interested family physicians may participate in research studies. Figure 13–3 illustrates a three-dimensional view of this spectrum incorporating three parameters: relevant disciplines, type of research, and level of involvement by the researcher.[36] By means of this grid, one can describe a particular study and level of involvement; for example, a clinical strategy study may draw especially from epidemiology and involve the family physician as a volunteer observer, as the principal investigator, in a collaborative way with peers, or as part of a multicenter regional or national study.

Collaborative studies offer ideal opportunities for interested family physicians without research experience to become involved with research. Two excellent examples of ongoing research networks involving medical schools and community-based physicians are the Primary Care Cooperative Information Project (COOP) conducted by the Department of Community and Family Medicine at Dartmouth and the WAMI Family Medicine Collaborative Research Group at the University of Washington.[37,38] Another example is the Ambulatory Sentinal Practice Network, sponsored by NAPCRG and funded by the Rockefeller Foundation. This network presently includes 38 sentinal practices in 14 states and 2 provinces of the United States and Canada for the purpose of surveillance of primary care problems and services.[39]

Departments of family practice in medical schools have both the opportunity and responsibility to develop active research programs involving their own faculty, residents, and students, as well as faculty from other disciplines and interested family physicians in the surrounding area. Active collaboration between academic centers and practicing family physicians is a vital linkage in the development of a sound foundation of empirical and experimental research in family practice.

COMMENT

Family practice is in the process of redefining traditional connotations of medical research as various kinds of research questions are being addressed in the clinical environment of the family physician. This process involves the development of some

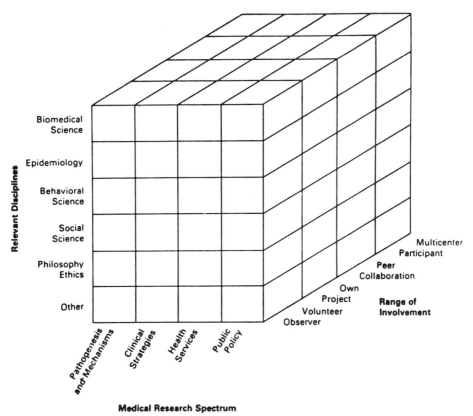

Medical Research Spectrum

Figure 13-3. Spectrum of involvement styles. *(From Phillips TJ: Research considerations for the family physician. J Fam Pract 7:121, 1978, with permission.)*

new investigative techniques, the modification of other established research methods to adapt to the family practice environment, and the potential collaboration of a wide range of related desciplines. The ultimate result of this process will be to convert family practice from an applied, derivative field drawing entirely from other disciplines to a clinical discipline basing its approaches to patient care and teaching more directly on the results of examined clinical experience in its own environment.

Research in family practice has a good start, but is still in a relatively early phase involving primarily descriptive studies. That various kinds of observational research collectively make up the major research effort to date in the field seems congruent with the major research issues, problems, and environment of research in family medicine settings. One would hope, however, that as research methods are further refined and adapted to the special needs of primary care, experimental research will occupy a somewhat more prominent role that it has to date in the development of new knowledge and evaluations of new techniques and interventions within the field.

Basic to the progress of research in family practice is an attitude of critical inquiry among family physicians. Questions need to be asked about the effectiveness of current clinical approaches in family practice. Documentation should be sought to validate current approaches, and those which lack demonstrated value should be rejected. Many related disciplines may be involved in the study of problems in family practice, but it is the family physician who must accept primary responsibility for asking and pursuing the questions needing study. The benefits of this process include expansion of the body of knowledge which family physicians will teach, an ongoing stimulus for continuing medical education, increased practice satisfaction, and most important, better health care for the patients and families of family physicians.

REFERENCES

1. Perkoff GT: Research in family medicine: Classification, directions, and costs. J Fam Pract 13:553, 1981
2. Haggerty RJ: The university and primary care. N Engl J Med 281:416, 1969
3. Ellenberg JH, Nelson KB: Sample selection and the natural history of disease: Studies of febrile seizures. JAMA 243:1337, 1980
4. Wood M, Stewart W, Brown TC: Research in family medicine. J Fam Pract 5:64, 1977
5. Byrne PS: Why not organize your curiosity? J Fam Pract 5:188, 1977
6. James G: The general practitioner of the future. N Engl J Med 270:1286, 1963
7. McWhinney IR: Family medicine as a science. J Fam Pract 7:54, 1978
8. The Random House Dictionary of the English Language. New York, Random House, 1967, p 277
9. Geyman JP: Climate for research in family practice. J Fam Pract 7:69, 1978
10. Froom J: An integrated medical record and data system for primary care. Part 2: Classifications of health problems for use by family physicians. J Fam Pract 4:1149, 1977
11. Froom J: ICHPPC-2: An improved classification system for family practice. J Fam Pract 10:791, 1980
12. Schneeweiss R, Stuart HW Jr, Froom J, et al.: A conversion code from the RCGP to the ICHPPC classification system. J Fam Pract 5:415, 1977
13. Tindall HL, Culpepper L, Froom J, et al.: The NAPCRG Process classification for Primary Care. J Fam Pract 12:309, 1981
14. Glossary for Primary Care. Report of the North American Primary Care Research Group (NAPCRG) Committee on Standard Terminology. J Fam Pract 5:633, 1977
15. Weed LL: Medical Records, Medical Education, and Patient Care. Cleveland, Ohio, Case Western Reserve University Press, 1970, p 13
16. Froom J: An integrated medical record and data system for primary care. Part 6: A decade of problem-oriented medical records: A reassessment. J Fam Pract 5:627, 1977
17. Hurst JW, Walker HK (eds): The Problem-Oriented System. New York, Medcom Inc., 1972, p 23
18. Froom J: An integrated medical record and data system for primary care. Part 1: The age-sex register: Definition of the patient population. J Fam Pract 4:951, 1977
19. Froom J, Culpepper L, Boisseau V: An integrated medical record and data system for primary care. Part 3: The diagnostic index: Manual and computer methods and applications. J Fam Pract 5:113, 1977
20. Froom J, Kirkwood R, Culpepper L, Boisseau V: An integrated medical record and data system for primary care. Part 7: The encounter form: Problems and prospects for a universal type. J Fam Pract 5:845, 1977
21. Culpepper L, Franks P: Family medicine research: Status at the end of the first decade. JAMA 249:63, 1983

22. Given CW, Simoni L, Gallin R: The design and use of a health status index for family physicians. J Fam Pract 4:287, 1977
23. Nelson E, Conger B, Douglass R, et al.: Functional health status levels of primary care patients. JAMA 249:3331, 1983
24. Horowitz GL, Jackson JD, Bleich HL: Paper chase: Self-service bibliographic retrieval. JAMA 250:2494, 1983
25. Gordon MJ: Research Workbook: A guide for initial planning of clinical, social and behavioral research projects. J Fam Pract 7:145, 1978
26. Parkerson GR, Gehlbach SH: Refining research questions. J Fam Pract 8:859, 1979
27. Geyman JP: Research in the family practice residency program. J Fam Pract 5:245, 1977
28. Spitzer WO: The intellectual worthiness of family medicine. Pharos Alpha Omega Alpha 40:2, July 1977
29. White KL: Primary care research and the new epidemiology. J Fam Pract 3:579, 1976
30. Cluff LE: A research agenda for family physicians. J Fam Pract 18:145, 1984
31. Ramsey CN: Family medicine: The science of family practice. J Fam Pract 17:767, 1983
32. Kleinman A: The cultural meaning and social uses of illness: A role for medical anthropology and clinically oriented social science in the development of primary care theory and research. J Fam Pract 16:539, 1983
33. Geyman JP, Berg AO: The Journal of Family Practice 1974–1983: Analysis of an evolving literature base. J Fam Pract 18:47, 1984
34. Wood M: What is NAPCRG? J Fam Pract 12:23, 1981
35. Parkerson GR Jr, Barr DM, Bass M, et al.: Meeting the challenge of research in family medicine: Report of the Study Group on Family Medicine Research. J Fam Pract 14:105, 1982
36. Phillips TJ: Research considerations for the family physician. J Fam Pract 7:121, 1978
37. Nelson EC, Kirk JW, Bise BW, et al.: The Cooperative Information Project: Part 2: Some initial clinical quality assurance, and practice management studies. J Fam Pract 13:867, 1981
38. Smith CK, Taylor TR, Gordon MJ: Community based studies of diabetes control: Program development and preliminary analysis. J Fam Pract 14:459, 1982
39. Green LA, Wood M, Becker L, et al.: The Ambulatory Sentinel Practice Network: Purpose, methods, and policies. J Fam Pract 18:275, 1984

14 Current Status of Family Practice

Since family practice had no formal place in medical education in the United States before 1969, a number of basic questions were understandably raised as the new specialty took root. Some of the more important questions were the following: Can viable teaching programs be organized and maintained at a high level of quality? Can faculty be recruited to teach in developing programs? Can interest among medical students in this emerging specialty be developed and sustained? Will graduates of family practice residencies locate in areas of need? Can the academic discipline of family medicine be defined and nurtured through ongoing research efforts?

Previous chapters have examined various aspects of these questions and documented substantial progress in all of these areas. A brief overview of several dimensions of the specialty's first 15 years of development is now of interest in order to measure the field's overall progress and principal needs.

SOME MEASURES OF PROGRESS

Organization of Teaching Programs

The development of teaching programs in family practice, at both predoctoral and graduate levels, has been the central concern of the specialty to date. The magnitude of this effort in just 15 years is remarkable. Figures 14–1 and 14–2 reflect impressive growth of medical school and residency programs, respectively.

As noted in the first chapter, the number of general/family physicians in the United States has been steadily declining for about 50 years. In 1976 this trend was reversed, with an increase in the number of general/family physicians in active practice observed for the first time over that period.[1] Gratifying as this progress is, the graduates of family practice residency programs have not yet increased sufficiently to make a major impact on the needs for primary care physicians in this country. More than any other specialty, family practice is presently characterized by a marked bimodal age distribution. For example, the two peak ages among the 55,000 plus members of the American Academy of Family Physicians is about 34 and 59 years of age. Over the next 10 years, family practice will shift from the oldest to the youngest specialty in American medicine in terms of its members' ages. Accordingly, expansion of the capacity of residency programs will continue as an important need well into the 1990s. The proportion of American medical school graduates entering family practice residency training has plateaued over the last 8 years at about 13 percent. There are more than 16,000 medical school graduates each year, and

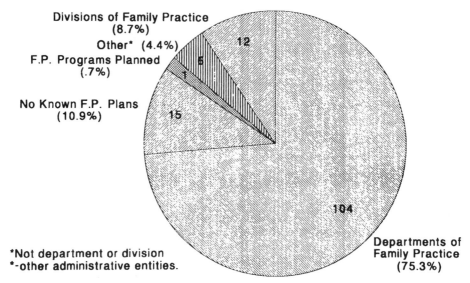

Divisions of Family Practice
(8.7%)

Other* (4.4%)

F.P. Programs Planned
(.7%)

No Known F.P. Plans
(10.9%)

*Not department or division
*-other administrative entities.

Departments of
Family Practice
(75.3%)

Figure 14-1. Family practice programs within the 138 U.S. medical schools and branches—1984.

cutbacks in class size have so far been small (usually no more than 10 percent). Since many advocate that family practice residencies should be able to accommodate at least 25 percent of U.S. medical graduates, considerable expansion would be required beyond today's level of 2500 first-year family practice residency positions if that goal is to be achieved.

The development of teaching programs in family practice to date has likewise been impressive in qualitative terms. As described in Chapters 6 and 7, excellent progress has been made in curriculum design, teaching techniques, and evaluation methods at both predoctoral and graduate levels. That family practice

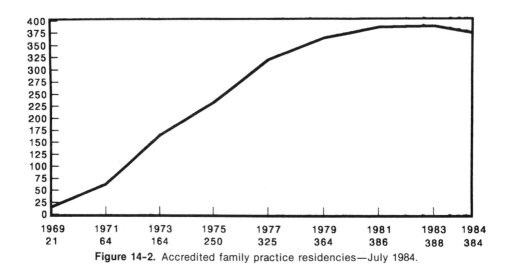

	1969	1971	1973	1975	1977	1979	1981	1983	1984
	21	64	164	250	325	364	386	388	384

Figure 14-2. Accredited family practice residencies—July 1984.

residencies have been found attractive by American medical graduates is reflected by fill rates of first-year family practice residencies of consistently over 95 percent (98.7 percent at this writing).* The proportion of foreign medical graduates in these programs has been quite low, usually on the order of about 10 to 15 percent. The attrition rate from family practice residency programs has also been low, and the majority of vacated positions have been promptly filled either by family practice residents transfering to another family practice residency or by other specialty residents transfering into family practice residencies. The net attrition rate for the class of 1985 (family practice residents starting training in 1982) was only 6 percent.

Especially noteworthy in terms of quality control in family practice teaching is the previously mentioned Residency Assistance Program.[2] A panel of experienced family practice educators has developed guidelines for quality graduate education in family practice that address such issues as curriculum content, teaching facilities, faculty supervision, and related subjects.[†] Consultations are provided to family practice residency programs on a voluntary basis and are intended to facilitate information sharing, identification of problems, and collaborative problem solving.

Faculty Recruitment

The recruitment of faculty for family practice teaching programs has been a challenging process because of the previous lack of an established teaching tradition in family medicine. The critical need has been to attract excellent clinicians from active family practice in the community with interest and skills in teaching and the capacity to serve as role models for students and residents. Many of these individuals have also been called upon to organize and administer teaching programs and contribute to the developing academic discipline of family medicine.

Significant progress has been made in faculty recruitment. In the 10-year period between 1971–72 and 1981–82, the number of full-time faculty in family practice in U.S. medical schools increased from 82 to 1012, and by 1983 there were 1148 such faculty.[3] A much larger number of full-time family practice faculty are now teaching in community-based teaching programs, but accurate estimates of this number are not available. Many thousands of additional family physicians have become involved in part-time teaching, often on a volunteer basis, in connection with residency teaching and student preceptorship programs.

A national study conducted in 1975 of 240 full-time family practice faculty characterized this group in terms of practice experience, previous training, and board-certification. The average age of these family practice teachers was 45 years, and about 85 percent were board-certified in family practice. Two-thirds had at least 10 years of practice experience, and a similar proportion had completed 2 or more years of graduate training, usually in general/family practice residencies.[4]

The development of teaching and research skills is by no means a spontaneous process, as is sometimes assumed in medical education. Considerable emphasis has been placed on faculty development programs to augment teaching skills of family practice faculty, and more recently some programs have been initiated for the pur-

---

*Data provided by the Division of Education, American Academy of Family Physicians, Kansas City, Missouri. Fill rates about 90 percent are generally considered complete filling, due to unavoidable logistical problems involved in the matching process.

†Copies of these guidelines are available by writing to the Project Director, Residency Assistance Program, 1740 West 92nd Street, Kansas City, Missouri, 64114.

pose of developing research skills. The Society of Teachers of Family Medicine and the American Academy of Family Physicians have sponsored a number of national and regional faculty development workshops. In addition, many federally funded faculty development programs have been established throughout the country ranging from short-term learning experiences to formal, 1-year fellowship programs. The Robert Wood Johnson Foundation has provided funds to establish 2-year fellowship programs in medical school departments of family medicine (presently operational at Case Western Reserve University, the University of Missouri, and the University of Washington). These programs often lead to a Master of Public Health degree, and emphasize the development of research and teaching skills.

Despite this progress, the recruitment of well-qualified family practice faculty to a sizable number of teaching programs remains a pressing need. A recent study by Jackson and MacInnes of promotion and tenure in family practice in U.S. medical schools has shown that the mean number of faculty members in each department is only about 12, that most of these are in junior ranks, and that it is difficult for many family practice faculty to qualify for tenure in their institutions.[5] It can be anticipated, however, that this problem will be relieved somewhat in coming years as the ranks of graduates of family practice residencies and fellowship programs continue to grow and as more of these young physicians opt for careers in teaching and research.

Student Interest

A question raised by some in the late 1960s, as family practice was first developing, was whether substantial student interest could be developed and sustained in this new specialty. Today this question can be answered strongly in the affirmative. Many medical schools report 15 to 30 percent of their graduates entering graduate training in family practice, with a few even higher (see Table 6–13). State medical schools report higher proportions of their graduating classes opting for family practice than private medical schools, as is also the case of medical schools with departments/divisions of family practice compared to institutions without established predoctoral teaching programs in family medicine.

Since there are not yet enough family practice residencies available to adequately meet student demand, a number of medical school graduates are entering flexible first-graduate year programs with the hope of obtaining a second-year position in a family practice residency thereafter. This creates a difficult problem which can only be resolved by expanding the capacity of family practice residency programs, since the total number of available second-year positions in family practice residencies is very small.

There is considerable evidence documenting the high caliber of medical graduates opting for family practice. In two classes of medical school seniors in one medical school, it was found that students selecting family practice attribute greater importance to "orientation to patient care" (e.g., helping, working with people, social change) and less importance to "orientation to the profession" (e.g., status, colleagues, challenge) than do those choosing traditional internal medicine.[6] Another study of attitudes of medical students showed that students opting for family practice and the other primary care disciplines hold more positive attitudes toward the elderly than are held by their peers entering nonprimary care fields.[7] One study of personality traits revealed that family practice residents from one medical school scored higher on affiliation need and lower on aggression and materialism than residents in four other major specialties.[8] In still another recent study, based on a

national survey more than 1200 third-year medical students in 1978, students planning to enter family practice demonstrated very competitive premedical academic
performance (Table 14–1). Those planning to enter one of the primary care specialties
were highly motivated to help people, were sensitive to psychosocial issues in health
care, were receptive to the need for change within the health care system, and were
not overly concerned with financial rewards or social status.[9]

Outcomes of Residency Training

The shortage of primary care physicians, especially of those trained in breadth to
care for the everyday problems of families, is a generalized phenomenon throughout
the country in urban, suburban, and rural locations. More than 17,000 family physicians have already graduated from U.S. family practice residency programs, and
the record to date shows that these graduates are entering practice in communities
of all sizes and types. Table 14–2 shows the distribution of intended practice locations of family practice residents graduating in 1984. It can be noted that 9.5 percent planned to enter practice in rural communities of less than 2500 population
more than 25 miles from large cities in 1984. It can also be seen that one-half of
1984 responding graduates planned to establish practice in communities smaller than
25,000 population, whereas almost one-third of these graduates planned to settle
in large metropolitan communities with populations more than 100,000 people. As
expected, family practice residency graduates settle outside of metropolitan areas
more readily than any other specialty; between 1970 and 1978, 38 percent of
graduates of family practice residencies located their practices outside of Standard
Metropolitan Statistical Areas. There is evidence, however, that the impact of family
practice upon low-income, inner-city communities with populations over 500,000
people has been relatively minimal, with only about 4 percent of graduates selecting practice sites in these settings.

In addition to contributing to improved geographic distribution of physicians
more effectively than any other specialty in medicine, family practice residency
graduates have reported themselves to feel generally well prepared for the needs
of their practices and to feel a high level of professional satisfaction in their practices.[10-13] Retention in family practice is close to 100 percent, and graduates are
more likely to be involved in teaching and to be interested in collaborative research
than their nonresidency-trained counterparts.

Patient Care

A number of important changes have taken place during the last 15 years in family
practice with respect to patient care. Earlier chapters have described refinements
in medical record systems, the increasing use of audit (including office-based audit
as part of recertification requirements by the American Board of Family Practice),
and the evolution of various kinds of team practice. The strong trend to partnership and group practice is another significant change evident in the last 15 years,
particularly among recent graduates of family practice residency programs. Annual
studies conducted by the American Academy of Family Physicians have shown a
consistent preference for partnership or group practice among residency graduates.
Table 14–3 shows the intended practice arrangements of 1984 family practice residency graduates.

A number of studies have been undertaken comparing the quality of patient
care in family practice with that of other specialties. Garg and colleagues, for example, found no significant difference in the quality of care provided by family

TABLE 14-1. MEASURES OF ACADEMIC ABILITY AND SPECIALTY CHOICE

	Undergraduate GPA[a]		MCAT Scores				
Specialty Choice	Mean	n	Science Mean	Quantitative Mean	General Information Mean	Verbal Mean	n
Male							
Family practice	3.50	117	613	623	563	538	125
Internal medicine	3.50	133	636	634	571	554	143
Obstetrics-gynecology	3.32	16	608	614	547	528	17
Pediatrics	3.54	34	624	630	573	562	38
Surgery	3.48	35	612	616	582	529	38
Other	3.40	71	610	621	572	559	72
Total	3.48	406	621	626	569	548	433
P (F test)	1.27		.143	.606	.684	.099	
Female							
Family practice	3.53	107	587	611	579	551	113
Internal medicine	3.54	128	602	608	599	562	138
Obstetrics-gynecology	3.46	61	586	600	565	545	66
Pediatrics	3.48	90	589	599	562	541	96
Surgery	3.53	22	594	612	586	559	26
Other	3.55	89	604	605	595	556	93
Total	3.52	497	594	606	583	552	532
P (F test)	.461		.462	.867	.005	.405	

[a]GPA = Grade point average.
(From Burkett GL, Gelula MY: Characteristics of students preferring family practice/primary care careers. J Fam Pract 15:505, 1982, with permission.)

TABLE 14-2. DISTRIBUTION OF INTENDED PRACTICE LOCATIONS OF 1984 GRADUATING RESIDENTS BY COMMUNITY SIZE

Character and Population of Community	Number of Reporting Grads	Percentage of Total Reporting Grads	Cumulative Percentage of Total Reporting Grads
Rural area or town (less than 2500) not within 25 miles of large city	146	9.5	9.5
Rural area or town (less than 2500) within 25 miles of large city	55	3.5	13.0
Small town (2500–25,000) not within 25 miles of large city	320	20.6	33.6
Small town (2500–25,000) within 25 miles of large city	265	17.0	50.6
Small city (25,000–100,000)	234	15.0	65.6
Suburb of small metropolitan area	37	2.4	68.0
Small metropolitan area (100,000–500,000)	158	10.1	78.1
Suburb of large metropolitan area	158	10.1	88.2
Large metropolitan area (500,000 or more)	112	7.2	95.4
Inner city/low income area (500,000 or more)	71	4.6	100.0
Total	1556	100.0	

(From Division of Education, American Academy of Family Physicians, Kansas City, Mo. These data are based upon a 68 percent response rate of 1984 graduates, with permission.)

physicians, internists, and cardiologists in the care of patients with congestive heart failure, transient ischemic attack, or recent stroke. They likewise found that the quality of care was comparable among family physicians and urologists in the care of patients with acute and chronic urinary tract infections.[14] In another study comparing process and outcomes of care for diabetic ketoacidosis by family physicians and internists in a teaching hospital, family physicians ordered a smaller number of laboratory and x-ray procedures while providing comparable outcomes of care as measured by complications, serum glucose levels, and urine sugar spillage.[15] Other studies have demonstrated comparable quality of obstetric care provided by family physicians and obstetrician–gynecologists.[16–19]

Other comparative studies have gone beyond quality of care to address patient satisfaction and cost effectiveness. Care by family physicians has been found to result in higher levels of patient satisfaction than alternative types of care in various settings.[20–22] Although a number of comparative studies have shown less resource utilization by family physicians in the diagnosis and management of selected clinical problems, most cost studies are marred by small numbers, sample biases, and difficulty in generalizing their results, so that the cost effectiveness issue by specialty is still not conclusively settled.

TABLE 14-3. INTENDED PRACTICE ARRANGEMENTS OF 1984 GRADUATING RESIDENTS

Type of Practice Arrangements	Number of Reporting Grads	Percentage of Total Reporting Grads
Family practice group	369	20.3
Multispecialty group	164	9.0
Two-person family practice group (partnership)	272	14.9
Solo	230	12.7
Practice (arrangement not specified)	75	4.1
Military	124	6.8
Teaching	43	2.4
USPHS	243	13.4
Emergency room	98	5.4
Hospital staff	19	1.5
Research	4	.2
Administrative	4	.2
Further training	42	2.3
Fellowship	30	1.6
None of the above	96	5.2
Total	1815	100.0

(From Division of Education, American Academy of Family Physicians, Kansas City, Mo. These data are based upon a 80 percent response rate of 1984 graduates, with permission.)

Another benchmark of clinical progress is the development of growing numbers of clinical departments of family practice in community hospitals. Guidelines have been developed by the American Academy of Family Physicians for the organization and operation of these departments, including an active role in the monitoring of quality of care by family physicians and the delineation of their hospital privileges conjointly with other departments.[23] One-half of the nation's short-stay hospitals more than 150 beds in size now have clinical departments of family practice.

The Academic Discipline and Research

An early chapter alluded to the evolution of family medicine as the academic discipline of family practice. What has evolved is a functional definition of family medicine based on the focus of the specialty's concerns in providing continuing, comprehensive care to patients and their families over time. This focus departs from the traditional reductionist view of disease of the biomedical model, and subscribes to the biopsychosocial model proposed by Engel[24] as applied to families, not just to individual patients.

With respect to the definition of family medicine as an academic discipline, some have looked for the unique aspects of the specialty not shared by the traditional specialties. That this is an unrealistic and illusionary approach is suggested by the following view of specialties expressed by Draper and Smits:[25]

> In fact there is nothing intrinsically rational or permanent about the way in which medical specialties are currently defined; all are more or less arbitrary. The first modern specialties, surgery and obstetrics–gynecology, were based on technic.

Subsequent fields depended for their definition on particular organs or systems, such as endocrinology or neurology, on the age of the patient, such as pediatrics or geriatrics, or on a specific aspect of medical technology, such as radiology. A specialty is essentially a social definition rather than a scientific or logical one; it is simply a social recognition of a grouping of practitioners who are carrying out similar work. Furthermore, the definitions of specialties are constantly changing, and the boundaries of few specialties are hard and fast: the nephrologist will need to be able to read kidney biopsies as well as or better than his colleague in pathology; specialists in respiratory diseases would not consider it appropriate to ask a radiologist to interpret chest x-ray films for them. Any clinical specialty is in fact a mixture of fields such as pathology, anatomy, physiology, biochemistry, pharmacology, and psychology; what defines the specialty is its focus rather than a unique kind of knowledge or skill.

Thus family medicine subsumes a range of content areas and an orientation distinctively different from the other specialties because of its functional role in medical practice. The last 15 years have described this range of content and orientation with some degree of specificity as noted in the chapters outlining predoctoral and graduate teaching programs. In fact, family practice has already developed more specific educational objectives than exist in many specialties. That there is overlap of content with many other specialties is undeniable, but substantial overlap exists among most specialties in medicine.

As summarized in the preceding chapter, considerable progress has been made in recent years in the definition of research goals and content areas, as well as in the development of research methods applicable in family practice. This progress can be measured in several ways, such as (1) the initiation of fellowship programs for faculty development of research skills; (2) the increasing participation of family physicians in the North American Primary Care Research Group; (3) the creation of a scientific journal in the specialty fostering and expanding literature base of original work in the field;[26] and (4) the growing awareness within the field that an active research base is the life blood of the specialty's clinical and teaching functions.

Organizational Development

Excellent progress has been made by several kinds of organizations over the past 15 years in support of the developing specialty of family practice. Perhaps most noteworthy is the American Board of Family Practice (ABFP), which with more than 30,000 diplomates has already become one of the largest American specialty boards. In recent years, only the American Board of Internal Medicine has certified more diplomates than the ABFP.[1] The first recertification examination was given in 1976, and more than 17,000 have been recertified since then. Table 14-4 presents a profile of the characteristics of diplomates who have been recertified through 1984.

The American Board of Family Practice (ABFP) has established high standards for training and competence in the field. In so doing, the ABFP has developed several innovative approaches that are likely to have considerable influence on the process of specialty certification in the United States. The ABFP, for example, was the first among American specialty boards to require all diplomates to pass the certification examination (no "grandfathering") and to impose compulsory periodic recertification (every 6 years).[1] The ABFP has also taken a leadership role by including a practice-audit component in the recertification process.

The American Academy of Family Physicians (AAFP) has played a principal role in the initiation and subsequent nurturing of family practice as a specialty. With

TABLE 14-4. PROFILE OF DIPLOMATES OF THE AMERICAN BOARD OF FAMILY PRACTICE WHO HAVE BEEN RECERTIFIED THROUGH 1984

72%	state that they are members of the American Academy of Family Physicians
50%	practice in communities of less than 50,000 population
62%	practice in communities of less than 100,000 population
38%	practice in communities of over 100,000 population
37%	are in independent (solo) practices
47%	practice in partnership or group
5%	are involved in family practice education
1.5%	are also board certified in another specialty

more than 55,000 members, the AAFP is second in size only to the American Medical Association (AMA) among medical organizations in the United States and is the largest medical specialty organization in the world. The AAFP has been involved in a wide range of activities, including faculty development; consultation to teaching programs; continuing medical education; liaison with other medical organizations, government and other groups; and related organizational functions. Starting in 1989, completion of family practice residency training will be required to become eligible for AAFP membership.

The Society of Teachers of Family Medicine (STFM) was established in 1968 as an academic organization concerned primarily with the development of the educational content of family medicine and the improvement of teaching skills among family practice faculty. This organization has grown to a membership of over 2400, including not only family physicians but also others involved in the teaching of family medicine, such as behavioral scientists, social workers, and other health care professionals. The STFM is represented on the Council of Academic Societies of the Association of American Medical Colleges (AAMC), and functions in a liaison capacity with a variety of academic, professional, and government organizations. The major activities of the STFM include faculty development, curriculum development, evaluation, and to a lesser extent, research.

The most recent family practice organization to develop is the Association of Departments of Family Medicine (ADFM). This group provides a forum for chairmen of medical school departments of family medicine to share information and address common issues and problems related to the academic and organizational development of the field in medical schools and affiliated community settings.

Although not exclusively a family practice organization, the North American Primary Care Research Group (NAPCRG), established in the mid-1970s, is playing an increasingly important role in the promotion of research in family practice. The annual meetings of this informal, apolitical organization are devoted to the presentation and critique of original work in the primary care disciplines, and provide meaningful faculty development experiences in terms of research methods and skills.

PRESENT STRENGTHS AND WEAKNESSES

Excellent progress has been made during the first 15 years of the development of family practice. Most of the initial organizational issues have been successfully addressed, and there is now general consensus that family practice is not only viable as a specialty but as an essential part of the changing health care system.

At the same time, however, it is clear that the development of any specialty is a long-term evolutionary process, and that some of its important needs cannot be approached or met until the more pressing initial organizational efforts have been completed. This is quite true of family practice, which has now embarked upon a second phase of further development and maturation.

Table 14–5 presents my personal assessment of the major strengths and weak-

TABLE 14-5. STRENGTHS AND WEAKNESSES OF FAMILY PRACTICE AFTER 15 YEARS

	Strengths	Weaknesses
Clinical	1. Breadth of patient care services 2. Continuity of ambulatory and hospital care 3. Demonstrated quality of care 4. Clinical departments of family practice in one–third of hospitals	1. Cost effectiveness suggested, but not yet widely accepted at policy level 2. Administrative departments of general practice in many hospitals
Education	1. Academic departments of family practice in 85 percent U.S. medical schools 2. Sustained student interest in family practice 3. High caliber of residents 4. Quality control of teaching programs 5. Congruence of residency training to practice needs 6. High practice satisfaction of residency graduates 7. Strong emphasis on continuing medical education	1. Many medical school departments below critical mass in size and resources 2. Shortage of qualified academic faculty 3. Funding instability of family practice teaching programs 4. Academic viability of family practice not yet demonstrated 5. Inadequate number of family practice residency positions
Research	1. Promising start of research development, including definition of overall goals, development of some methods, and initiation of literature base	1. Limited research base 2. View among many family physicians of family practice as a "derivative" specialty, not an academic and scientific clinical discipline in its own right
General	1. High quality process of board certification and required recertification 2. Regional variations of practice patterns of family physicians based on community needs 3. Demonstrated geographic distribution to communities of all sizes 4. Public and governmental support 5. Organizational development with complimentary roles (e.g., ABFP, AAFP, STFM)	1. Family practice with fractional role in nation's primary care sector (e.g., 13 percent of total residency positions, bimodel distribution in family practice, unclear "contract" for primary care in health care system; persistent emphasis in medical education more on tertiary care than on primary care, with inertia in redistribution of residency positions by specialty)

nesses of family practice after 15 years of development as a specialty in the United States. Others may argue for addition or deletion of specific items, but most will probably agree that these items are of considerable value when charting the course for the future development of family practice.

CHALLENGES FOR FURTHER DEVELOPMENT

As made clear by earlier sections of this book, the issues today are quite different from those encountered by the emerging specialty in the late 1960s and 1970s. The most urgent needs today can be summarized as follows:

1. Increase numbers of family practice faculty: Many of the family practice teaching programs in operation today are still short of qualified faculty, and this shortage is exacerbated by the need to further expand the capacity of these programs at both predoctoral and graduate levels. It can be anticipated, however, that a variety of faculty development efforts now underway, combined with a steadily growing pool of potential teachers trained in family practice residencies, will gradually alleviate this problem in coming years. In addition to the need for more family practice faculty, continued emphasis must be directed to various kinds of faculty development programs especially oriented to teaching and research skills. In general, in future years it can be anticipated that family practice faculty will assume an increasing proportion of the overall teaching carried out in family practice programs.

2. Strengthen the family practice base in medical schools: Although some of the departments of family practice are quite well established, many are still short of faculty, funding, space, and curriculum time. The development of a strong base in medical schools will invariably call for additional resources as are essential to the mission of these departments and to their effective interface with other departments and with affiliated programs in the community. The successful development of university programs is absolutely essential to the further development of family medicine as an academic discipline, to the vitality of research in family practice, and to the attainment of academic credibility as a clinical and scientific discipline.[27] The long-term viability of family practice requires that these goals be met, and the burden for achieving them falls largely to the university programs. We have only to recall the fate of the general practice residency effort in the 1950s and 1960s (almost all community based without a university base) to realize how important this is.

3. Expand family practice teaching programs: As previously discussed, the present national goal calls for expansion of the capacity of family practice residencies to accommodate 25 percent of U.S. medical graduates. Even this goal may ultimately fall short of the public's need for primary care services by broadly trained family physicians. It is clear that today's health care system is in a state of rapid flux and uncertainty. It is equally clear, however, that whatever path the future health care system takes, a major increase in the number of practicing family physicians will be required. More family practice teaching programs are still needed together with the expansion of many existing programs.

4. Develop quality control and outcome measures of primary care: We have

seen earlier that the present health care system lacks a clear definition of who should provide primary care, and that a "hidden system" of partial primary care services by other specialties exists to a considerable extent. The future expansion of various prepaid health care programs based on the gatekeeping concept may clarify primary care responsibilities. However, family practice remains as the only specialty with an undivided focus on primary care, since internal medicine and pediatrics embrace variable combinations of primary care and consultant roles. Because of the need to assure quality of primary care by various providers in an era of cost containment, there is an urgent need for improvement of clinically useful quality of care measures (including functional outcomes) in primary care, and family practice should take the lead in this effort.

5. Demonstrate cost effectiveness compared to other primary care approaches: Many studies have shown that family physicians use less laboratory and x-ray services in reaching a diagnosis and managing clinical problems, and that their style of practice emphasizes ambulatory services. It is likely that widespread recognition of family practice as the cost-effective approach to primary care can be demonstrated to the point of shaping health care policy, but this has not yet been accomplished due to various problems with cost studies to date. This is a matter of utmost importance to the health care system, and will require a full participation of family physicians.

6. Expand the number of clinical departments of family practice in community hospitals: Only one-third of the nation's short-stay hospitals now have functioning clinical departments of family practice. Excellent guidelines are now available to assist in the development and operation of these departments, which are vital to the monitoring of quality of hospital care by family physicians and the maintenance of appropriate standards. There is therefore a pressing need to convert the traditional administrative departments of general practice to active clinical departments of family practice throughout the country.

7. Increase funding for family practice programs: Present funding of family practice teaching programs is a somewhat unstable combination of federal, state, and local support together with revenue from patient care. Since the clinical income of family practice programs is relatively low compared to the more procedure-oriented specialties, and because the teaching commitments of these programs are quite high, there is an urgent need to stabilize their funding. This will require ongoing state and federal support, as well as a revision of reimbursement policies to more adequately cover the range of services provided by family physicians.

8. Further develop the research base of family practice: Although some progress has been made in the definition of research goals and the development of research methods applicable to family practice, visible and respected examples of research programs and researchers have not yet emerged in most family practice settings in the United States. This deficit has been partly due to the overriding initial priority of organizational and teaching efforts in developing programs, and partly due to the lack of experience and skills in research among most family practice faculty and practitioners. As stressed in the preceding chapter, the development of a vigorous research base in family practice is absolutely essential to the future of this specialty and to the quality of its teaching and patient care functions.

TABLE 14-6. RECOMMENDATIONS OF AD HOC COMMITTEE FOR FAMILY PRACTICE (WILLARD COMMITTEE)

Original Recommendation 1: Major efforts should be instituted promptly to encourage the development of new programs for the education of large numbers of family physicians for the future, as described in the body of this report. The educational programs should relate to all levels of medical education, including premedical preparation, medical school education, internship and residency training, and continuing medical education. Keynotes should be excellence comparable with programs in other specialties and flexibility to permit the design of programs that will meet the needs and interests of individual physicians.

New Recommendation: Major efforts should continue to increase the number and size of modern educational programs for family practice at all levels of medical education. It is particularly important to develop strong family practice programs in medical schools, because medical school experience usually exerts a strong influence on the career choices of medical students. Without a strong department, many students may fail to consider family practice as a career choice because they know nothing about it. The keynotes for such programs should continue to be excellence and flexibility. A goal should be established to have 25 percent of the graduates of U.S. medical schools enter residency training in family practice by 1985.

Original Recommendation 2: Medical schools and teaching hospitals should be urged to explore the possibility of developing models of family practice, in cooperation with the practicing profession.

New Recommendation: Every family practice program, whether in an urban or a rural setting, should provide the opportunity for experience in a model of family practice. The model of family practice continues to be an absolute essential for a family practice program; without a satisfactory model, the family practice program is not worthy of the name. Flexibility in the design of the model should be permitted, provided that the essential characteristics of the model are maintained, as described in the original Ad Hoc Committee report.

Original Recommendation 3: New sources of financial assistance should be developed for the support of family practice teaching programs. Substantial funds should be made available for all aspects of the programs, including the conduct of the educational program, the recruitment and training of full-time faculty, the development of facilities and models of family practice, and the conduct of research in patient care and community medicine.

New Recommendation: Adequate, sustained financial support should be provided for the development of new programs and for the maintenance and expansion of existing educational programs in family practice. The financial support is necessary at both undergraduate and graduate levels, for the development of facilities and models of family practice, for the stipends of residents, for the recruitment and training of faculty, and for the conduct of appropriate research. The sources of financial support should be diversified, and the use of the funds should be as unrestricted as possible to permit flexibility and originality in the design of educational programs.

TABLE 14-6 *(cont.)*

Original Recommendation 4: Recognition and status equivalent to other medical specialties should be given to family practice. An appropriate system of specialty certification should be provided for those who have completed approved educational programs and have demonstrated their competence as family physicians. The graduate program, i.e., internship-residency program, should be an integrated whole and evaluated for accreditation by one body rather than two.

Original Recommendation 5: Careful attention should be given to other factors that should make the environment for family practice more favorable and serve as incentives to medical students and young physicians to enter this field.

Reimbursement policies of third-party payers should be modified to permit full funding of health care services in ambulatory settings and particularly in models of family practice.

New Recommendation: The Committee believes that the ABFP satisfies the need for recognition of those who take specialty training in family practice and that the board has achieved status comparable with that of other specialty boards. The Committee has no new recommendation to offer in this area.

New Recommendation: Continued attention should be given to factors that will make the environment for family practice more favorable and increase the attractiveness of the field to medical students, residents, and faculty members. The AMA, the American Hospital Association, and the Joint Commission on Accreditation of Hospitals should take steps to ensure that family physicians can obtain practice privileges commensurate with their education and demonstrated competence and without arbitrary restrictions.

There should be further study of the use of physician extenders by family physicians and of the function of family physicians with other allied health personnel, with particular reference to compensation for services provided and the possibility of reduction in the cost of medical care. Improvement of the academic environment for family practice will require that the status and recognition of family practice faculty be enhanced through the development of appropriate areas for scholarly investigation, probably in the social and behavioral sciences. Assistance should be provided to family practice faculty with limited teaching and research experience to develop competence and confidence in these important activities.

(Continued)

TABLE 14-6 *(cont.)*

Original Recommendation 6: Careful study should be made of the effect of premedical programs and the admission procedures, curricula and student evaluation policies of medical schools upon the production of family physicians.	*New Recommendation:* No additional recommendation.
Additional Recommendations Preceptorships	*New Recommendation:* Further emphasis should be given to the development of well-planned and well-conducted preceptorship programs in family practice at both undergraduate and graduate levels of medical education. The possibility should be explored of developing residency programs that make extensive use of preceptorships with group practices of good quality and with highly qualified individual physicians, as a basic part of the educational experience.
Regulation of Residencies	*New Recommendation:* There should be full and free access to residency training in all specialty fields of medicine. It would not be in the public interest or in the interest of the field of family practice to restrict entrance to residency training or to have regulation of the number, type, and location of residency programs or positions, either by a federal agency or by an agency in the private sector.
Geographic Distribution of Physicians	*New Recommendation:* The Committee commends the AAFP for carrying out careful studies of the distribution and function of graduates of family practice residency programs and recommends that such studies be continued and expanded in the future to provide an evaluation of the impact of the family practice movement.

CONCLUSION

As mentioned in an earlier chapter, the 1966 report of the Ad Hoc Committee for Family Practice, established by the American Medical Association, was instrumental in the genesis and early development of family practice as a specialty. Eleven years later, this group met again in 1977 to reconsider the progress, problems, and needs of the specialty. All of the initial recommendations were reviewed, and new recommendations were made for the specialty's further development. Table 14–6 lists both the original and new recommendations of this group.[1] At this writing, some of these recommendations have been effectively implemented while others are still short of the mark and point to the directions and priorities for future development.

In summary, the progress made by family practice during the last 15 years has been quite remarkable. Family practice has already demonstrated its viability as an essential and major specialty in medicine, and its future is one of promise and further maturation.

REFERENCES

1. Willard WA, Ruhe CHW: The challenge of family practice reconsidered. JAMA 240(5):454, 1978
2. Stern TL, Chaisson GM: The Residency Assistance Program in family practice. J Fam Pract 5:379, 1977
3. Higgins E: Personal communication. Association of American Medical Colleges, Dec. 6, 1984
4. Longenecker DP, Wright JC, Gillen JC: Profile of full-time family practice educators. J Fam Pract 4:111, 1977
5. Jackson M, McInnes I: Promotion and tenure in family practice in U.S. medical schools. J Fam Pract 18:435, 1984
6. Plovnick MS: Career orientations in the primary care specialties. J Med Educ 54:655, 1979
7. Holtzman JM, Toewe CH, Beck JD: Specialty preference and attitudes toward the aged. J Fam Pract 9:667, 1979
8. Collins F, Roessler R: Intellectual and attitudinal characteristics of medical students selecting family practice. J Fam Pract 2:431, 1975
9. Burkett GL, Gelula MY: Characteristics of students preferring family practice/primary care careers. J Fam Pract 15:505, 1982
10. Ciriacy EW, Bland CJ, Stoller JE, et al.: Graduate follow-up in the University of Minnesota Affiliated Hospitals Residency Training Program in Family Practice and Community Health. J Fam Pract 11:719, 1980
11. Mayo F, Wood M, Marsland DW, et al.: Graduate follow-up in the Medical College of Virginia/Virginia Commonwealth University Family Practice Residency System. J Fam Pract 11:731, 1980
12. Geyman JP, Cherkin DC, Deisher JB, et al.: Graduate follow-up in the University of Washington Family Practice Residency Network. J Fam Pract 11:743, 1980
13. Black RR, Schmittling G, Stern TL: Characteristics and practice patterns of family practice residency graduates in the United States. J Fam Pract 11:767, 1980
14. Garg ML, Mulligan JL, Gliebe WA, Parekh RR: Physician specialty, quality and cost of inpatient care. Soc Sci Med 13:187, 1979
15. Hamburger S, Barjenbruch P, Soffer A: Treatment of diabetic ketoacidosis by internists and family physicians: A comparative study. J Fam Pract 14:719, 1982
16. Ely JW, Ueland K, Gordon MJ: An audit of obstetric care in a university family medicine department and an obstetrics–gynecology department. J Fam Pract 3:397, 1976
17. Phillips WR, Rice GA, Layton RH: Audit of obstetrical care and outcome in family medicine, obstetrics and general practice. J Fam Pract 6:1209, 1978
18. Wanderer MJ, Suyehira JC: Obstetrical care in a prepaid cooperative—A comparison between family practice residents, family physicians, and obstetricians. J Fam Pract 11:601, 1980

19. Shear CL, Gipe BJ, Mattheis JK, et al.: Provider continuity and quality of medical care. A retrospective analysis of prenatal and perinatal outcome. Med Care 21:1204, 1983
20. Nice DS, Butter MC, Dutton L: Patient satisfaction in adjacent family practice and non-family practice Navy outpatient clinics. J Fam Pract 17:463, 1983
21. Farrell DL, Worth RM, Mishina K: Utilization and cost effectiveness of a family practice center. J Fam Pract 15:957, 1982
22. Schroeder RE: Satisfaction of patients in two Air Force family practice programs. J Fam Pract 4:731, 1977
23. Family Practice in Hospitals. Kansas City, Mo., American Academy of Family Physicians, 1977
24. Engel GL: The need for a new medical model: A challenge for biomedicine. Science 196:129, 1977
25. Draper P, Smits HL: The primary-care practitioner—specialist or jack-of-all trades. N Engl J Med 293(18):904, 1975
26. Geyman JP, Berg AO: The Journal of Family Practice 1974–1983: Analysis of an evolving literature base. J Fam Pract 18:47, 1984
27. Goodale F: Academic credibility: Can your department of family medicine meet the challenge? J Fam Pract 18:471, 1984

15 Future Projections:

Primary Care and Family Practice in a New Era

These are times for physicians to reflect upon why we came into medicine in the first place, and perhaps to consciously rededicate ourselves to the ideas and ideals that inspired us in our earlier years when, for most of us, things were very different. . . . The heart of medical practice is a physician, a patient, and what takes place when one seeks help and the other tries to help, using knowledge, skills, care, and understanding that have been learned through training and experience. . . . the more the practice of medicine changes, the more it remains the same.

Malcolm S.M. Watts[1]

This book has sketched some of the major problems of today's health care system in the United States. Within this context, the development of family practice over its first 15 years has been examined, for this phenomenon can only be understood by reference to the specialty's larger environment. It is now useful to further broaden our view in order to gain perspective of the anticipated future roles of primary care and family practice in a new era. This chapter will first focus broadly on the overall health care system, followed by more specific consideration of future projections for primary care in general, and finally for family practice in particular.

HISTORIC PERSPECTIVE

Medical education in the United States is over 200 years old. Since the first medical graduate in 1770, the medical profession in this country has grown to over 520,000 physicians. Specialism is little more than 65 years old, and family practice as a primary specialty is only 15 years old.

In a recent presentation at the Fall 1984 meeting of the Society of Teachers of Family Medicine in Chicago, Dr. Richard Wilbur, Executive Vice President of the Council of Medical Specialty Societies, outlined an historic overview of the development of American Medicine in four distinct periods.[2]

	Typical Features of Period
1867–1945	Dominance of fee-for-service and solo practice
	Infectious disease main cause of death, especially in young
	Hospitals for poor, often for terminal care

	Surplus of physicians in early 1900s
1945–1966	Rapid increase in specialization, decline of general practice
	Increasing insurance coverage, initially for surgery and hospitalization, later for medical and ambulatory care
	Increasing technology and emphasis on hospital care
1966–1982	Passage of Medicare and Medicaid (1966)
	Perception of physician shortage (1960s), with increased demands for care
	Expansion of medical schools and physician supply
	Influx of foreign medical graduates
1982 to present	Passage of TEFRA legislation (September 1982)
	Prospective Payment System (DRGs) (October 1983)
	Procompetition with increased diversity of health care plans (many on prepayment basis)
	Industrialization of medicine
	Increasing role of corporate business
	Cutbacks in federal and state health care programs

The last two periods were ushered in by sudden events, and have led to irreversible changes in medical practice. The current period, which started just 3 years ago, is certain to produce more sweeping changes in medical practice in 5 years than any other change in the history of American medicine. Of special interest is the fact that the revolutionary changes evolving from the TEFRA legislation in 1982 (passed rapidly as an innocuous-appearing amendment to Social Security legislation) have not come about through the leadership or even the backing of any of the major parties involved (i.e., organized medicine, academic medicine, hospital organizations, even insurance companies). Dr. Paul Elwood views the inevitability of this phenomenon as due to widespread public reaction to unabated cost escalations in health care and to the fact that the current changes fit today's culture while the previous system no longer does.[3]

A paradox now exists as a result of the vast development in medical technology and increasing specialization in the post-World War II years. Despite the potential availability of a remarkable level of technical excellence and a high quality of medical care, such care cannot be provided to all of the country's expanding population. The process of health care is proceeding rapidly in the direction of fragmentation and depersonalization. As Freidson has observed,[4] with the decline of the general practitioner

. . . the layman has had less and less chance to gain responsiveness from professionals to his own views. And as the state comes to intervene more and more—a state which has become so large and formal as to be rather distant from the lives of its citizens, and whose notions of public good are guided largely by professionals—the individual has even less opportunity to express and gain his own ends. Some way of redressing the balance must be found.

The major effect of the expansion of medical education programs during the last 20 years has been to increase the total number of physicians, to the point of surplus, without redressing the imbalance between primary care and nonprimary care fields. It is clear that simply increasing the total number of physicians available for patient care is not enough. An oversupply of physicians exists in many fields, yet there are acute shortages in other fields. The more specialized in a narrow field that physicians become, the less productive they are in terms of patient care. As Millis has observed, ". . . The more sophisticated, the higher the level of competence of anyone of us, the less productive we are. . . . The fact is that medicine year-by-year becomes less productive."[5] And further, as Pellegrino notes,[6] "Human ills are too personalized and individualized to fit the tight frame of any specialty for long. The more technically confined the specialty, the more it needs the generalist, since the patient's problems can extend so readily beyond its categorical perimeters."

FUTURE PROJECTIONS FOR THE HEALTH CARE SYSTEM

First, it is of interest to briefly review, 15 years later, the accuracy of future projections made in 1969 by Dr. John Millis, Chairman of the Citizens Commission on Graduate Medical Education which was so influential in the creation of family practice as a specialty. He foresaw a fundamental future shift in the role of the consumer of health care from the user to buyer. Other developments which he predicted included the following:[7]

- Acceptance of health care as a right, not as a privilege
- Increasing sophistication of patients, corporate officers, government and union officials
- Increasing specialization among physicians, including subspecialization and subsubspecialization
- Increasing institutionalization and organization of health care
- Rapid rise of group practice
- Decreasing productivity of physicians
- Increasing emphasis on preventive health care
- Increased public concern about access, cost, and quality of health care

The extent to which these projections were on target in forecasting today's events is remarkable.

The rapidly evolving present events in health care can be best understood in the context of four dynamic and interrelated themes: (1) industrialization of medicine (from virtually a cottage industry); (2) cost containment, including changes in reimbursement from dominant fee-for-service and cost-based systems for physicians and hospitals, respectively, to prepayment and prospective reimbursement of physicians and hospitals; (3) increasing numbers of physicians and other health care providers; and (4) increasing competition among physicians (within and between specialties) and between physicians and nonphysicians.

The rapidity of change, and the extent to which the future health care system has already been shaped, is reflected by the following examples:

- Hospital Corporation of America (HCA), the country's largest for-profit hospital chain, now owns more than 400 hospitals worldwide, with a total of more than 58,000 beds[8]
- Almost one-third of the nation's long-term renal dialysis is provided by one corporation[9]
- By the end of 1983, almost three-fourths of California's fee-for-service physicians had been approached by one or another preferred provider organization to consider some form of contract[10]
- In a contracting battle in 1984 in California, Blue Cross under its Prudent Buyer Plan, signed contracts with almost one-third of California's acute care facilities and one-quarter of the state's physicians, with average reductions in hospital rates of 23 percent and of physicians fees of 10 to 15 percent[11]
- The proportion of the population on some form of prepaid health care in Madison, Wisconsin, increased from 20 percent to 57 percent between 1983 and 1984[3]
- Chrysler Corporation, which paid $375 million in health insurance premiums in 1983 ($600 per car or more than 10 percent of the cost of the Omni) has initiated various kinds of cost containment programs, including a foot screening program and an audit of hospital admissions for low back pain and obstetrical care[12]
- A 1984 survey of 2000 U.S. hospitals showed a 4 percent decrease in seasonally adjusted hospital admissions compared to 1983, with one-third of hospital beds empty and 60,000 fewer hospital employees[13]
- In the last 5 years, the South Florida Health Action Coalition, Inc. has grown to encompass 32 corporate and government employers representing more than 380,000 employees and dependents in a three-county area[14]
- Early in 1984, there were 600 applicants for one cardiology position at Kaiser Permante[15]
- In the one-third of New Jersey hospitals under contract to HMO of New Jersey for the care of 82,000 enrollees, radiology, laboratory services, podiatry, and mental health care are already reimbursed on a capitation basis; coronary artery bypass surgery was put out to bid in Philadelphia hospitals, the costs of the procedure have been thereby reduced by one-half and all of the services of the hospital and hospital-based physicians are included in the bid figure[16]
- By 1983, almost one-half of the country's physicians (excluding residents in training) were salaried, and physicians' unions had between 40,000 and 50,000 members[17]

The magnitude of these changes has prompted many close observers of the health care system to make various assessments and projections for the future. Elwood sees the likelihood that just 20 huge medical care organizations will control the majority of the nation's health care services within the next 10 to 15 years, and that a majority of Americans will decide where to seek care largely on the basis of cost (presently only 7 percent decide on this basis) and availability of services. He sees employers intervening directly in the health care of their employees, mainly by efforts to decrease the volume of services. He observes that the effect of DRGs will be to turn hospitals into insurance companies, and that hospitals will no longer be able to tolerate retaining physicians on their staffs who are not cost effective. He also foresees national instead of regional competition for tertiary care (e.g., the Mayo clinic "went national" in 1984 by opening up satellite facilities in Florida and Arizona), all of the big multispecialty clinics developing new primary care programs, and primary care systems typically involving satellites of three to five primary care physicians about 4 miles apart.[3]

Relman has described the trends and problems associated with the "medical–industrial complex,"[18] and recently called for the following actions by the medical profession as an agenda:[17]

1. Deal with the problems of physician oversupply, including shifting the balance toward the primary care specialties.
2. Restructure the relative value scale for medical fees, reducing the incentives to procedures and use of technology and favoring primary care services.
3. Increase emphasis on controlling the quality of health care.
4. Encourage the development of a national program of technology assessment.
5. Support experiments in health care delivery which reduce unnecessary hospitalization and foster more efficient practice.
6. Support improvements in the hospital reimbursement system, including prospective reimbursement and cost containment efforts.
7. Adopt an ethical code which separates the medical profession per se from the health care industry (i.e., physicians should derive income from their own professional services, not through entrepreneurial interests in the health care industry).

Pellegrino views today's trends as raising three basic options for the future role of the physician vis-a-vis the patient: (1) the physician as scientist, with the ethical imperative being competence (i.e., a craftsman's ethic, the predominant one today); (2) the physician as businessman, with medical care a commodity transaction reduced to contract or business ethics; and (3) the physician as healer, involving concern for the patient as a human being; concern for illness, not just disease; and ethics based on obligation to the patient's needs. Pellegrino makes a clear and timely plea to address these issues in favor of the third alternative (covenantal model), and provides an eloquent portrayal of the risks of the first two models.[19]

Where does all of this leave us in terms of forecasting the future of medical practice? It has been said that the occupational hazard to gazing in crystal balls is an encounter with ground glass. Despite this risk, the following elements seem rather certain to be fully established in the nation's health care system by the year 2000, with many probably well in place by the late 1980s or 1990s:

- Vertical integration of health care services (e.g., ambulatory care, hospitalization, nursing home and home care, hospice care)
- Horizontal integration of health care services (e.g., consortia of acute care hospitals)
- Improved access to care and geographic distribution of physicians
- Assured basic level of health care for entire population
- Indirect rationing of services through exclusions of insurance coverage
- Increased competitive bidding for health care contracts by government agencies, business and corporate groups, etc.

- Increased networking of both primary and nonprimary care services
- "Unbundling" of selected hospital services to ambulatory setting (e.g., diagnostic and imaging centers, laboratory services, surgery)
- Increasing joint ventures between physician groups and hospitals
- Predominance of group practice, including increase in size and number of groups and near-disappearance of solo practice
- Decrease in physician autonomy, with shift of control from physicians to insurance companies, conglomerates, government, etc.
- Predominance of prepayment through capitation and negotiated fees
- Increased emphasis on geriatrics, decrease in surgical services
- Widespread application of microcomputers for clinical, administrative, teaching, and research purposes
- Reduction in size of medical school classes and number of residency positions
- Substitution of full-time staff for housestaff in selected surplus specialties
- Increase in underemployed physicians, especially in nonprimary care fields
- Increase in numbers of physicians involved in various levels of the delivery system
- Strong influence of consumer groups, including political alliance of employers and unions
- Increased conflict between physicians and managers; between academic medical centers and community hospitals; between local and corporate needs; between agencies of government at local, state, and federal levels

Zirkle summarizes the reasons underlying these changes in Figure 15–1 and graphically displays some of these trends in Figure 15–2.[20]

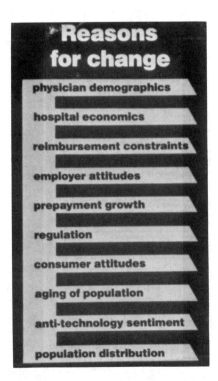

Figure 15-1. Reasons underlying changes in health care system. *(From American Medical News at 25: Looking back, ahead. Am Med News, Sept. 23, 1983, pp 12–13, with permission.)*

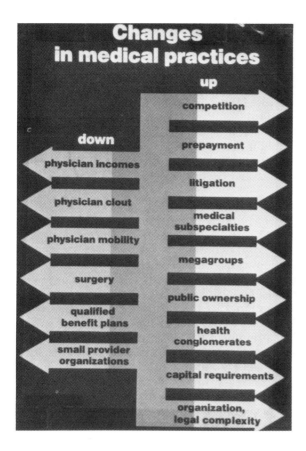

Figure 15-2. Overall trends in medical practice. *(From American Medical News at 25: Looking back, ahead. Am Med News, Sept. 23, 1983, pp 12–13, with permission.)*

FUTURE PROJECTIONS FOR PRIMARY CARE

Present trends and priorities seem to be leading toward a stronger primary care base. There is widespread recognition today of the importance of primary care, as witnessed by continued federal funding for teaching programs in the primary care specialties; the current initiatives of many previously nonprimary care-oriented multispecialty groups to establish primary care programs; the new interest in primary care networks by hospitals; and the growing trend toward various types of alternative health care systems based upon the primary care physician serving in a gatekeeper role.

As pointed out in Chapter 4, a major and still unresolved issue is the matter of who should provide primary care. A heated debate is still in progress concerning the relative contributions of the so-called "hidden system" and the designated primary care specialties to primary care.

Several years ago Aiken and colleagues explored the role of nonprimary care physicians in the provision of primary care services, and concluded that they serve such a substantial primary care role that the nation no longer is faced with a significant shortage of primary care physicians.[21] This conclusion has come under sharp criticism on several counts (e.g., incomplete definitions of primary care;[22,23] lack of information on the training, motivations, competence, and practice satisfaction of specialists serving in "primary care" roles).[24]

Recently the work of Weiner and Starfield has produced objective measures of the extent to which various specialties contribute to primary care. Table 15–1, for example, summarizes their findings of a study of Baltimore physicians on the basis of the Empirical Primary Care Index (EPCI). This is derived from information obtained from patients whereby each encounter is classified into one of four categories: (1) principal care (ongoing care for preventive and acute day-to-day problems); (2) first contact (visit not by referral); (3) specialized care (nonreferral care for a particular problem or set of problems only); and (4) consultative care (referral by another physician). A score of 100 for the EPCI indicates only principal care, while a score of 0 indicates entirely referral care. On this basis, it can be seen that only family practice, internal medicine, and pediatrics qualify as major providers of primary care.[25]

The recent work of Spiegel and colleagues provides further evidence that the contributions of the "hidden system" to primary care have been greatly overestimated. They object to the "majority of care" criterion as not sufficiently specific to define bona fide primary care, and warn that patients' perceptions are essential to making judgments of the contributions of the various specialties to primary care. Table 15–2, for example, compares the extent to which particular kinds of physicians were named to receive the results of multiphasic screening tests in a study of more than 2700 people enrolled in the Rand Health Insurance Experiment.[26]

The shift of emphasis to primary care in recent years has posed a vexing conceptual and educational problem to a number of the traditional specialties, particularly internal medicine, pediatrics, and obstetrics–gynecology. These specialties have faced the dilemma of clarifying their present and future roles as consultants or generalists. This is a somewhat schizoid task, for excellence in both roles simultaneously is a conflictual goal. In the case of internal medicine, for example, the extent of this ambivalence is reflected in the 1982 recommendation by the Federated Council for Internal Medicine that the time allocated to continuity experience in internal medicine clinic be reduced from 25 percent to only 15 percent in general internal medicine residencies;[27] in the negative attitudes of internal medicine subspecialty fellows toward primary care;[28] and in the finding by a recent national survey of internal medicine graduate training programs that more than one-half of the residents are entering subspecialty fellowship training and that the ratio of subspecialty internists to general internists continues to increase.[29]

As a specialty in breadth, family practice is neither encumbered by the generalist:consultant dilemma nor limited by age or sex with respect to its patient population. Earlier chapters have documented the extent to which family practice is meeting the needs of the public for primary health care. The Ad Hoc Committee for Family Practice of the American Medical Association views this issue as follows:[30]

The Committee is aware that efforts are being made to emphasize residency education in general internal medicine, general pediatrics, and general obstetrics and gynecology, in preference to subspecialty education in those disciplines, in the hope that this will meet the need for more physicians prepared specifically to provide primary care. While these efforts are commendable, the Committee believes that there is a greater probability that the graduates of family practice residencies will function as family physicians providing primary care than that this function will be assumed by the graduates of other kinds of residency pro-

TABLE 15-1. EMPIRICAL PRIMARY CARE MEASURES BY SPECIALTY[a]

					Specialty			
Measure	Internal Medicine (n = 65)	Pediatrics (n = 20)	Ob/GYN (n = 46)	Family Practice (n = 42)	General Surgery (n = 38)	Psychiatry (n = 21)	Medical Sub-specialties (n = 19)	Surgical Sub-specialties (n = 17)
Principal Care	75.2	81.0	44.6	76.7	27.8	4.0	9.6	1.5
First Encounter Care	5.0	7.3	7.2	8.4	5.6	2.9	14.8	4.7
Specialized Care	5.8	2.8	31.4	11.9	14.4	13.7	29.2	16.6
Consultative Care	13.9	4.8	16.2	3.1	52.2	79.3	46.3	77.1
Empirical Primary Care Index (EPCI)[b]	70.9	79.9	46.7	73.3	26.2	10.1	34.8	11.2
SD	18.2	17.3	16.6	16.0	25.2	11.0	24.7	16.3

[a]The figures in the top four rows represent the percentage of all specialty's encounters that can be classified into each category. n represents the number of office-based physicians in each specialty who completed the encounter log. The results of 18 physicians, in specialties other than those listed, are not reported.
[b]The EPCI is a weighted index that combines the four encounter categories, where 100 is indicative of primary care.
(From Weiner JP, Starfield BH: Measurement of the primary care roles of office-based physicians. Am J Publ Health 73:666, 1983, with permission.)

TABLE 15-2. TYPES OF PHYSICIANS NAMED TO RECEIVE MULTIPHASIC SCREENING RESULTS, AS COMPARED WITH DISTRIBUTION OF PHYSICIANS IN THE COMMUNITY

Type of Physician	No. of People Naming Each Type (%)		No. of Physicians in the Community (%)
Generalists (total)	1419	(88)	524 (39)
General practitioners	793	(49)	272 (20)
Internists	265	(16)	187 (14)
Pediatricians	361	(22)	65 (5)
Specialists (total)	201	(12)	828 (61)
Internal-medicine subspecialists	36	(2)	51 (4)
Obstetrician– gynecologists	79	(5)	92 (7)
Surgeons	60	(4)	260 (19)
Others	19	(1)	358 (26)
Unknown specialty	7	(0.4)	67 (5)
Totals	1620	(100)	1352 (100)

(From Spiegel JS, Rubenstein LV, Scott B, et al.: Who is the primary physician? N Engl J Med 308:1208, 1983, with permission.)

grams. Consequently, the Committee believes that the needs of the public for more family physicians are most likely to be met by increasing the number of residents in family practice.

Pellegrino sees the evolution of primary care in similar terms:[31]

> General internal medicine itself has a problematic future. I believe it has a unique and legitimate role in secondary and tertiary care under special circumstances.[32] The general internist certainly can also function as a personal physician for adults, and the general pediatrician can do so for children. But if the general internist and the pediatrician intend to assume the care of the family, they must augment their skills as generalists with special knowledge of the care of the family and the age groups each now excludes. Under these circumstances, they become de facto family physicians. It is more likely that general internal medicine and pediatrics will merge gradually with family medicine, and that much of the current stress among them will be slowly dissipated.

As we have seen in earlier chapters, the extent of actual change in redressing the country's maldistribution of physicians by specialty has been cosmetic to date. No fundamental change has yet been implemented (e.g., the primary care:nonprimary care ratio still lies heavily in favor of the latter, particularly in view of the continued active trend toward subspecialization in internal medicine and pediatrics. As noted by Somers:[33]

> Rather than increase the ratio of primary to specialist physicians, we have continued in just the opposite direction. The ratio of family and general practitioners to all active physicians fell from about 50 percent at the end of World War II to about 13 percent in 1981 without any sign of a turnaround. Even if one ac-

cepts the concept of "primary care potential," including all internists and pediatricians as well as family and general practitioners, which is obviously unrealistic, the drop was from 60 percent to about 34 percent. However defined and calculated, it is probable that no more than one-fourth of all U.S. physicians today are really primary care physicians. Is it realistic to ask this fourth to be gatekeepers for the other three-fourths? If not, how do we change these ratios? It's not as though strenuous efforts have not already been made, for example, through federal support of family practice residencies.

The inertia in organized medicine and academic medicine in seriously addressing this basic problem has raised the question whether this is indeed possible without external pressure. In my view, external forces will be required if any significant resolution of this problem is to occur. The most important mechanisms might well be through long-term preferential funding policies by government for bona fide primary care residency training together with the pressure of changing practice opportunities in a vastly different marketplace. The latter is extremely likely in view of the increasing shift to alternative health care systems based on primary care physicians as the gatekeeper. In order for such systems to be successful, these physicians must be well trained for a comprehensive primary care role, enjoy this type of practice, and be competent and willing to provide more rather than less in the range of services to patients. The ultimate bankruptcy of United Healthcare (SAFECO), for example, was in large part due to the relative lack of selectivity initially of the participating primary care physicians (e.g., even surgeons were invited to participate), as well as the fact that new (i.e., tighter) referral systems were not established.[34] Today HMOs and similar prepaid health care systems are far more rigorous in the initial selection of primary care physicians, and are in a position to require board-certification in a primary care specialty as well as demonstrated competence and interest in primary care per se.

The experience of primary care physicians (mostly family physicians) at Group Health Cooperative of Puget Sound is a interesting case in point. With the total patient enrollees approaching 400,000, only recently was a second rheumatologist hired. Primary care physicians at Group Health provide most of the care for rheumatologic problems, as is true of other areas (e.g., normal obstetrics, nonoperative orthopedics); other specialists serve exclusively as consultants without primary care roles. The expansion of alternative health care systems based on primary care is certain to drastically reduce practice opportunities in the limited specialties. Dermatology (with acne comprising one-half of the dermatologist's practice) and allergy, for example, are already being affected by these changes.

Based upon these trends, the following projections can be made with some confidence for the future of primary care in the United States:

1. Changing marketplace to precipitate major shift from nonprimary care to primary care specialties
2. Continued pluralism of primary care roles
   a. Family practice with growing proportion of primary care
   b. Increasing differentiation among internists (i.e., toward an "either-or" approach to the consultant versus primary care role)
   c. Similar increased differentiation among pediatricians, with an increasing tendency to subspecialization in hospital-based practice
3. Increasing exclusion of nonprimary care fields (i.e., the "hidden system") from primary care roles

4. Tendency for most primary care to emphasize continuity of care, with episodic care services (e.g., the Urgicare model) limited to certain settings (e.g., the inner city)

5. Increased conflict between nonprimary care specialties (the "hidden system") and primary care specialties, as well as between the three primary care specialties; in both instances this conflict is likely to diminish after 1990 as the new health care system establishes itself and as the roles of the respective specialties become clarified.

FUTURE PROJECTIONS FOR FAMILY PRACTICE

As already suggested by the above projections for the health care system and for primary care, the future of family practice appears bright. As the only specialty in U.S. medicine with an undivided interest and commitment to primary care, it represents a solid base upon which to build a new health care system. As documented in the last chapter, family practice has already demonstrated itself equal to the task based upon its demonstrated performance over the past 15 years in patient care, teaching, and responsiveness to the public interest.

The timing and development to date of family practice as a specialty is by no means coincidental, but is a logical outgrowth of a changing society. Family medicine fits the new culture, and is a logical extension of a number of the "megatrends" that have been described by Naisbitt:[35]

Centralized society	⟶ Decentralized society
Institutional medicine	⟶ Personal responsibility
Sickness orientation	⟶ Wellness orientation
Quantitative information	⟶ Qualitative knowledge

Family medicine represents a compensatory human response to the increasing technologic development of the society.

In spite of the above points, however, family practice is still relatively small in numbers and resources compared to the magnitude of the task before it. As a young specialty, it must overcome the developmental problems and successfully address the challenges identified in the last chapter. For family practice to reach its full potential in serving as the kind of foundation needed for a new health care system, fundamental changes must take place in medical education and medical practice in favor of primary care.

At this time, based again on current trends, the following future projections for family practice seem likely:

- Family practice as an expanding foundation of the new health care system
- Strengthened medical school base
- Expanded predoctoral and graduate training programs
- Dominance of various types of group practice, including primary care networks
- Gatekeeper role well established (I hope an improved name can be coined that avoids the negative connotations of "gatekeeper" or "case manager")
- Continued active hospital practice

- Improved information management systems, including the advent of "computer-assisted practice"
- Strengthened clinical departments of family practice in hospitals
- High number of varied practice opportunities
- Salaries much closer to those of other specialties
- Oldest to youngest specialty in U.S. medicine (because of present biomodel age distribution)
- Continued public support
- Increased conflict among specialties in next 5 to 10 years, then decreasing conflict
- Probable eventual political alliance with other primary care specialties

The remainder of the 1980s seems certain to be more conflicted and chaotic than any other period in American medicine. Family practice will be in the cross-fire among interspecialty and hospital–physician struggles, and is at the forefront of change as the health care system is rebuilt on a new kind of primary care base. It will be important for family physicians to keep the long view during these turbulent years, for the 1990s should see reduction in uncertainty, confusion, and the negative aspects of competition within medicine. In this context, a recent observation by Pellegrino is on target:[36]

> Family medicine, if it is to be true to its commitment to integral medicine and to its concern for healing the human person scientifically yet compassionately, can only choose the covenantal model. Family medicine, authentically practiced and taught, can lead to the reformation of the family of medicine—nuclear and extended.

CLOSING COMMENT

It is only natural that many physicians view the current changes in medicine with bewilderment, frustration, and concern. For older physicians, these changes represent a faster rate of change than has ever occurred in American medicine; for many, the "good old days in medicine" may seem over. For medical students and residents in training, the changes may provoke confusion and uncertainty about their future practice.

It is useful to keep in mind, however, that the heart of medicine—the special therapeutic relationship between physician and patient—will remain regardless of the shape of the future health care system. Further, there are major problems and inequities in the present health care system which could well be improved by the trends in progress. The present changes in medicine provide a new opportunity to create a better health care system than exists today.

The challenge now before medicine is to participate actively and to provide leadership in the reassessment and remodeling of the health care system to extend the highest possible quality of care to the entire population at a cost that can be afforded in a society approaching the limits of what can be allocated from its gross national product to health care. Although by no means a panacea for all the problems of this country's health care system, the continued successful development of family practice as the foundation of primary care in the United States is an important part of this remodeling process, and represents an effective and proven response to existing and projected deficits in primary health care.

REFERENCES

1. Watts MSM: On measuring both quality and costs in patient care. West J Med 141:237, 1984
2. Wilbur R: Issues, problems, and opportunities, facing family medicine. Presentation at Fall Meeting of Society of Teachers of Family Medicine, Chicago, Ill., Oct. 28, 1984
3. Elwood P: The changing health care system. Presentation at Advanced Forum in Family Medicine, Keystone, Colo., Sept. 22, 1984
4. Freidson E: Profession of Medicine: A Study of the Sociology of Applied Knowledge. New York, Dodd, Mead, 1970, p 352
5. Millis JS: The future of medicine. JAMA 210(2):500, 1969
6. Pellegrino ED: The academic viability of family medicine: A triad of challenges. JAMA 240(2):132, 1978
7. Millis JS: The future of medicine: The role of the consumer. JAMA 210:498, 1969
8. HCA to purchase psychiatric hospitals. Am Med News, Oct. 19, 1984, p 26
9. Seward EW, Gallagher EK: Reflections on change in medical practice: The current trend to large-scale medical organizations. JAMA 250:2820, 1983
10. Iglehart JK: Cutting costs of health care for the poor in California. N Engl J Med 311:745, 1984
11. Contracting battle escalates in California. Am Med News, Feb. 10, 1984, p 1
12. Califano JA: Chrysler perspective. Group Practice J, 6 May/June 1984
13. Hospital use dropping sharply. Am Med New, Oct. 12, 1984, p 18
14. Colasanto RM: Coalition perspective. Group Practice J, 16, May/June, 1984
15. Lee P: Personal communication, Jan. 17, 1984
16. Kane T: Personal communication, Dec. 6, 1984
17. Relman AS: The future of medical practice. Health Affairs 12:4, Summer 1983
18. Relman AS: The new medical-industrial complex. N Engl J Med 303:963, 1980
19. Pellegrino ED: The family of medicine, broken or extended? The need for moral cement. J Fam Pract 19:287, 1984
20. American Medical News at 25: Looking back, ahead. Am Med News, Sept. 23, 1983, pp 12–13
21. Aiken LH, Lewis CE, Craig J, et al.: The contribution of specialists to the delivery of primary care: A new perspective. N Engl J Med 300:1363, 1979
22. Peterson ML: The place of the general internist in primary care. Ann Int Med 91:305, 1979
23. Phillips TJ: Letter to the editor: The delivery of "primary care" by specialists. NEJM 301:893, 1979
24. Mull JD: Sound and fury in perspective: Comments on the primary care backlash. J Fam Pract 10:333, 1980
25. Weiner JP, Starfield BH: Measurement of the primary care roles of office-based physicians. Am J Publ Health 73:666, 1983
26. Spiegel JS, Rubenstein LV, Scott B, et al.: Who is the primary physician? N Engl J Med 308:1208, 1983
27. Federated Council for Internal Medicine. Ambulatory training in internal medicine residencies. Ann Int Med 96:526, 1982
28. Earp JA, Fletcher SW, O'Malley MS, et al.: Attitudes of internal medicine subspecialty fellows toward primary care. Arch Int Med 144:329, 1984
29. Schleiter MK, Tarlov AR: National Study of Internal Medicine Manpower: VIII. Internal medicine residency and fellowship training: 1983 update. Ann Int Med 99:380, 1983

30. Willard WR, Ruhe CHW: The challenge of family practice reconsidered. JAMA 240(5):455, 1978
31. Pellegrino ED: The academic viability of family medicine: A triad of challenges. JAMA 240(2):132, 1978
32. Pellegrino ED: Internal medicine and the functions of the generalist: Some notes on a new synergy. Clin Res 24:252–257, 1976
33. Somers AR: And who shall be the gatekeeper? The role of the primary care physician in the health care delivery system. Inquiry 20:301, Winter 1983
34. Moore SH, Martin DP, Richardson WC: Does the primary-care gatekeeper control the costs of health care? Lessons from the SAFECO experience. N Engl J Med 309:1400, 1983
35. Naisbitt J: Megatrends: Ten New Directions Transforming Our Lives. New York, Warner Books, 1982
36. Pellegrino ED: The family of medicine, broken or extended? The need for moral cement. J Fam Pract 19:287, 1984

Index